Risk Management in Orthodontics:

Experts' Guide to Malpractice

RISK MANAGEMENT IN ORTHODONTICS:
Experts' Guide to Malpractice

Edited by

Thomas M. Graber, DMD, MSD, PhD

Theodore Eliades, DDS, MS, Dr Med, PhD

Athanasios E. Athanasiou, DDS, MSD, Dr Dent

Quintessence Publishing Co, Inc

Chicago, Berlin, Tokyo, Copenhagen, London, Paris, Milan, Barcelona, Istanbul, São Paulo, New Delhi, Moscow, Prague, and Warsaw

Library of Congress Cataloging-in-Publication Data

Risk management in orthodontics : experts' guide to malpractice / edited by Thomas M. Graber, Theodore Eliades, Athanasios E. Athanasiou.
    p. ; cm.
 Includes bibliographical references and index.
 ISBN 0-86715-431-4 (hardcover)
 1. Orthodontics—Practice. 2. Risk management. 3. Dentists—Malpractice.
 [DNLM: 1. Malpractice—United States. 2. Orthodontics—legislation & jurisprudence—United States. 3. Legislation, Dental—United States. 4. Risk Management—United States. WU 44 AA1 R595 2004] I. Graber, T. M. (Thomas M.), 1917- II. Eliades, Theodore. III. Athanasiou, Athanasios E.

 RK521.9.R576 2004
 617.6'43—dc22

                          2004002202

©2004 Quintessence Publishing Co, Inc

Quintessence Publishing Co, Inc
551 Kimberly Drive
Carol Stream, IL 60188
www.quintpub.com

Editor: Lisa C. Bywaters
Cover design: Dawn Hartman
Production: Susan Robinson

Printed in China

Table of Contents

Section 2   Malpractice and Risk Management

Preface

Over the last two decades, a new and complex pseudo-discipline has evolved: litigation and malpractice. This unlikely blend of principles, derived from the broader health and law sciences, is man-made; it cannot be defined by natural rules, and its implications vary greatly. Although the risk of litigation due to medical and dental malpractice is much higher in the United States than in any other part of the world, fears regarding medicolegal involvement and risk management plague health service providers everywhere. Today, practitioners devote a significant amount of time and effort, probably equivalent to half of that devoted to education, to avoiding legal entrapment arising from often trivial omissions, such as failing to record on the patient file that the parents of the adolescent patient had "ample time to study the treatment plan" and that they "definitely have no question or concern." This development has transformed the health care provider into a record-keeper *homo malpracticus*! To paraphrase Mark Twain: "Adam and Eve had many advantages besides escaping teething: the main one was that there were no malpractice cases at that time."

It would be interesting to review the malpractice cases of the last decade and record the direct involvement of the clinician, conscious or involuntary, that resulted in harm to the patient's well-being. It is difficult to explain the paradox that the delirious proliferation of malpractice cases in the US has been accompanied by an equally tremendous increase in fatal iatrogenic incidents, reaching the shocking number of 100,000 per annum! Logic would tell us that malpractice litigation would lead to higher standards of care by eliminating careless or reckless practitioners. Since this does not seem to be the case, perhaps future studies can critically analyze these indices to identify the underlying causes for both incident increases. Furthermore, the practitioner's need for legal protection has led to an increase in the number of diagnostic procedures prescribed to comprehensively evaluate the pretreatment health status of the patient, thereby increasing malpractice coverage insurance premiums and the application of complicated, legalistic informed consent protocols.

In orthodontics, where the risk of harm is considerably limited compared to surgery or other invasive medical therapies, malpractice has taken on significant dimensions over the past decade, thus compelling the scientific community to issue guidelines to avoid the unfortunate incidents. This book has been written for the orthodontic community to achieve two basic aims:

1. To explore the *etiopathology* of various conditions that have been described to emanate from orthodontic treatment, and
2. To define the risk factors associated with the induction of pathologies, in an effort to isolate and eliminate them from the standard practice.

The first aim corresponds to Section 1 of the book, comprising 10 chapters that exhaustively review current knowledge on the association between orthodontic treatment procedures and materials and several adverse tissue or system reactions. These include the dental hard and soft tissues and systemic reactions. As these sections make clear, there is no consensus established on the direct association between any procedure or material and a potential harmful situation. To put it in lay terms, one can find evidence to substantiate both positive and negative involvement of specific procedures in pathology, and varying degrees of severity can be found in the condition induced. Several factors have contributed to what has become a very chaotic situation: contradicting studies; case reports describing severe effects that are nevertheless rare; variability in approaching research questions; and statistical or methodological flaws in studies that have found their way into publication, often because of less-than-qualified reviewing processes. Because of this situation, contingency fee plaintiff attorneys can manipulate the literature so that it will appear to substantiate their case to an uninformed jury—"It's written in the journal." Although the current litigious trend displays geographical and geopolitical boundaries, limited mainly to the US and Canada, the implications are that the editors of orthodontic journals should make every effort to seek the opinion of the best-qualified experts for the manuscript review process. Furthermore, an effort should be made to eliminate personal opinions that are not directly related to the results of the study. Unfounded and undocumented anecdotal statements too often serve as the basis for legalistic arguments and, when taken out of context, could alarm the public unnecessarily. The final chapter in this section offers specific examples of how to manage orthodontic problems in the presence of other disorders or abnormalities.

Section 2 addresses the first part of the title of the book, that is, risk management. Again, this is the first nontechnical guide to avoiding malpractice written from diverse perspectives: that of an orthodontist who is also an expert in litigations; an orthodontist-periodontist who has specialized in dental malpractice for more than two decades; an insurance specialist; and an attorney who has specialized in professional liability for the past 20 years. The chapters in this section are based on a program in Philadelphia in 2001, by the American Association of Orthodontics, which was sponsored by the AAO Insurance Company (AAOIC). The material summarizes cases tried in the past, tells you the dos and don'ts of treating patients, and formulates a risk-management plan for a safe practice, presenting simple steps that could prevent future complications. This section alone warrants a place on your reference library shelf.

To bring this volume to print, a team of 21 specialists has been assembled from 6 countries on two continents, representing different professional, academic, and research backgrounds and interests. We extend our gratitude to all the eminent scholars involved in this team effort for their contributions and to Quintessence for being the first publisher to realize the impact that risk management imposes on the average practitioner.

Contributors

Athanasios E. Athanasiou, DDS, MSD, Dr Dent
Professor and Chairman
Department of Orthodontics
Dean, School of Dentistry
Aristotle University of Thessaloniki
Thessaloniki, Greece

Marianne Bergius, DDS
Senior Consultant
Department of Orthodontics
Faculty of Odontology
Göteborg University
Göteborg, Sweden

Samir E. Bishara, BDS, DDS, D Ortho, MS
Professor
Department of Orthodontics
College of Dentistry
University of Iowa
Iowa City, Iowa

T. Gerard Bradley, BDS, MS
Assistant Professor and Director
Division of Developmental Sciences
School of Dentistry
Marquette University
Milwaukee, Wisconsin

William A. Brantley, PhD
Professor, Section of Restorative Dentistry,
   Prosthodontics and Endodontics
Director, Graduate Program in Dental Materials
   Science
College of Dentistry
The Ohio State University
Columbus, Ohio

Heinz Duschner, Dr rer nat, Dr Med Dent
Professor
Department of Applied Structure and Microanalysis
Johannes Gutenberg–Universität Mainz
Mainz, Germany

George Eliades, DDS, Dr Dent
Associate Professor
Section of Basic Sciences and Oral Biology
Director, Biomaterials Laboratory
School of Dentistry
University of Athens
Athens, Greece

Theodore Eliades, DDS, MS, Dr Med, PhD
Honorary Research Fellow
Biomaterials Science Unit
Turner Dental School
University of Manchester
Manchester, United Kingdom

Adjunct Scientist
Houston Biomaterials Research Center
University of Texas, Houston Dental Branch
Houston, Texas

Adjunct Clinical Assistant Professor
Division of Developmental Sciences
School of Dentistry
Marquette University
Milwaukee, Wisconsin

Carla A. Evans, DMD, DMSc
Professor and Head
Department of Orthodontics
College of Dentistry
University of Illinois at Chicago
Chicago, Illinois

Elizabeth Franklin, MA
Claims Manager
AAO Services, Inc
St Louis, Missouri

Thomas M. Graber, DMD, MSD, PhD, Odont Dr
 (hc), DSc (hc), ScD (hc), MD (hc), FRCS (Edin)
Professor
Department of Orthodontics
College of Dentistry
University of Illinois at Chicago
Chicago, Illinois

Aphrodite Kakaboura, DDS, Dr Dent
Associate Professor
Department of Operative Dentistry
School of Dentistry
University of Athens
Athens, Greece

Stavros Kiliaridis, DDS, Odont Dr
Professor and Head
Department of Orthodontics
School of Dentistry
University of Geneva
Geneva, Switzerland

Eva Levander, DDS, Odont Dr
Senior Consultant
Department of Orthodontics
Eastmaninstitutet
Stockholm, Sweden

Olle Malmgren, DDS, Odont Dr
Former Head
Eastmaninstitutet
Stockholm, Sweden

Claude Matasa, D Chem Eng, D Tech Sci
Lecturer
Department of Orthodontics
College of Dentistry
University of Illinois at Chicago
Chicago, Illinois

Adjunct Assistant Professor
Department of Orthodontics
College of Dental Medicine
Nova Southeastern University
Fort Lauderdale, Florida

Bjørn Øgaard, DDS, Dr Odont
Professor and Head
Department of Orthodontics
Faculty of Dentistry
University of Oslo
Oslo, Norway

Stavros Papaconstantinou, DDS, MS, Dr Dent
Private Practice
Athens, Greece

Birgit Thilander, DDS, Odont Dr
Professor
Department of Orthodontics
Faculty of Odontology
University of Göteborg
Göteborg, Sweden

David Thomas, JD
Attorney-at-law
Detroit, Michigan

Robert L. Vanarsdall, DDS
Professor and Chair
Department of Orthodontics
School of Dental Medicine
University of Pennsylvania
Philadelphia, Pennsylvania

Classification of Undesirable Tissue, Organ, and System Effects Hypothetically Linked to Orthodontics:
An Introduction

Thomas M. Graber, Theodore Eliades,
Athanasios E. Athanasiou

Orthodontic treatment involves the application of various materials and procedures that can have local effects on the teeth and surrounding tissues as well as systemic complications. Despite a lack of incontrovertible evidence of a direct connection between treatment and specific pathologic sequelae, studies have attempted to link orthodontically induced variables, such as treatment longevity, force magnitude, temporomandibular joint (TMJ) complaints, periodontal problems, allergic responses, and even post-treatment relapse, with the occurrence of various deleterious effects.

The intense interest of investigators in this area is evidenced by the plethora of articles, organized symposia, and special issues of journals devoted exclusively to the role of integral parameters of orthodontic therapy in specific iatrogenic effects. Thus:

- New materials have been introduced to minimize the enamel involvement in bonding and the associated increased potential for enamel damage following debonding;

- Emphasis has been placed on introducing alternatives for standard polymeric adhesive materials and appliances to eliminate such disadvantages as monomer leaching and allergies;
- The significance of applying light forces and avoiding extensive tooth movement has been stressed to decrease the prevalence of root resorption; and
- Claims have been made concerning the role of orthodontic therapy as a predisposing factor for the development of craniomandibular dysfunction.

Recently, professional organizations have urged universal use of carefully crafted informed consent forms, and even governmental agencies have begun requiring that patients should be informed of the "potential" or "possible" hazardous effects of biomaterials, including orthodontic materials.[1]

From a different perspective, the desire of the scientific and clinical communities to effectively limit undesirable effects is reflected in the introduction by the industry of various materials that purportedly carry

Table 1-1 Observed and hypothesized side effects of orthodontic treatment and the corresponding mechanism that has been proposed

Procedure/ material	Tissue/ system involved	Observed or hypothesized reaction	Proposed mechanism*
Bonding	Enamel	Tooth discoloration, decalcification, caries	Inhibition of remineralization; colonization by streptococcal species
Prolonged therapy*	Cementum-dentin	Root resorption	Unknown (several predisposing factors have been proposed)
Tooth movement*	Periodontal apparatus	Periodontal complications*	Unknown (no direct association has been shown)
Treatment*	Stomatognathic system*	Craniomandibular dysfunction*	Unknown (no direct association has been shown)
Polymeric adhesives	Immune system	Allergic reaction; estro-genicity of Bis-GMA monomer	Leaching of monomer or other material components
Ni-containing wire alloys	Immune system	Hypersensitivity; chronic fatigue syndrome*	Ni-induced elevation of cytokines (in vitro)

*Information insufficient at present; literature shows no direct correlation between complications and orthodontically induced variables.

less risk relative to their predecessors. It is interesting to note that the potential risks that the new materials claim to avoid were never mentioned in the original release of products that are now being replaced!

Whereas the issue of iatrogenic response has attracted the attention of the medical community, as evidenced by the formation of organizations such as the American Iatrogenic Association, only recently has the dental community expressed interest in hazards associated with certain procedures, materia technica, and various therapeutic modalities. Several new textbooks deal with risk factors in implant prostheses,[2] as well as iatrogenic sequelae in endodontics and associated clinical procedures.[3]

Within the past two decades, some unfortunate incidents involving patients who showed signs of generalized root resorption or who claimed signs or symptoms of TMJ dysfunction have led to litigation and instigated further investigation of the actual involvement of orthodontics in the expression of these side effects.[4,5] Malpractice suits (eg, *Thomas v Price*[6]) have followed,

claiming that orthodontic therapy produces periodontal problems and loss of alveolar bone.

Periodontal complaints against orthodontists are increasing as well. One well-known risk-management attorney has said, while deposing one of the authors as an expert witness in a malpractice case, "Periodontal cases are easy to win. It's like taking candy away from a baby." Table 1-1 lists the side effects often claimed to be linked to orthodontic treatment.

Within the same period, increased emphasis has been placed on the possible relationship between craniomandibular dysfunction along with other potential iatrogenic sequelae and orthodontic treatment, leading the American Association of Orthodontists Foundation to fund many investigations into the problems. In 1995, the National Institutes of Health (NIH) conducted an international multidisciplinary symposium to assess all possible associations between TMJ sequelae and the stomatognathic system. In 1997, a full report of the orthodontic implications was published by McNamara.[7]

Currently, as the McNamara article shows, the orthodontic literature lacks consensus about the role of orthodontic treatment in the effects shown in Table 1-1. A small number of case reports that attempt to link various pathologies with orthodontics have appeared in the literature. Often, conditions have mistakenly been assigned to treatment despite the presence of serious systemic diseases or metabolic dysfunction that could partially account for the appearance or progression of symptoms. On the other hand, systematic approaches to investigating a cause-effect relationship between orthodontic therapy and certain local or systemic side effects present several methodologic problems that compromise the soundness of the conclusions.

The purpose of this introductory chapter is to briefly list and discuss the wide variety of pathologic conditions that have been assigned to orthodontics. A more thorough analysis of each subject is provided in the following chapters, where the currently available evidence linking orthodontic treatment and conditions is exhaustively investigated and scrupulously scrutinized. Generally, the content of the succeeding chapters pertains to the following:

A. Analysis of physiologic phenomena associated with orthodontic mechanotherapy and materia technica employed and discussion of the variables that could result in deviation of the process from normality and an expression of pathology;

B. Investigation of fundamental flaws existing in several methodologic approaches that have led to studies assigning a cause-effect relationship to certain orthodontic treatment parameters;

C. Comprehensive review of the state-of-the-art experimental and clinical procedures and instrumentation to study the phenomena analyzed; and

D. Formulation of guidelines for the prevention and management of potential complications for the practicing orthodontist.

Classification of Risk Factors

A classification of risk factors associated with orthodontic therapy is a cumbersome and complex task. As shown in Table 1-2, which summarizes the methods of classification, three major courses may be followed

in this process. The first categorization pertains to the localization of the effect, within which general-systemic and local development of a pathology are the main discriminating variables. (An alternative method is based on the biologic domain affected, involving tissue, organ, and system entities.) A second classification is related to the involvement of the clinician and induction of certain conditions, regardless of the apparent magnitude of the pathology induced. The third one, based on the severity of the induced condition, is of limited practical value since the seriousness of the medical implication is not always related to the treatment procedures.

Classification based on the localization of a condition or disease

As noted above, a classification based on the localization of a condition or disease does not allow for differentiation of the clinician's intervention because it indiscriminately groups dissimilar entities derived from various procedures and/or factors within the same class. However, it may facilitate a brief overview of the multiplicity of the conditions possibly associated with orthodontic treatment.

1. Generalized or systemic conditions

This category includes conditions that affect the organism as a whole and may derive from the operator's manipulations or the procedure itself. A systemic reaction to a material component is a typical example of this type of condition. The chapter by Claude Matasa is a well-documented, historically based analysis of one category of the materials we use in the fabrication of functional appliances, retainers, TMJ splints, etc. A number of legal cases against orthodontic suppliers and orthodontists claiming culpability because of adverse reactions on both hard and soft tissues are winding their way through the courts. Although at first glance the development of a temporomandibular disorder (TMD) may not be listed under this category, the fact that the pathology may affect more than one tissue (bone, cartilage, muscles, and tendons-ligaments) suggests that it should be included in the generalized pathologic entities. This can be done without arbitrarily assigning a causative factor.

Table 1-2 Classification of risk factors based on the localization severity and operator's intervention in the induced condition*

Localization of effect	Operator's intervention	Severity of effect
Systemic	***Standard risk***	***Severe irreversible***
Allergic reaction to material component (latex or nickel)	Allergic reactions	Multiple caries-decalcifications
TMD syndrome (see text)	TMD syndrome	Severe TMD involvement
	Root resorption (treatment free of possible predisposing variables such as force magnitude and duration)	Loss of periodontal attachment (>4 mm)
		Severe generalized root resorption (>5 mm)
	Enamel surface alterations due to acid etching–mediated bonding	
Local	***Patient-related or intrinsic***	***Moderate irreversible***
Decalcification-caries	Medical history predisposing to defects of tissues not disclosed to clinician (calcium homeostasis)	TMD symptoms
Root resorption		Fracture or accidental grinding of enamel during debonding
Periodontal tissues (bony isolated support, attachment, gingivitis)	TMD syndrome	Apical root resorption of teeth <3 mm
Enamel color changes		Loss of attachment <3 mm
Enamel fractures during debonding and resin grinding		
	Passive intervention	***Moderate reversible***
	Impaired monitoring of early signs of root resorption, caries, gingiva status	Fracture of a ceramic crown or veneer on debonding
		Gingivitis
	Enamel cracking during debonding (if appropriate instruments and techniques are used)	
	Wrongful judgment	***Light reversible***
	Proclining of mandibular incisors	Inflammation of periodontal tissues
	Loss of attachment in maxillary teeth due to overexpansion	
	Enamel loss during debonding (if inappropriate instruments or techniques are used)	
	Functionally unfavorable and esthetically unpleasing treatment result	

*The association of a condition with orthodontic sequelae does not imply a cause-effect relationship and serves only for classification purposes. The reliability of several orthodontics-related variables as predisposing factors for induction of pathologic conditions is examined in the corresponding chapters.

2. Local effects

Local effects include mainly enamel involvement during bonding and debonding, as discussed in Chapter 3; periodontal complications; and root resorption. While the latter involves two tissues—cementum and dentin—the localization of the effect in the vicinity of the root apex supports the rationale for grouping this condition with local effects.

Classification based on operator intervention

The term *iatrogenic*, which describes conditions induced by the treatment provider as a result of negligence or wrongful judgment, is from the Greek word *iatrogenis*, which means medicine or medical practitioner. In its original use, the term denotes the result of a medical action performed by a therapist. Therefore, side effects associated with patient-related factors or specific allergic reactions should be described not as iatrogenic but rather as undesirable or side effects. Moreover, this term does not differentiate between pathology induced by a procedure that may be in accordance with the standards of practice and that induced by an unacceptable or wrongful judgment. For example, development of root resorption during treatment for which all treatment guidelines were followed is inappropriately but routinely included in the iatrogenic effects.

This understanding of the term contrasts with traditional beliefs, which, under the medicolegal meaning of the term, denotes procedures resulting from the operator's intervention that are not included in mainstream models advocated by the standards of orthodontic practice. In medicine, the incorporation of the foregoing sense of "standard practice" introduces a degree of subjectivity in the meaning of the term. However, the prerequisite for a consensus in our field and the associated necessity for introducing a universally accepted set of principles may outweigh the importance of objectivity.

While it is recognized that differentiating the involvement of a practitioner in a medical procedure imposes legal implications and cannot be viewed exclusively from a scientific perspective, a basic classification is provided in the following section. The reader is cautioned that the structure of the succeeding classification serves only as a working tool to thoroughly analyze the contribution of each category to the induced pathology. Therefore, it should not be viewed as a reference for a medicolegal treatment of the subject, nor should the conclusions derived be used as arguments in clinical cases.

1. Standard risk factors

This category involves the exposure of a patient to conditions that may be induced during treatment and are operator-irrelevant—normally associated with the placement of alloys, metals, resins, and acrylics in the oral cavity. In this category, the clinician's involvement does not extend beyond the standard procedures suggested for the treatment of the malocclusion. Thus, the onset of a condition occurs randomly, probably a reaction of the patient's organism to the constituent component of therapy, ie, materials. An example could be the allergic reaction of a patient to latex elastics or nickel-containing alloys, for which no previous history was disclosed to the clinician, due either to absence of knowledge on behalf of the patient or the patient's failure to respond appropriately to relevant questions during examination. These cases are covered by a consent form recently suggested by the California state legislators.[1] In general, the literature has not been supportive of a direct association between exposure of the oral mucosa to orthodontic materials and pathologic conditions, while minimal risk has been confirmed for patients or operators who follow standard precautions. For a thorough review of this important issue and an analysis of factors possibly eliciting an allergic reaction in patients or operators, the reader is referred to the extensive work of the Scandinavian Institute of Dental Materials (NIOM) group, led by Hensten-Pettersen.[8–16] For an ex vivo treatment of the subject, the work by Wataha and colleagues is suggested for a systematic examination of the role of metal ions in the physiology of cell cultures.[17–22]

2. Patient-related or intrinsic risk factors resulting in the establishment of a condition

Metabolic diseases not disclosed during the examination or in the history, probably unknown even to the patient, and for which no sign or early symptom can be detected before the onset of a condition are included in this category. Normally, this section involves systemic conditions, and the potential responsibility of the practitioner is confined to the lack of proper monitoring of the development of pathologic symptoms. For example, poor oral hygiene may result in severe decalcification of multiple dental units and multiple caries. Although oral hygiene is basically a responsibility of the patient, monitoring and continual encouragement of patient compliance, as well as possible discontinuation of therapy, may be exercised by the orthodontist. The same holds true for the onset of root resorption. Assuming that the application of forces is performed at appropriate intervals and that they are not of exceedingly high magnitude, induction of root resorption may not be related to the treatment provider but represents rather a response of an organism to an exogenous stimulus. In the foregoing case, the responsibility of the clinician cannot extend beyond the proper monitoring and possibly discontinuation of treatment as needed. A review of the possible etiology factors predisposing to this pathology are listed in Chapter 4.

3. Passive operator intervention resulting in the progression of a condition

This category represents cases where the developing condition is allowed to progress through lack of proper monitoring. It includes the pathologic entities described in the previous section in an advanced stage along with other incidents such as enamel fractures upon debonding of ceramic brackets. Again, this category includes cases where the developing pathology is not the result of a wrongful judgment but rather may be related to instantaneous manipulation of an otherwise proper procedure. Alternatively, it may be an implication of a clinician's passive failure to do something that he or she should have done (eg, monitoring of a sign or symptom). Unfortunately, litigious action is brisk here also.

4. Active operator involvement: Wrongful judgment

This category involves the cases of wrongful judgment that necessitate the active involvement of the clinician in the development of the effect. For example, excessive labial proclination of mandibular incisors that results in decreased bony support, or buccal movement of posterior segments that leads to loss of attachment may be erroneously incorporated in the treatment plan or result from inappropriate mechanics.

It is interesting to note that a wrongful treatment plan may have consequences of decreased severity relative to the development of conditions for which no direct cause-effect has been shown for the patient, as listed in the foregoing categories. Thus, the seriousness of the side effect developed seems not to be directly associated with the manipulations of the clinician. Often, a relatively trivial negligence of monitoring, as in the case of improper control of oral hygiene or radiographic examination of root apices, may induce far more serious conditions (eg, multiple caries or advanced root resorption). Conversely, an indisputable wrongful judgment, such as intentionally moving a tooth into a region of decreased bone support, may result in a loss of attachment of 3 to 4 mm, a condition far less alarming than that of generalized root resorption.

Classification based on the severity of the condition

Classification of the risk factor based on the severity of the condition involves the pathologies listed in Table 1-2. In general, systemic side effects are not always the most severe, although they affect an expanded area of the organism. Also, to what degree the condition has advanced may be of paramount significance in assessing its impact on the health status of the patient. Systemic conditions presenting slight to moderate signs or symptoms, such as developing gingival proliferation, may have a decreased impact on the patient's health relative to localized but severe conditions, such as excessive root resorption of two maxillary anterior teeth.

Conclusions

An approach to investigating the reliability of assigning various effects to orthodontic treatment variables should follow the course of associated medical disciplines. In the latter, the reported effects are meticulously recorded and analyzed, and studies are designed to investigate the cause-effect relationship of conditions and treatment. When a direct association between a variable and an effect is established, a warning is issued to the scientific community; when no association is detected and the flow of incoming reports on occurrence of a side effect persists, an alternative procedure or material is suggested. This approach, which is far from the commonly followed "I saw it first" type of report that often appears in the literature, is a prerequisite for a reliable and effective means of identifying the source of an unfavorable sequence of events occurring in our patients' health.

An overemphasized litigation component of the iatrogenic or side effect sequelae may have an unpredictable impact on the process of minimizing the exposure of patients to risk factors as well as identifying the risk sources present among various treatment procedures and/or materials. This phenomenological paradox may be because reports of side effects and the concomitant optimization of treatment modalities may be disturbed by the probability that the practitioner is exposed to malpractice risk. Thus, the clinician does not perform what he/she thinks would be most beneficial for the patient's health but tries to combine this with the least possible risk of litigation. Therefore, in the treatment of marginal cases that present a high degree of complexity, treatment strategies include a clinician's safety factor, which depends on the legislation and litigation status of the country in which the procedure is performed at a given time. Elimination of unnecessary risk of a practitioner being involved in a litigation turmoil may lead to decreased risk of patients who may be treated more "aggressively" and effectively.

References

1. Turpin DL. California proposition may help patients in search of better oral health [editorial]. Am J Orthod Dentofacial Orthop 2001;120:1.
2. Renouard F, Rangert B. Risk Factors in Implant Dentistry. Chicago: Quintessence, 2000.
3. Lambrianidis T. Risk Management in Root Canal Treatment. Thessaloniki, Greece: University Studio Press, 2001.
4. Woodside DG. The $4.4 million case. World J Orthod 2001;2:10–20.
5. Graber TM. Pimples, dimples, and chad [editorial]. World J Orthod 2001;2:5–6.
6. Thomas versus Prince, Circuit Court, 13th District, Ottawa, IL, Case 85, L159, Nov 1995.
7. McNamara JM. Orthodontic treatment and temporomandibular joint disorders. Oral Med Oral Pathol Oral Radiol 1997;83:107.
8. Kerosuo H, Kullaa A, Kerosuo E, Kanerva L, Hensten-Pettersen A. Nickel allergy in adolescents in relation to orthodontic treatment and piercing of ears. Am J Orthod Dentofacial Orthop 1996;109:148–154.
9. Jacobsen N, Hensten-Pettersen A. Occupational health problems and adverse patient reactions in orthodontics. Eur J Orthod 1989;11:254–264.
10. Hensten-Pettersen A, Jacobsen N, Grímsdóttir MR. Allergic reactions and safety concerns. In: Brantley WA, Eliades T (eds). Orthodontic Materials: Scientific and Clinical Aspects. Stuttgart: Thieme, 2001:287–299.
11. Hensten-Pettersen A. Nickel allergy and dental treatment procedures. In: Maibach HI, Menne T (eds). Nickel and the Skin: Immunology and Toxicology. Boca Raton: CRC Press, 1989:195–205.
12. Kerosuo M, Moe G, Hensten-Pettersen A. Salivary nickel and chromium in subjects with different types of fixed appliances. Am J Orthod Dentofacial Orthop 1997;111:595–598.
13. Grímsdóttir MR, Gjerdet NR, Hensten-Pettersen A. Composition and in vitro corrosion of orthodontic appliances. Am J Orthod Dentofacial Orthop 1992;101:23–30.
14. Hensten-Pettersen A. Skin and mucosal reactions associated with dental materials. Eur J Oral Sci 1998;106:707–712.
15. Hensten-Pettersen A, Helgeland K. Evaluation of biologic effects of dental materials using four different cell culture techniques. Scand J Dent Res 1977;85:291–296.
16. Hensten-Pettersen A. Casting alloys: side effects. Adv Dent Res 1992;6:38–43.
17. Wataha JC, Hanks CT, Sun ZL. Effect of cell line on in vitro metal ion cytotoxicity. Dent Mater 1994;10:156–161.
18. Wataha JC, Hanks CT. Biocompatibility testing–What can we anticipate? Trans Acad Dent Mater 1997:109–120.
19. Wataha JC, Lockwood PE, Nelson SK. Initial versus subsequent release of elements from dental casting alloys. J Oral Rehabil 1999;10:798–803.
20. Wataha JC, Lockwood PE, Marek M, Ghazi M. Ability of Ni-containing biomedical alloys to activate monocytes and endothelial cells in vitro. J Biomed Mater Res 1999;45:251–257.
21. Wataha JC, Sun ZL, Hanks CT, Fang DN. Effect of Ni ions on expression of intercellular adhesion molecule 1 by endothelial cells. J Biomed Mater Res 1997;36:145–151.
22. Wataha JC. Principles of biocompatibility. In: Brantley WA, Eliades T (eds). Orthodontic Materials: Scientific and Clinical Aspects. Stuttgart:Thieme, 2001:271–287.

Potential Iatrogenic Responses

Dental Tissues

Periodontal Tissues

Systemic Unfavorable Responses

Neuromuscular and Aberrant Growth Involvement

CHAPTER 2

Enamel Color Alterations Associated with Orthodontics

Theodore Eliades, Aphrodite Kakaboura, George Eliades, T. Gerard Bradley

The question of color alteration in dentistry is usually related to the study of tooth chromatometric parameters as well as the appearance of restorative materials designed to replace missing tooth structures. Maxillofacial prosthetics and ceramic and composite restorative materials are the concerns of most of the research efforts in the field. Variation in tooth color is of profound importance because alterations encountered over a lifetime may be attributed to aging or trauma or to the recent popularity of whitening procedures. The color stability of various restorative materials is of paramount importance because they must appear natural but also change with time relative to tooth aging.

Following a review of the fundamentals of color science, including color variables and their significance in color perception, this chapter will describe essential research in the direction of tooth color and alterations and the basics of applied restorative material color alterations. Reports of changes in enamel color induced by orthodontic bonding will be summarized based on the limited literature in the field, along with those of interesting recent clinical applications of whitening to orthodontically treated teeth. These changes have potential litigious implications.

Color Science: Terminology, Background, and Applications in Dentistry

Light is a form of electromagnetic radiant energy that can be detected by the human eye. The "visible spectrum" of this band is the portion that can stimulate the receptor cells of the retina, thus initiating the response known as vision. The eye is sensitive to a range extending from approximately 400 nm (violet) to 700 nm (dark red) wavelengths of the spectrum, as shown in Fig 2-1. The combined intensities of the wavelengths in a beam of light determine the property termed *color*.[1]

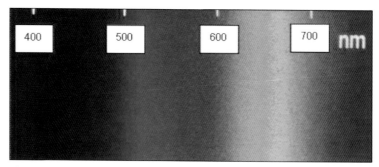

Fig 2-1 The region of visible spectrum.

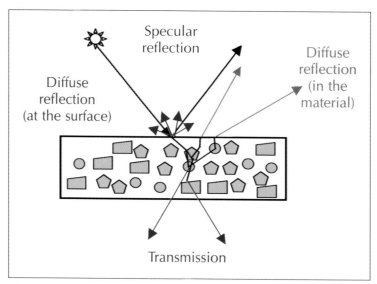

Fig 2-2 Schematic representation of reflected and transmitted forms of light when ray strikes the surface of a material.

Vision, as stated earlier, is the response of the human eye to light coming from an object. Light is concentrated to the retina and converted into nerve impulses, which are transmitted to the brain. Thus, since the sensation of color takes place only in the human brain, all objects are actually colorless.[2,3] Therefore, color is not a physical property of an object but rather the capacity of the object to modify the incident light. As such, color is influenced by the characteristics of the light source and the degree of absorption, transmittance, and reflection of the object.[4] When an incident light strikes a surface, spectral absorption, reflection, and transmission are obtained (Fig 2-2).[4] Opaque bodies absorb and reflect light, while translucent structures absorb and transmit light.

Albert Henry Munsell created a numeric system of color notation,[5] which is divided into three parameters: hue, chroma, and value. *Hue* is the attribute of color most frequently confused with color itself[6]; it refers to the dominant wavelengths present in the spectral distribution.[7] Hue is also the name of the color. For convenience, the hues of the spectrum are described by the acronym "Roy G. Biv": *red, orange, yellow, green, blue, indigo,* and *violet. Chroma* is the degree of hue saturation and therefore can only be present with hue; it also better represents the quality of hue. Pale colors are of low chroma, while strong colors have a high chroma. *Value* describes the brightness of a color by expressing its relative whiteness or blackness. Since the human eye is more sensitive to

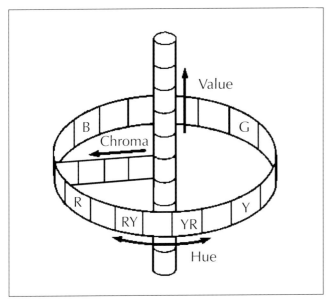

Fig 2-3 Representation of coordinates value, hue, and chroma in the Munsell system of color notation.

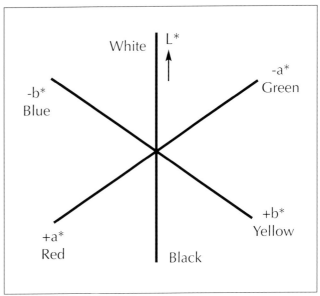

Fig 2-4 Representation of coordinates L*, a*, and b* in the CIE L*a*b* color measurement system.

value changes than it is to hue and chroma, differences in tooth value may be more noticeable. The appearance of an object is strongly dependent on the nature of the light under which the object is viewed.[8] Thus, two colors that may have the same hue under a specific light source possess unmatched hues under a different light source. This phenomenon is known as *metamerism*. In addition, the same object under different lighting conditions can give the impression of having different colors in the eyes of the same observer because each of the eyes may create a different picture. This phenomenon is termed *metatrophy*. Moreover, the steady staring at an object for more than 5 seconds complicates the perception of color because an accommodation effect takes place, and the process of perception is biased because of eye sensitivity.

Theory and essentials of color measurements

In the Munsell system of color notation, the three dimensions are expressed with capital letters (H, C, V). Munsell's color solid can be visualized as a series of nine stacked wheels, each being lighter than the next from bottom to top. The hue is arranged sequentially around the rims, while the intensity of the color or chroma is represented by the decreasing intensity (increasing grayness) of the spokes toward the achromatic central axis, as illustrated in Fig 2-3.

In 1931, the Commission Internationale de l'Eclairage (CIE) developed a system that enabled color perception to be quantified based on standard observer curves and standard illuminants, which represented average daylight over the spectral range of 300 to 830 nm and a color temperature range of 4,000 to 25,000 K.[9]

Another CIE color system (L*a*b*) uses the three parameters L*, a*, and b* to define colors. This system may be represented by three axes that intersect at right angles (Fig 2-4). In this system, L* is a measure of lightness similar to "value" in the Munsell system. The a* and b* values represent positions on a red/green and yellow/blue axis, respectively. The hue angle can be calculated as $\tan^{-1}(b^*/a^*)$ and chroma as $(a^{*2} + b^{*2})^{1/2}$.

The Munsell system is useful for dental applications of color research because it is a psychologically ordered system.[10] When colors are digitalized, color differentials of the same object, after time or due to storage conditions, are expressed by the equation $\Delta E = (\Delta L^{*2} + \Delta a^{*2} + \Delta b^{*2})^{1/2}$. It has been determined that color differences of less than three CIE L*a*b* units represent clinically acceptable color matching.[11]

Tooth color

Incident light follows regular light paths through the tooth. The degree of absorption along these paths may be associated with the lengths of the paths and the absorption coefficient of tooth structure; multiple light scattering inside the tooth may also be a contributing factor. The average length of light path into the tooth can be up to 3 mm, and the average distance between point of light entrance and point of exit may range from 1 to 2 mm.[12]

In the natural dentition, light passes through the translucent enamel and reflects from the deeper zones of the relatively opaque dentin. The enamel in this case behaves as a light filter over the dentin, inducing scattering at wavelengths within the blue range.[13] The enamel surface is a micromorphologically and chemically complex region.[14–16] The mineral prisms or rods of the enamel have the appearance of a crystalline structure embedded in an organic matrix and surrounded by water as hydration shells.[17–19]

Several studies have recognized that the color along the surface of a tooth is not uniform.[20–22] The color of the middle third of a tooth represents the color of the entire tooth structure because the incisal site is translucent and therefore is affected by its own background, while the cervical color is influenced by the scattered light from the gingiva. In general, the chroma of teeth increases with age.[23] Teeth tend to become yellow with age beginning at the cervical site; this may be attributed to exposure of the yellow root surface through gingival recession. After the age of 35, teeth become more reddish, dark, and saturated. Also, the lightness (L*) at the center, center-cervical, and cervical sites decreases with age, while the translucency decreases as a result of occlusal wear.[24] "Deepening" of tooth color with age may be attributed to increased nitrogen content and cracking of enamel and to deposition of colored blood products in the dentin.[25]

Color of esthetic dental materials

When a light beam penetrates a composite dental material, reflection and refraction phenomena may affect the composite filler particles. As a result, a portion of the light is absorbed while the remainder of the light is transmitted or reflected from the inside.[26] Translucent materials allow some light to pass through and some of the light to be absorbed.[27] On the other hand, opacity depends on the scattering coefficient, the light reflection from an infinite depth of material, and the material thickness[28,29]; it is defined as the ratio of the light reflected from a material placed on a black background (Ro) to that when it is placed on a white background (Rr), Cr = Ro/Rr, where r is the reflectivity of the white surface.[30] In composite materials, color changes take place after setting because of a slight difference in the refractive index between the monomer and the polymer, which makes the material less translucent due to increased light scattering.[31]

Exogenous discoloration of the materials may arise from a superficial absorption of color pigmentation from food dyes, colored mouth rinses, plaque, and the development of colored degradation products.[32,33] Endogenous discoloration is irreversible since it is caused by changes in the chemical structure of the material. Resistance to external staining is largely dependent on the surface finish and the material stability[34] since surface texture can influence the light reflection and thus the color of the material.

Enamel Color Alterations Associated with Orthodontics

In general, orthodontic bracket bonding and debonding (see Chapter 3)[35,36] have been shown to cause enamel loss caused by etching; enamel alterations during fixed orthodontic treatment caused by inhibition of remineralization and leading to decalcification and, possibly, caries development; and enamel microcracks, scratches, and abrasions caused by adhesive debonding and cleaning procedures. These alterations may also lead to decalcification in the form of white spot formation and discoloration.

Despite the relatively extensive evidence available on decalcification, the incidence of enamel color changes associated with orthodontic bonding has not been investigated. Enamel color alterations may result from the irreversible penetration of resin tags into the enamel structure at depths reaching 50 μm.[37] Since resin impregnation in the enamel structure cannot be reversed by debonding and cleaning procedures, enamel discoloration may occur by direct absorption of food colorants and products arising from the corrosion of the orthodontic appliance.[38] Alternatively, the invasive procedures of resin grinding following debonding may adversely affect the color variables of enamel by altering its surface properties.

Recently, resin-modified glass-ionomer adhesives have been tested for orthodontic bonding based on their higher survival probability relative to conventional glass ionomers. These materials carry a mechanism involving the formation of chemical bonding to enamel and thus do not require etching in their application.[39]

Very limited information is available on the enamel color changes induced by orthodontic bonding. A search of the relevant literature lists a single study using an acid etching and a non–acid etching mediated bonding technique to reveal their effects on enamel color alterations.[40] Specifically, a no-mix (one-phase) adhesive resin and a glass-ionomer adhesive were used to bond brackets to extracted premolars, employing a configuration involving a method to maintain a 3-mm-diameter enamel window to standardize the area intended for analysis. Two groups of 15 teeth each were bonded to brackets with the two adhesives, and the enamel surfaces were colorimetrically evaluated at three time intervals: *(a)* before bonding (baseline), *(b)* following debonding and cleaning, and *(c)* after artificial photo-aging for 24 hours. The CIE color parameters (L*, a*, b*) were recorded and averaged for each material-interval group, and the corresponding color differences (ΔE) were calculated. The largest differences were observed for both resin and glass-ionomer adhesives at the baseline-debonding interval whereas the smallest differences were observed at the debonding–photo-aging interval.

The larger differences observed at the baseline-debonding interval relative to the debonding–photo-aging interval for both materials may be explained by the invasive nature of the debonding and cleaning-related procedures. For the resin adhesive, the post-debonding and adhesive cleaning enamel surface is mainly composed of cut enamel infiltrated by resin tags occupying the sites of enamel rods dissolved from acid etching. Because the depth of resin-infiltrated enamel usually reaches 30 to 50 μm, the refractive index of the region may be altered, thus modifying the diffusely reflected light component and influencing the color parameters. Conversely, for the glass-ionomer adhesive, where no enamel conditioning is performed, the predominating surface features following debonding and cleaning are those of unaffected enamel. This is because the mechanical retention facilitated by these materials is limited to the flow characteristics of the cement, which allow for adequate enamel wetting and establishment of a reversible hydrolytic molecular bond mechanism between ionized glass-ionomer carboxyl groups and enamel calcium.

The lack of statistically significant differences with respect to ΔE between the baseline and debonding mechanisms implies that the effect of the surface roughness induced by cleaning and polishing procedures may outweigh any differences in the compositional pattern of enamel surfaces subjected to debonding. This observation is of importance to orthodontists, who may adversely affect the roughness of the bonding surface by grinding the enamel during adhesive removal. A recent $80,000 settlement of such a case illustrates the clinician's culpability. The enamel-cleaning technique adopted in this study involved the use of low-speed rotary instruments to limit the influence of the process on tissue integrity.

The specularly reflected light component, a surface roughness–dependent parameter, is highly sensitive to cleaning and polishing procedures, thus influencing the L* values of the substrate.[42] Even though the dependence of color on surface texture and roughness has been clearly demonstrated, it must be emphasized that the pattern of this relationship is currently unknown. Recently, a direct relation has been found for opacity and L* in resin composite and resin-modified glass ionomers.[43] Opacity depends partially on surface roughness since roughly finished surfaces demonstrate whitish appearance due to increased contribution of surface-localized random specular reflections. However, the correlation between opacity and roughness is yet unknown.

Discoloration of the resin tags may account for the ΔE values recorded in the resin adhesive specimens. This color instability has been attributed to the formation of oxidation byproducts containing chromophore groups such as carbonyls arising from the additional reaction to the pendant carbon-carbon double bonds of the crosslinked network.[44] Moreover, for chemically activated systems, oxidation of auxochrome groups present in amine accelerators and inhibitors, such as tertiary amino or hydroxyl groups, may modify the color at a rate determined by the type of substitution of the aromatic ring.[33,44,45] Decomposition of the initiators has been found to be consistent with discoloration linked with changes in b* values toward yellow.

The mechanism underlying the post-debonding photo-aging of the enamel samples bonded with glass-ionomer adhesives is currently unknown. Possibly, the initial low pH of the glass ionomer, which induces local dissolution of apatite and redeposition of calcium fluoride salts, may alter the color characteristics of enamel.

While the foregoing considerations indicate that the color of the substrate may be affected by a multifactorial set of parameters that can be identified in all stages of appliance bonding and removal, it seems that some alterations in enamel color are inevitable. This may be due to the irreversible nature of microstructural modifications associated with enamel bonding and debonding procedures, as well as the low tolerance of color variables to induced variations.

Whitening of Orthodontically Treated Teeth

After the removal of orthodontic appliances, a residual amount of adhesive usually remains on the surface of the teeth.[47] Although a layer of enamel is removed,[48] some may be left intact since resin tags extend a distance of 30 to 50 μm into the enamel, and this could obstruct the natural movement of a bleaching/whitening agent. In addition, excess resin is removed by a mechanical process that can result in varying amounts of enamel being removed, affecting the reflection of light. A recent study[49] compared the response to whitening of teeth that were untreated and those that were orthodontically bonded and debonded. Both groups were subjected to 4-hour whitening and 20-hour hydration sessions for 30 days. Color change readings were taken before and after each 4-hour whitening session. Additional readings were taken at 48-hour intervals for 30 days following the cessation of active whitening.

A mean clinical color difference was found for enamel surfaces subjected to orthodontic bonding/debonding of attachments relative to control sites after whitening. Bonding and debonding procedures resulted in a significant color difference between orthodontic bonded and control sites at the end of the active period, which became insignificant at the end of the 30-day period of monitoring. Both the control and debonded sites responded to whitening; however, the control sites initially responded to a greater extent, whereas the orthodontic debonded sites did not respond until after 2 weeks of continuous whitening. After the 2-week period, the improved response of the debonded sites decreased the color difference between the two groups.

There are three possible variables in the debonding procedure that may be responsible for the differences seen on the experimental surfaces. The saturation of enamel by resin tags and the amount of residual adhesive may vary substantially for each test surface. This could lead to different degrees of color reflectivity as a result of the implication of the resin color and the material left on the tooth surface. The debonding procedure also may alter the morphology of the enamel, as reported in previous studies.[36,48] Changes in morphologic condition can affect the degree of light reflected from the test surface and analyzed by the colorimeter. In addition, the amount of enamel lost by the debonding procedure[35] could be different for each surface, resulting in a color difference not only between the individual experimental surfaces but also between the experimental and control surfaces.

The lack of initial response by the experimental group supports the speculation that tags affect the penetration of the whitening agent or delay the penetration into the enamel rod. Once a path of penetration is established, the ability of the whitening agent to remove stain from the enamel improves. This delayed response is reflected in the finding that no significant color difference was present between the treated and untreated groups at the end of the 30-day monitoring period.

The clinical relevance of the finding pertains to the potential need for modification of bleaching protocols on teeth previously subjected to orthodontic bonding and debonding. It must be noted, however, that in vitro tests may not be a reliable reflection of the clinical situation, and therefore randomized clinical trials are necessary to further verify the findings of this study in vivo.

References

1. Lynch D, Livingston W. Color and Light in Nature. Cambridge: Cambridge University Press, 1995:31–47.
2. Wandell B. Foundations of Vision. Sunderland: Sinaner, 1995:33–43.
3. Ronchi V. Optics. The Science of Vision. New York: Dover, 1991:205–260.
4. Layet G. Light, the eye, and the tooth. A divertissement in 3 acts (1). Rev Fr Prosthet Dent 1989;9:21–28.
5. Munsell A. A Color Notation, 11th ed. Baltimore: Munsell Color, 1961:15–20.
6. Sproull R. Color watching in dentistry. Part I. The three-dimensional nature of color. J Prosthet Dent 1973;29: 416–424.
7. Billmeyer F, Saltzman M. Principles of Color Technology. New York: John Wiley & Sons, 1966:292–504.
8. Kaiser P, Boynton R. Human Color Vision. Washington, DC: Optical Society of America, 1966:492–504.
9. CIE Colorimetry. Official Recommendations of the International Commission on Illumination. Publication CIE (suppl 21). Paris, France: Bureau Central de la CIE, 1978.
10. Ragni F. Color in dentistry. Dent Cosmos 1984;52:13–42.
11. Johnston M, Kao C. Assessment of appearance match by visual observation and clinical colorimetry. J Dent Res 1989;68:819–822.
12. Vaarkamp J, ten Bosch J, Verdonschot E. Propagation of light through human dental enamel and dentine. Caries Res 1995;29:8–13.
13. Spitzer D, ten Bosch J. The absorption and scattering of light in bovine and human dental enamel. Calcif Tissue Res 1975;17:129–137.
14. Gwinnet A. Structure and composition of enamel. Oper Dent 1992; Suppl 5:10–17.
15. O'Brien J. Double layer effect and other optical phenomena related to esthetics. Dent Clin North Am 1985a;29: 667–672.
16. van der Burgt T, ten Bosch J, Borsboom P, Kortsmit W. A comparison of new and conventional methods of qualification of tooth color. J Prosthet Dent 1990;63:155–162.
17. ten Bosch J, Coops J. Tooth color and reflectance as related to light scattering and enamel hardness. J Dent Res 1995;74:374–380.
18. Borsboom P, ten Bosch J. Fiber optic scattering monitor for application on bulk biological tissue, paper and plastic. SPIE 1983;369:417–421.
19. Schwabacher W, Goodkind R, Lu M. Interdependence of the hue, value and chroma in the middle site of anterior human teeth. J Prosthet Dent 1994;3:188–192.
20. Goodkind R, Schwabacher B. Use of a fiber-optic colorimeter for in vivo color measurements of 2,830 anterior teeth. J Prosthet Dent 1987;58:535–541.
21. Hasegawa A, Ikea F, Kawaguchi S. Color and translucency of in vivo natural central incisors. J Prosthet Dent 2000; 83;418–423.
22. Winter R. Visualizing the natural dentition. J Esthet Dent 1993;5:102–117.
23. Solheim T. Dental color as an indicator of age. Gerodontics 1988;2:114–118.
24. ten Gate A, Thompson G, Dickinson J, Hunter H. The estimation of age of skeletal remains from the color of root of teeth. Can Dent Assoc H 1977;43:83–86.
25. Bhussry B, Emmel V. Changes in the nitrogen content of enamel with age. J Dent Res 1955;34:627–631.
26. O'Brien W. Color and appearance. In: Dental Materials. Properties and Selection. Chicago: Quintessence, 1989: 51–69.
27. Brodbelt R, O'Brien W, Fan P. Translucency of dental porcelains. J Dent Res 1980;59:70–75.
28. Crisp S, Abel G, Wilson A. The quantitative measurement of the opacity and aesthetic dental filling materials. J Dent Res 1979;58:1585–1596.
29. Johnston W, O'Brien W, Tein T. The determination of optical absorption and scattering in translucent porcelain. Color Res Application 1986a;49:1431–1436.
30. Powers J, Dennison J, Lepeak P. Parameters that affect the color of direct restorative resins. J Dent Res 1978;57: 876–880.
31. Kap A, Sim C. Loganathan V. Polymerization color changes of esthetic resoratives. Oper Dent 1999;24:306–311.
32. Inokoshi S, Burrow M, Kataumi M, Yamada T, Takatsu T. Opacity and color changes of tooth-colored restorative materials. Oper Dent 1996;21:73–80.
33. Leibrock A, Rosentritt M, Lang R, Behr M, Handel G. Colour stability of visible light-curing hybrid composites. Eur J Prosthodont 1997;5:125–130.
34. Chung K. Effects of finishing and polishing procedures on the surface texture of resin composites. Dent Mater 1994; 10:325–330.
35. van Waes H, Matter T, Krejci I. Three-dimensional measurement of enamel loss caused by bonding and debonding of orthodontic brackets. Am J Orthod Dentofacial Orthop 1997;112:666–669.
36. Sandisson R. Tooth surface appearance after debonding. Br J Orthod 1981;8:119–201.
37. Silverstone LM, Saxton CA, Dogon IL, Fejerskov O. Variation in the pattern of acid etching of human dental enamel examined by scanning electron microscopy. Caries Res 1975;9:373.

38. Maijer R, Smith DC. Corrosion of orthodontic bracket bases. Am J Orthod 1982;81:43–48.

39. Fricker J. A new self-curing resin-modified glass-ionomer cement for the direct bonding of orthodontic brackets *in vivo*. Am J Orthod Dentofacial Orthop 1998;113:384–386.

40. Eliades T, Kakaboura A, Eliades G, Bradley TG. Comparison of enamel colour changes associated with orthodontic bonding using two different adhesives. Eur J Orthod 2001;23:85–90.

41. Wilson AD, Prosser HJ, Powis DR. Mechanisms of adhesion of polyelectrolyte cements to hydroxyapatite. J Dent Res 1983;62:590–592.

42. Inokoshi S, Burrow MF, Katanni M, Yamada T, Tekatsu T. Opacity and color changes of tooth-colored restorative materials. Oper Dent 1996;21:73–80.

43. Omomo S, Inokoshi S, Pereira PNR, Burrow M, Yamada T, Tagami J. Initial opacity and color changes of resin-modified glass-ionomer cements. In: Sano H, Umo S, Inoue S (eds). Modern Trends in Esthetic Dentistry. Osaka: Kuraray, 1998;15–125.

44. Ruyter IE, Svedsen SA. Remaining methacrylate groups in composite restorative materials. Acta Odontol Scand 1978;36:75–82.

45. Davis BA, Friedl KH, Powers JM. Color stability of hybrid monomers after accelerated aging. J Prosthodont 1995;4:111–115.

46. Kinch AP, Taylor H, Warltier R, Oliver RG, Newcombe RG. A clinical study of amount of adhesive remaining on enamel after debonding. Comparing etch times of 15 and 60 seconds. Am J Orthod Dentofacial Orthop 1989;95:415–421.

47. Årtun J, Thylstrup A. Clinical and scanning electron microscopic study of surface changes of incipient enamel caries lesions after debonding. Scand J Dent Res 1986;94:193–210.

48. Hintz JK, Bradley TG, Eliades T. Enamel colour changes following whitening with 10% carbamide peroxide: A comparison of orthodontically bonded/debonded and untreated teeth. Eur J Orthod 2001;23:411–415.

Enamel Effects During Bonding-Debonding and Treatment with Fixed Appliances

Bjørn Øgaard, Samir E. Bishara, Heinz Duschner

Historically, the practice of bonding attachments to dental enamel has significantly improved orthodontic treatment while at times causing irreversible changes to the tooth surface. During the early development of the acid-etching technique, strong acids were applied to the enamel surface for relatively long periods in an attempt to achieve sufficient bond strength. In addition, materials with large filler particles were used to provide high bond strength. Over the years, many reports of decalcification in association with fixed appliance therapy have been published. Furthermore, during debonding, variable amounts of adhesive material are inadvertently left on the enamel surface. This material must be removed mechanically to avoid the risk of discoloration and plaque accumulation. Severe damage to enamel surfaces during debonding of ceramic brackets has also been reported in the literature. In spite of these potential complications,

bonding represents an important advancement as an orthodontic treatment technique. The success of this procedure is the result of significant improvements in orthodontic materials and techniques and the growing acceptance of preventive dentistry principles.

This chapter presents principles and techniques for bonding and debonding orthodontic attachments to the enamel surface along with measures to help clinicians minimize damage to the enamel surface during treatment. It is organized into four parts:

1. Enamel changes associated with bonding attachments to enamel surfaces
2. Enamel changes associated with fixed appliance therapy
3. Enamel changes associated with the debonding of attachments
4. Clinical guidelines

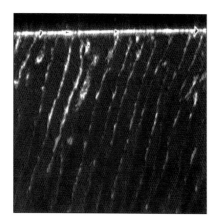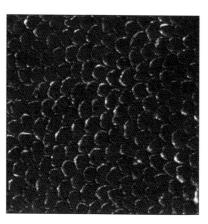

Fig 3-1 Confocal laser scanning microscopic (CLSM) image of sound enamel. The interprismatic enamel appears as light colors and the prism centers as dark colors. Note the typical keyhole or honeycomb structure of the prisms. *Left:* Optical section perpendicular to the surface. *Right:* Optical section parallel to the surface.

Enamel Changes Associated with Bonding Attachments to Enamel Surfaces

The enamel surface

Enamel is characterized by a high mineral content (96 wt%) and a low content of organic matter (0.4 to 0.8 wt%) and water (3.2 to 3.6 wt%). The mineral phase is generally described as calcium hydroxyapatite, which belongs to an isomorphous series of compounds known as *apatites*. The enamel is extremely heterogeneous from a chemical point of view, and it has been shown to contain a large number of impurities, particularly in the caries-susceptible areas. The tightly packed, hexagonal, needle-shaped crystallites of the hydroxyapatite are the real units of enamel, and these are arranged in prisms. The appearance of the "keyhole"-shaped prisms radiating from the dentinenamel junction toward the outer surface is the result of differences in the orientation of the crystallites (Fig 3-1). In the interprismatic area, the crystallites are more randomly oriented and loosely packed, and consequently this area contains more water and organic matter than the area within the prisms.[1]

Under scanning electron microscopy (SEM), surface enamel exhibits large variation, probably due to age and location on the surface in the oral cavity. Macroscopically and with SEM, the surface enamel of newly erupted teeth exhibits so-called perikymata or imbrication lines (Fig 3-2). It has been found that perikymata represent geometrically closed circles.[2] Subsequent to tooth eruption, the perikymata are progressively worn away as a result of normal function and toothbrushing. Perikymata are thus rarely seen in adults. Bonding and debonding procedures associated with orthodontic treatment will contribute to loss of the perikymata. Studies using orthodontic bands to induce plaque on premolars destined to be extracted for orthodontic treatment have shown that the initial caries process starts along the perikymata lines by exposing the prism endings and then progressing along the interprismatic areas. The areas where the perikymata overlap have the ability to act as a reservoir for fluoride after topical treatment.[3]

Principles of bonding

Etching the enamel surface

Successful bonding of orthodontic attachments was first reported in the 1960s.[4] Modern bonding systems for resin-based materials are based on a micromechanical retention principle. To achieve this, an acid is used to clean the surface and dissolve the minerals. Since the dissolution rate in acids differs on various parts of the enamel structure, particularly between interprismatic and prismatic enamel, a very subtle, uneven surface topography is created (Fig 3-3).[5] It is important that the bonding material reach these etched areas and poly-

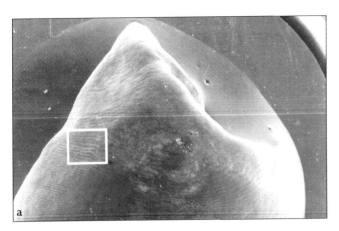

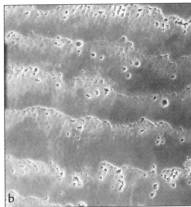

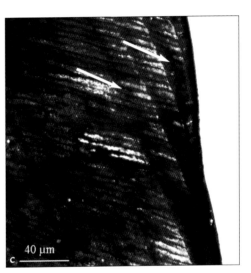

Fig 3-2a Scanning electron microscope (SEM) micrograph of sound enamel from a newly erupted premolar.

Fig 3-2b Higher magnification of the area outlined in Fig 3-2a. Note the typical perikymata pattern.

Fig 3-2c CLSM image of sound enamel with the optical section perpendicular to the surface. Note the incremental lines, or striae of Retzius (arrows), which end at the surface in the perikymata grooves.

merize to give retention (Fig 3-4). The bonding material must therefore be able to wet the surface, either by the surface having a higher energy/tension than the bonding material or by using material that is sufficiently "soluble" in the components of the surface. Because of this property, acid etching of the enamel creates a high surface energy that almost "sucks" the resin material into the rough surface (Fig 3-5). The principle of bonding resin materials to the enamel surface is markedly less complicated than is bonding to dentin.[6]

Crystal growth on the enamel surface

Another principle of retaining adhesives to enamel is by inducing the growth of crystals on the surface.[7-11] Crystal bonding on the enamel can be obtained through application of a polyacrylic solution containing phosphate ions. This causes the formation of calcium sulfate dihydrate crystals (gypsum), which can retain the adhesive. Crystal bonding produces lower bond strengths than conventional acid etching and has therefore not grown in popularity.[12]

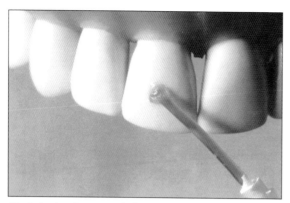

Fig 3-3a Application of phosphoric acid gel.

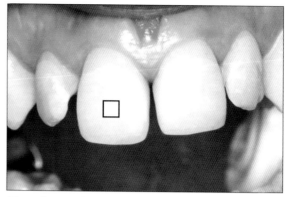

Fig 3-3b Typical frosty white appearance of enamel surface etched with 37% phosphoric acid.

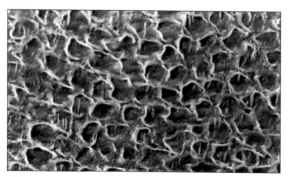

Fig 3-3c SEM micrograph of enamel surface exposed to phosphoric acid. Note the etch pattern where the prism centers have been dissolved.

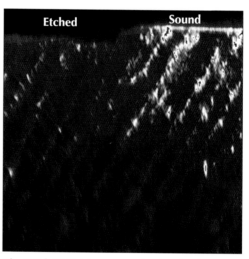

Fig 3-3d CLSM image at the border between etched and sound enamel. The optical section is perpendicular to the surface.

Laser conditioning Recently, laser devices for enamel surface conditioning prior to bonding have been tested and found to provide acceptable bond strength. A Nd:YAG (neodymium:yttrium-aluminum-garnet) laser creates a honeycomb-like enamel microstructure similar to that of acid etching.[13] One advantage of using lasers is that by selecting appropriate power, frequency, and time settings, the enamel surface pattern can be planned. However, concerns have been raised about the effects of increased pulpal temperatures following the use of lasers. More research is needed before routine clinical use can be recommended.

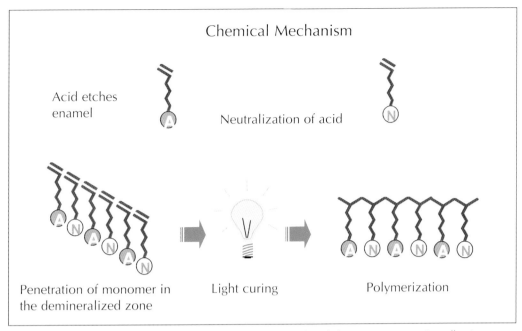

Fig 3-4 The chemical mechanism of bonding brackets with a light-curing composite adhesive to an enamel surface etched with phosphoric acid. (Printed with permission of 3M Unitek.)

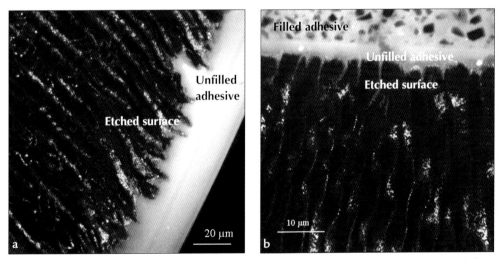

Fig 3-5 CLSM images showing the interface between enamel and *(a)* an unfilled resin and *(b)* a small, unfilled resin layer covered by a filled resin. The optical section is perpendicular to the enamel surface. The penetration of resin into enamel is the result of etching with phosphoric acid. The depth of penetration is dependent on the acid used, the prism directions, and the etching pattern, which is not homogenous within one tooth. (Courtesy of Dr Thomas Pioch, University of Heidelberg, Germany.)

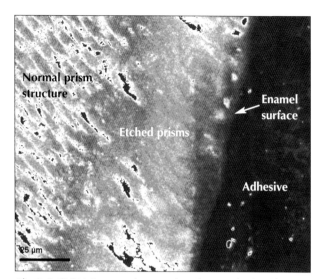

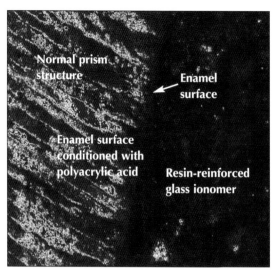

Fig 3-6 CLSM image of enamel surface etched with 37% phosphoric acid for 30 seconds and bracket bonded with a conventional light-curing composite adhesive (Transbond). The optical section is perpendicular to the surface. Note destruction of prism structures to a depth of at least 50 μm.

Fig 3-7 CLSM image of enamel surface conditioned with polyacrylic acid for 30 seconds and bracket bonded with a light-curing resin-reinforced glass-ionomer cement (GC Fuji Ortho). The optical section is perpendicular to the surface. Note dissolution of prism structures at the outer few microns.

Bonding materials

Composite resins

The two types of composite adhesives used in orthodontics are acrylic and diacrylic resins. Acrylic resins contain a methylmethacrylate monomer and can form only linear polymers, whereas the diacrylic adhesives (which are based on Bowen's proposed resin, bisphenol a glycidyl dimethacrylate [Bis-GMA]) may polymerize by crosslinking into a three-dimensional network, contributing to far greater strength of the material. Inorganic materials like quartz or silica glass may be added to adhesives to increase strength.[12,14] Large filler particles (3 to 20 μm) produce higher strength but also retain more plaque compared to microfilled adhesives (0.2 to 0.3 μm), which penetrate more easily into the etched enamel surface (Fig 3-6).[15]

Compomers

Compomers, or polyacid-modified resin composites, are composite resins with fluoride-releasing potential that have been designed for bonding orthodontic attachments.[16-23] Fluoride can be incorporated into composite resins in several ways: as a mixture of water-soluble agents, as dispersions of sparingly water-soluble agents, or as chemically bound agents. Whereas early attempts to incorporate fluoride into composites resulted in weaker bond strength, more recent research has shown no such effects. However, most of the fluoride from composites is released during the first few days or weeks, leading some to question the long-term cariostatic effect.[24,25]

Glass ionomers

Glass ionomers are the materials of choice for cementing orthodontic bands to teeth; they have practically eliminated the problem with decalcification associated with bands.[26] This is most likely due to the strong bond of the glass ionomers to both enamel and metal as well as to the substantial release and uptake of fluoride.[27-30] Glass-ionomer cements have also been introduced for bonding brackets to the enamel surface because initially no etching was thought to be required and because of the advantage of the fluoride effect.[31-43] Glass ionomers bond chemically to enamel through calcium bridges, hydrogen bonds, or van der Waal forces, but the bond strength is clearly weaker than that of resin composites. To increase bond strength, resin components have been added to the glass ionomers. These resin-modified glass ionomers contain components both of the conventional glass ionomers and of the resin composites. The setting chemistry of resin-modified glass-ionomer cements differs from that of conventional glass ionomers, requiring both an acid-base reaction and polymerization.[44]

Resin-reinforced glass ionomers have shown higher tensile bond strengths and lower failure rates than conventional glass ionomers, though their initial bond strength is clearly weaker than that of resin composites.[45–53] These hybrid-type products release at least as much fluoride in vitro as conventional glass-ionomer cements. Photopolymerizable monomers have also been incorporated in resin-reinforced glass ionomers. Although acid etching of the enamel surface is not necessarily required to bond glass ionomers to enamel, application of a conditioner (usually polyacrylic acid) is recommended. Preconditioning the enamel surface with a polyacrylic acid and bonding brackets with resin-reinforced glass ionomers produces less damage to the enamel surface than conventional procedures with phosphoric etching and composite adhesives (Figs 3-6 and 3-7). Relatively high bond strength has been reported when using resin-modified glass ionomers with conventional phosphoric acid conditioning.[50,52,53]

Bond strength

The bond strength should be high enough to withstand the forces from the arch wires, auxiliary components, masticatory forces, and occlusion. Bond strength is given in megapascals (MPa = N/mm^2) (1 kp is equivalent to 9.8 N). Assuming a maximum shear force on the bracket of 120 N and an average bracket base of 15 mm^2, materials and procedures that can resist shear debonding forces of 8 MPa are considered adequate for orthodontic use. This is significantly less than the 20 to 25 MPa forces required to retain composite fillings in operative dentistry as a result of the contractile forces in the material.[54,55]

Enamel can resist relatively high forces before fracturing. Forces applied along the long axis of the enamel prisms must exceed 25 to 30 MPa to induce fractures. However, when occurring at an angle to the prisms, forces as low as 13 MPa may fracture the enamel.[12] Testing of the shear or tensile forces of materials in the laboratory can be useful for screening purposes, but only clinical testing will determine their true effectiveness.

In a recent longitudinal study of more than 300 patients treated by experienced clinicians with fixed orthodontic appliances, the average failure rate of metal brackets bonded with a no-mix adhesive was 7.2%,[56] similar to the rates found by many other recent studies on bond failure.[57–66] The highest failure rates were associated with the mandibular second premolars; on average every fourth bracket bonded to these teeth failed, often several times, during treatment. Variation in the strength of attachments bonded to different teeth has been attributed to differences in the microtopography of the buccal enamel and may be one of the factors that explains why posterior teeth experience more bond failures than anterior teeth.[67,68] Clearly, bonding of brackets to mandibular second premolars represents a challenge and requires improvement. Interestingly, development of white spot lesions during treatment was commonly associated with a high rate of bond failure. Complex appliance design was also associated with frequent bond failures.[56]

Influence of bonding on the enamel surface

Bonding is a rather complicated process but generally consists of the following steps: First, the enamel surface is cleaned with a pumice, rinsed, and dried before an acidic agent is applied. Another rinse then removes the etchant, and care is taken to avoid contaminating the surface with saliva. Application of a sealant prevents recontamination with saliva, and the surface is dried before the bracket is bonded. Preparation of the tooth surface may induce irreversible changes to both the outer enamel surface and to the underlying structures. Moreover, it can create conditions adjacent to the attachment favoring plaque accumulation and possibly decalcification of the enamel surface.

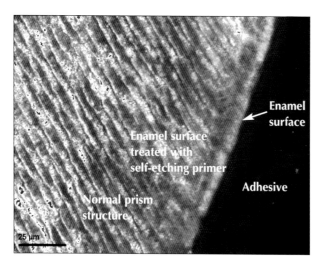

Fig 3-8 CLSM image of enamel surface exposed to self-etching primer (Transbond Plus self-etching primer) and bracket bonded with a conventional light-curing composite adhesive (Transbond). The optical section is perpendicular to the surface. Note slight dissolution of prism structures at the outer few microns.

Etching

Routine etching with phosphoric acid removes several microns of the enamel surface, although not at a uniform depth. Alterations in the enamel structure can be observed microscopically up to 100 to 200 μm beneath the surface, although the actual loss is 10 to 50 μm (see Fig 3-6). It should be pointed out that etched enamel that is not covered with resin remineralizes within a few days of exposure to saliva.[69–71]

As noted above, it is the opening up of the interprismatic areas during etching that causes the mechanical retention of the attachment. The enamel on primary teeth often appears prismless on the outer surface. Therefore, when bonding attachments to primary enamel, microetching with aluminum oxide prior to acid etching has been recommended to remove the outer prismless enamel.[14]

Sealants/primers

When fillers are added to the sealants, the adhesive's ability to penetrate deep into the etched enamel surface is limited. Sealants or primers penetrate more easily into the micropores of the etched enamel surface and may therefore increase bond strength. It has been shown that resin tags from the unfilled sealants may be present as deep as 60 to 80 μm. Some authors suggest etching the entire labial enamel surface rather than only the area required for the attachment to apply a caries-protective sealant on the surface.[14] Such a sealant also prevents saliva from interfering with the etched surface before bonding. Moisture-insensitive or hydrophilic bonding systems have also been introduced.[72,73] One problem with the thin layer of sealant is that oxygen can penetrate it to inhibit polymerization.[74] With photo-induced polymerization, this appears to be a minor problem compared with the use of chemically cured sealants. Recently, bonding without applying a sealant was shown to have no influence on bond strength,[75] although some authors contradict this finding.[12]

Self-etching primers

The relatively new self-etching or acidic primers have attracted considerable interest. A self-etching primer combines the etching and priming steps into one (Figs 3-8 to 3-10), eliminating the need to rinse and possibly avoiding damage to the gingival tissue. The active ingredient of most of the self-etching primers is a methacrylated phosphoric acid ester. Phosphoric acid and a methacrylate group are combined into a molecule that etches and primes simultaneously. The phosphate group on the methacrylated phosphoric acid ester dissolves the calcium and removes it from the hydroxyapatite. The primer molecules penetrate the enamel rods concurrent with etching. The etching process is effectively stopped because the phosphoric

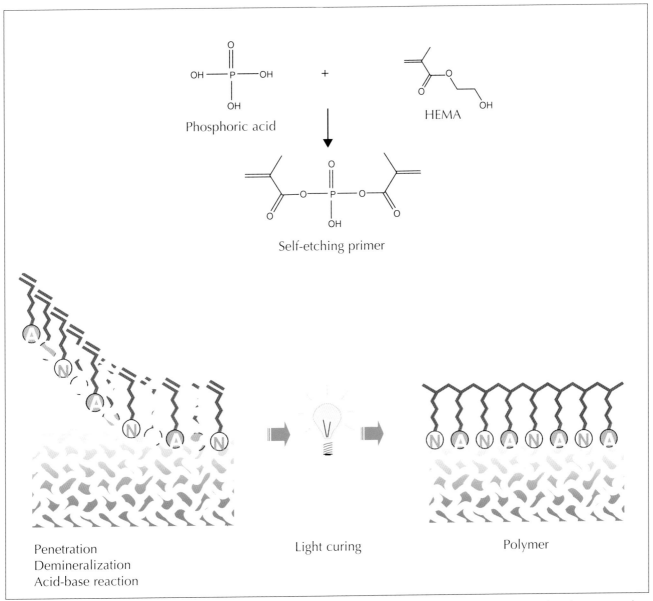

Fig 3-9 The chemical mechanism of bonding brackets with a light-curing composite adhesive to an enamel surface exposed to a self-etching primer. (Courtesy of 3M Unitek.)

acid forms a complex with the dissolved calcium. Furthermore, the solvent is driven from the primer during the air burst step, and the primer monomers polymerize during light curing.[76] Although the etching pattern is claimed to be identical to conventional etching, the short application time of a few seconds does not dissolve as much hard tissue or produce the same damage to the underlying structures (see Fig 3-8). Bond strength appears to be comparable but not as strong as with conventional etching.[77,78] However, bonding brackets with self-etching primers clearly produces less injury to the enamel surface (compare Figs 3-6 and 3-8).

Fig 3-10 Clinical management of self-etching primers. (Courtesy of 3M Unitek.)

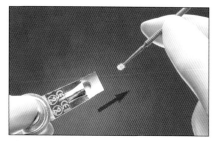

Fig 3-10a Disposable applicator.

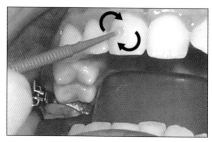

Fig 3-10b The liquid on the applicator is rubbed onto the enamel for only 3 seconds.

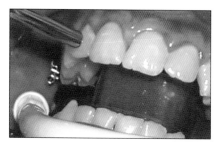

Fig 3-10c When all the teeth in an arch are primed, the surfaces are gently dried with compressed air.

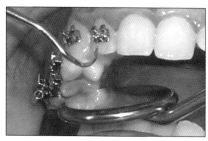

Fig 3-10d The bracket is bonded, and excess material is removed with a scaler.

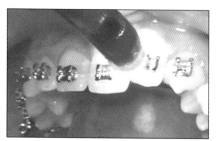

Fig 3-10e Light curing.

Enamel Changes Associated with Fixed Appliances

The use of orthodontic appliances can create conditions leading to iatrogenic effects on the tooth, namely excessive wear of opposing teeth from ceramic attachments and decalcification of the enamel surface.

Excessive tooth wear from ceramic attachments

Ceramic materials are the third hardest type of material known to humans. Therefore, when ceramic attachments come into contact with opposing teeth, they can cause wear of the relatively softer enamel.[12,14] Accordingly, placement of ceramic brackets is contraindicated on the mandibular anterior teeth in den-

titions with deep overbite and minimal overjet. In such cases, sufficient overjet must be created before the mandibular incisors can be bonded. Similarly, during maxillary incisor retraction, the overbite should be reduced first so that the maxillary incisors do not contact the mandibular ceramic brackets. Care should also be taken to bond ceramic brackets on the mandibular canines when they are in a Class II relationship.

Decalcification of the enamel surface

Decalcification of the enamel surface is by far the most important iatrogenic effect of fixed orthodontic appliance therapy (Fig 3-11).[79–84] To prevent the development of lesions and assure proper treatment, the clinician must be familiar with the major aspects of the caries process and current principles of preventive dentistry.

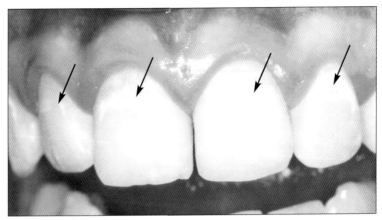

Fig 3-11 Severe decalcifications (white spot lesions) on the maxillary anterior teeth after treatment with a fixed orthodontic appliance.

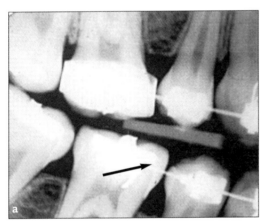 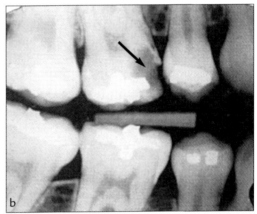

Fig 3-12 Large caries lesion *(arrow)* on maxillary first molar detectable only after debanding *(b)*. Note that the archwire in the mandibular dentition masks the proximal surfaces *(arrow)* *(a)*.

Orthodontic treatment and caries development

Orthodontic treatment is generally carried out during childhood and adolescence, a period when caries incidence is relatively high. Because of visual obstruction by the appliance, lesion development and progression in the proximal surfaces may be difficult to diagnose. Bands protect the proximal surfaces, but they also make radiographic examination more difficult (Fig 3-12).

Individuals with malocclusions often have many retention sites as a result of irregularities in their teeth. More retention sites are then introduced when orthodontic appliances are bonded or banded to the teeth. Oral hygiene is thus markedly more difficult to carry out for orthodontic patients than for individuals with a normal dentition. Studies have shown that fixed orthodontic appliances induce a rapid increase in the volume of dental plaque and that the plaque in orthodontic patients has a lower resting pH than that in nonorthodontic subjects.[85,86] The plaque-retentive properties of the appliance thus impose a severe cariogenic challenge on the labial surfaces, where caries usually does not develop. This may explain the strong relationship between oral hygiene and caries incidence in orthodontic patients.[87] The increased amount of plaque associated with orthodontic appliances also rapidly induces gingival inflammation, especially in areas adjacent to bands. This gingival inflammation is thought to be a result of unspecific bacteria in plaque and is usually reversed after debonding and debanding.[88]

There is a rapid shift in the bacterial flora of plaque following the introduction of orthodontic appliances. Unlike gingival inflammation, caries is associated with acidogenic bacteria. Plaque and salivary levels of *Streptococcus mutans* become significantly elevated after insertion of orthodontic appliances. Both *S mutans* and lactobacilli are often associated with caries development. The association between caries and bacteria is not a simple one, and prediction of caries development based on bacterial counts is uncertain and of little clinical significance.[89–92]

A number of studies have investigated the relationship between orthodontic treatment with fixed appliances and caries development. Whereas some earlier studies showed increased caries frequency and a higher prevalence of fillings in subjects receiving orthodontic treatment, more recent investigations do not confirm this correlation.[79,83,93–97] Several reports have, however, shown an increased incidence of early enamel caries (white spot lesions) on the labial enamel surface during orthodontic treatment (Figs 3-11 and 3-13).[80–82,84,91] These white spot lesions rarely progress to caries and generally are not registered as caries lesions requiring restorative treatment in the DMFT/S indices. Studies have shown that more than 50% of subjects may experience an increase in the number of white spot lesions with fixed orthodontic appliances when no preventive fluoride programs are used.[80] The first molars and maxillary lateral incisors are most significantly affected. Even with regular use of a fluoride dentifrice, enamel dissolution may occur around orthodontic brackets, but probably at a lower rate.[98] With specially designed orthodontic bands, visible white spot lesions can be induced within 4 weeks, ie, within the time period between one clinical appointment and the next.[99] Initial caries developed in the cariogenic environment of an orthodontic appliance may thus become a rapidly progressing process.

Of clinical importance is the observation that pH in the plaque on bonded maxillary incisors is generally lower than in other parts of the bonded dentition, presumably as a result of the low clearance of saliva in this area. Accordingly, any reservoirs of fluoride are rapidly lost. This loss of fluoride and the limited cariostatic effect of fluoride in the low pH in plaque perhaps explains in part why white spot lesions frequently develop on bonded maxillary incisors (Fig 3-14).[100]

Rational caries prophylactic measures for orthodontic patients

It is logical to differentiate between prevention of caries lesion development during orthodontic treatment and treatment of lesions found on labial surfaces at the time of debonding. Since fluoride is the most important agent in caries prevention, the greatest emphasis will be given to different forms of fluoride prophylaxis.

Prevention of caries lesion development during orthodontic treatment

Fluoride dentifrices Fluoride dentifrice is the basis for all caries prevention.[101,102] Most dentifrices contain either sodium fluoride, monofluorophosphate, stannous fluoride, amine fluoride, or a combination of these. Although fluoride concentrations may vary, the maximum allowed is 0.15% in the European community and 0.11% in the US. Fluoride concentrations below 0.1% in dentifrices are not recommended for orthodontic patients.

The cariostatic potential of fluoride dentifrices is most likely larger than generally shown in short-term clinical studies. This is due to a cumulative effect of fluoride through remineralization as a function of time. Furthermore, the cariostatic effect will improve significantly if oral hygiene also is improved (eg, by preventing pH in plaque from dropping under the critical limit for remineralization).[103] Good oral hygiene is thus important in orthodontic patients treated with fixed appliances. Stannous fluoride has a plaque-inhibiting effect as well as an anticaries effect.[104,105] Stannous ions interfere with the adsorption of plaque bacteria to enamel by being bound to the phosphate polymer lipoteichoic acid present on

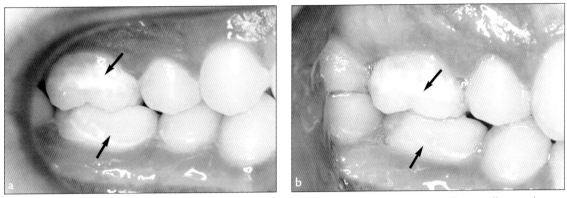

Fig 3-13 White spots (demineralized or hypomineralized enamel) on the labial surfaces of the maxillary and mandibular right first molars *(arrows)* prior to orthodontic treatment *(a)* and at debonding *(b)*. This is an illustration of how important it is to have good photos of the dentition prior to bonding orthodontic attachments.

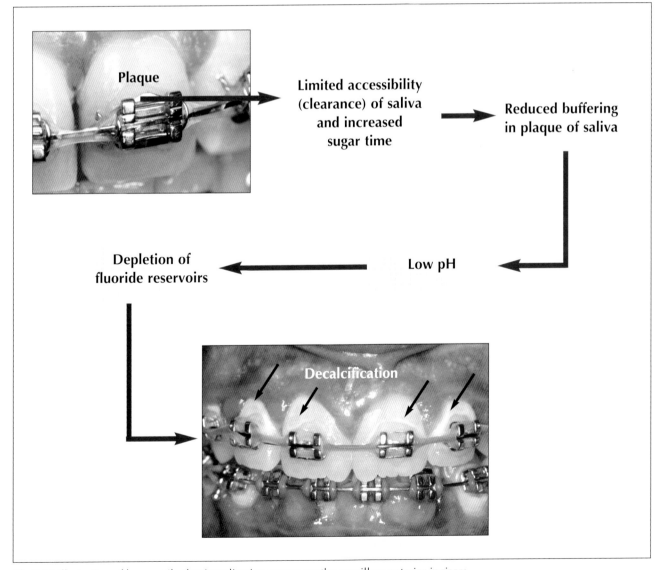

Fig 3-14 Illustration of how easily demineralization occurs on the maxillary anterior incisors.

the surface of gram-positive bacteria. Stannous fluoride also interferes with the acidogenicity of plaque. It is possible that tin atoms bound to the surfaces of the bacteria also block the passage of sucrose into the cell and inhibit acid formation. Stannous fluoride may therefore offer beneficial effects not only against caries, but also against plaque-induced gingival diseases during orthodontic treatment. One disadvantage, a tendency to discolor the enamel, has been reported after the use of stannous fluoride in high concentrations.

Detergents are surface-active agents and are incorporated into dentifrices and mouthrinses to lower the surface tension of the fluid environment in the mouth, to penetrate and loosen surface deposits on the teeth, and to emulsify and suspend the debris removed from the tooth surfaces. Detergents are responsible for the foaming properties and the taste of the dentifrices, and thus they play a major role in the acceptance of the dentifrice by consumers. Detergents also exhibit antimicrobial activity due to their interference with membrane structures and various biologic processes in microorganisms. The anionic agent sodium lauryl sulfate (SLS) is the most popular detergent in dentifrices. It has been shown, however, that the permeability of the oral mucosa is increased in the presence of SLS.

Exposure of the oral mucosa to SLS may therefore potentiate the effect of an allergen. Guinea pigs became sensitized to nickel and chromium ions only when these agents were mixed with SLS. In patients with allergic stomatitis who were sensitized to various food proteins, a significant decrease in the number of oral ulcers was reported when SLS-containing dentifrice was avoided. The ulcerogenic effect of SLS was a result of its denaturing influence on glycoproteins in the oral mucin layer, which induced increased mucosal exposure to food proteins.[106–108] Dentifrices without SLS may therefore be a good choice for orthodontic patients who develop ulcers from their appliance, for those who are potentially allergic to nickel and chromium, and for those who suffer from recurrent aphthous ulcers.

Supplementation of fluoride For the average orthodontic patient, dentifrice alone is ineffective in preventing the development of lesions.[98] Orthodontic patients are therefore instructed to use a fluoride mouthrinse

(0.05% sodium fluoride) daily in addition to fluoride dentifrice. Experimentally, it has been shown that conventional fluoride mouthrinses significantly reduce lesion development beneath bands, although complete inhibition may not be obtained if the cariogenic challenge is severe. An improved cariostatic effect of fluoride mouthrinses has been obtained by combining fluoride with antibacterial agents such as chlorhexidine (CHX), triclosan, and zinc.[30] CHX inhibits plaque formation but has limited clinical applicability because it discolors the teeth and tongue and has a metallic taste. Triclosan has an antibacterial effect and is often combined with zinc to increase the latter agent's antiplaque effect. Furthermore, triclosan has an anti-inflammatory effect. The addition of triclosan to SLS reduced pain and desquamation caused by exposure to this agent. The new fluoride mouthwashes containing triclosan may therefore offer potential benefits for orthodontic patients as a supplement to fluoride dentifrice during treatment.

Although fluoride mouthrinsing has been recommended as a supplement to fluoride dentifrice during fixed appliance therapy,[109] Geiger and coworkers showed that less than 15% of the orthodontic patients rinsed daily with fluoride as instructed.[110] Given the strong and long-lasting cariogenic challenge imposed by fixed orthodontic appliances, a more continuous form of fluoride supplementation is needed independent of patient cooperation. Therefore, topical fluoride in the form of varnishes, solutions, or gels is recommended, especially on the maxillary anterior teeth. Despite large variations in fluoride concentrations, there is no distinct difference in the caries-preventive effect of these different methods of fluoride application. Thus, the choice of method depends on cost, convenience, patient acceptance, and safety. The use of fluoride varnishes has proven to be a safe and feasible method of fluoride application. With fluoride varnishes, the amount of fluoride exposure can be controlled and a minimum amount of chair-time is required compared to conventional solutions and gels. A dose-response effect to concentrated fluoride agents is not readily apparent, and the benefit of frequent application has not been clearly established. If caries activity remains high despite the regular use of dentifrice and topical fluoride applications, additional preventive methods that aim at reducing the challenge

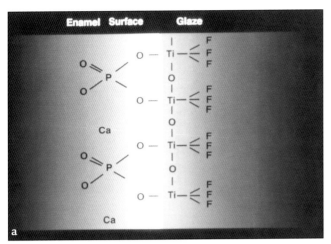
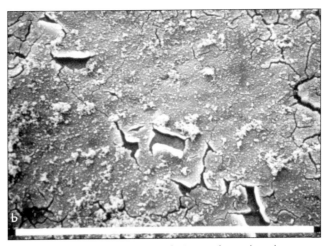

Fig 3-15 *(a)* The mechanism of interaction of titanium tetrafluoride with enamel. Strong Ti–O–Ti–O chains are formed on the enamel surface. *(b)* A titanium-rich, glaze-like coating formed on the enamel surface following application of titanium tetrafluoride.

(improved oral hygiene, use of antimicrobials and other agents that deposit acid-resistant coatings) should be applied instead of increasing the level of fluoride exposure.[111]

Several recent efforts have been made to enhance the cariostatic potential of current fluoride agents and procedures for orthodontic purposes. An improved cariostatic effect of topical fluoride was demonstrated in an orthodontic appliance model of a fluoride solution with low pH and by topical application of a titanium tetrafluoride solution.[112,113] Such procedures produce coatings on the enamel surface that may protect the surface from a lower pH than that for fluorapatite (Fig 3-15). Stannous fluoride has a similar effect.

Fluoride-releasing materials for orthodontic purposes
As explained earlier, glass ionomers have the ability both to release and to take up (recharge) fluoride from the environment. Fluoride-release data from these materials have shown them to be pH dependent; moreover, laboratory experiments probably underestimate their long-term effects.[27] Short-term clinical experiments involving bonding of brackets with glass-ionomer cements have shown that fluoride release significantly inhibits lesion formation when compared to the use of a non-fluoride adhesive. Clinicians who use resin-reinforced glass ionomers to bond brackets usually report fewer problems with enamel decalcification.

Recently, however, Millett et al reported the low cariostatic effects of a glass-ionomer cement.[114] Still, such bonding materials may be of some help in patients with increased risk of decalcification, especially in bonding attachments to the maxillary anterior teeth. However, the major disadvantage of these materials is the low shear bond strength during the first 30 minutes when the archwire is tied.

The long-term cariostatic effect of composite fluoride-releasing adhesives has been questioned since the fluoride concentration is relatively low compared to that of glass ionomers and because most of the fluoride is released shortly after bonding.[24] The ability of compomers to take up fluoride is also limited. Fluoride-releasing composite resins therefore cannot be recommended unless other prophylactic measures are implemented. Fluoride-releasing sealants and elastomeric modules have also been introduced to minimize decalcification. Fluoride-containing sealants can be combined with conventional bonding agents, though the cariostatic effect appears minor.[115] Recently, it was reported that fluoride-releasing elastomeric modules reduced but did not eliminate the incidence of decalcification following orthodontic treatment.[116] Since these modules need to be changed frequently to maintain adequate force, they periodically have a fresh source of fluoride for release.

Treatment of caries lesions developed during orthodontic treatment

Debonding the orthodontic appliance reduces or eliminates the cariogenic environment on the labial surfaces, especially on the maxillary anterior teeth. However, resin remnants are found on almost all teeth after debonding regardless of the finishing technique used (Fig 3-16). This presents another potential risk for plaque to accumulate on the labial surface after debonding, perhaps in particular on the mandibular premolars and molars where brackets are bonded close to the gingival margin. Lesions in these locations may thus progress after debonding if plaque is allowed to accumulate. Treatment of lesions that develop during appliance therapy in the different sites of the dentition represents a clinical challenge.

It has been well established that small carious lesions can heal or remineralize. Fluoride increases the initial rate of remineralization of early enamel lesions and slows the caries process by reacting with the minerals present in the surface of the lesion. This reaction results in the arrest of the lesion.[117] These arrested lesions, which exhibit a white color or become yellowish or dark brown due to exogenous uptake of stains, will persist for life (Fig 3-17). Whether complete remineralization occurs or not seems to be related to the type of lesion present. Initial, surface-softened lesions that develop rapidly (ie, within weeks) can remineralize in saliva if they are kept plaque-free even without concentrated fluoride treatment.[118] Similarly, lesions of the subsurface type that developed over a longer time period may remineralize to some extent in saliva. However, since lesions associated with orthodontic appliances develop during months of treatment, they may be several hundred microns deep and thus are less likely to undergo complete remineralization. Furthermore, it is unlikely that the minerals in these lesions are deposited in the same manner as in sound enamel. Consequently, light scattering from the partly remineralized lesion may not necessarily be identical to that of sound enamel. Most likely, the reduction reported by some researchers in the depths of these lesions is due mainly to surface wear rather than redeposition of minerals.[119,120] Therefore, direct topical application of fluoride on white spot lesions on the maxillary anterior teeth is probably not advisable immediately after debonding.

It has been suggested that acid etching of white spot lesions may increase the surface porosity and hence remineralization.[121] The rate of remineralization in etched and non-etched white spot lesions in either the presence or absence of fluoride has been investigated longitudinally.[122] Typically, the lesions persisted at the end of the experiment, and complete remineralization was not attained irrespective of the treatment. The rate of remineralization varied significantly between the groups at the beginning of the experiment. Etched enamel exhibited more pronounced lesion reduction than non-etched enamel, especially in the absence of fluoride. Later the remineralization process slowed down, and at the end of the experiment no significant differences were found between the groups. The etched lesions retained a porous structure of their surface layer even after a long period of remineralization in vitro.[123] Also, in vitro remineralization is known to proceed more rapidly than in vivo remineralization. Therefore, at this time there is insufficient evidence to recommend etching of white spot lesions to enhance remineralization.

Bonded retainers and space maintainers

Stability following treatment is one of the most important issues in orthodontics. Fixed bonded retainers (Fig 3-18) have gained popularity because of their ease of fabrication, flexibility, esthetics, and need for minimal patient compliance. Several types of bonded retainers and space maintainers have been developed, but they are beyond the scope of this chapter.[14] The most popular bonded retainers are the mandibular and maxillary canine-to-canine retainers. Retainers can be fabricated from thin (0.0195 inch) or thick (0.032 inch) round plain or spiral/multistrand wires. Clinical studies have shown no difference between these wires in terms of plaque and calculus accumulation.[124,125] Based on a thorough analysis and evaluation, the clinician may choose to bond the retainer to each tooth using a thin wire or to the canines only using a thick wire. Oral hygiene in the embrasures is maintained by dental flossing and requires some skill

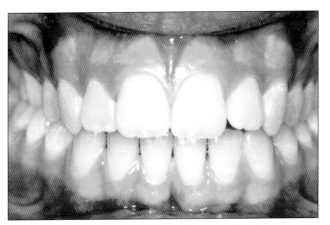

Fig 3-16a Patient with a distal occlusion and a large overjet prior to orthodontic treatment with fixed appliances.

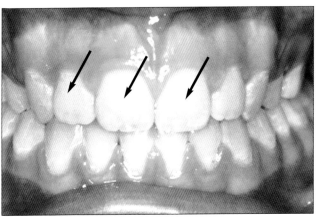

Fig 3-16b Same patient 6 months after debonding. Unesthetic yellow discoloration of resin remnants are visible in the enamel.

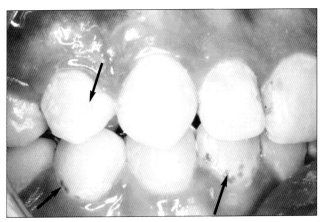

Fig 3-17 Discolored caries lesions *(arrows)* that formed during orthodontic treatment, recorded several years after debonding.

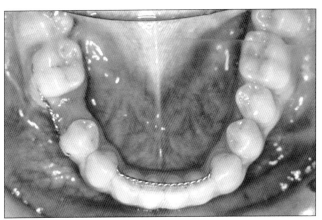

Fig 3-18 Bonded mandibular lingual retainer and space maintainer made from 0.032-inch spiral wires.

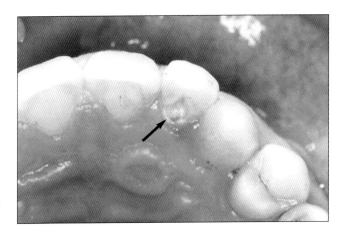

Fig 3-19 Discolored caries lesion *(arrow)* that formed beneath a bonded lingual retainer on the maxillary incisors. Photo taken after debonding.

on the part of the patient. As with brackets, bond failure occurs with retainers, especially with those bonded on the lingual surface of the maxillary anterior teeth. Failure of retainers bonded on the canines only is easier for the patient to detect than when each tooth has been bonded. Loose bonds rapidly create a local cariogenic environment with a greater risk of decalcification (Fig 3-19). The patient must be informed about this potential danger and advised to contact the orthodontist immediately following bond failure.

Enamel Changes Associated with the Debonding of Attachments

Debonding orthodontic attachments and removing residual bonding material from the enamel surface represent critical steps in the overall orthodontic management.[126–130] The debonding and removal of ceramic brackets, in particular, has generated much discussion because of the potential for fracture (Fig 3-20), flaking, and cracking of the enamel as well as the risk of pulp damage. Also, debanding compromised molars may constitute a risk of tooth fracture if the bands have increased retentive properties (ie, are microetched) and have been cemented with glass ionomers.[12,14]

With metal brackets, clinicians worry that the bond is too weak to withstand the forces of orthodontic treatment. With ceramic brackets, clinicians are concerned about whether the bond is too strong for safe debonding. The forces needed to remove an attachment will depend on a number of factors: the bracket type and its retention mechanism, the method of debonding, the composition of the adhesive, and the method of enamel conditioning. As already mentioned, debonding forces above 13 MPa may produce enamel fractures or tears, especially if the forces occur at an angle to the prisms. Fortunately, most debonding techniques result in forces below this level. However, the use of conventional debonding pliers on ceramic brackets that are chemically retained to the enamel surface and that also have been conditioned with phosphoric acid may produce forces far above the limit for safe debonding.

Enamel cracks

Enamel cracks often are difficult to detect without the use of special transillumination techniques (Fig 3-21); that is, they generally are not visible on routine examination or in intraoral photographs. As a result, documentation of enamel cracks before treatment is difficult except perhaps those on the anterior teeth. The prevalence of enamel cracks after debonding has been found to be as high as 50%, of which vertical cracks are the most common. However, cracks oriented in an oblique direction are also frequently observed. A clear correlation has been found between enamel cracks and debonding forces, and a large number of horizontal cracks after debonding may indicate improper bonding/debonding techniques.[12]

Debonding metal brackets

Metal brackets can usually be debonded relatively easily by applying forces that peel the bracket base away from the tooth. Often such forces cause bond failure at the adhesive-bracket interface, leaving most of the adhesive on the enamel surface. Pliers are available that place the sharp edges at the enamel-adhesive interface and apply a slow, gradual squeezing force until the bracket fails. The gentlest method is to use a Weingart type of pliers to squeeze the bracket wings (Fig 3-22).[14] This deforms the bracket and peels it off the enamel surface. One of the authors (BØ) prefers to use a band remover and simply squeeze one of the bracket wings (Fig 3-23). This induces stress in the adhesive and removes the bracket without discomfort to the patient. The same pliers can then be used to remove the bands.

Debonding ceramic brackets

Over the last decade, ceramic brackets have become increasingly popular as patients demand more esthetic orthodontic appliances. Ceramic brackets are made of polycrystalline or monocrystalline forms of aluminum oxide, which is an inert material; as a result, they cannot chemically adhere directly to any of the currently available bonding resins. For this reason, two basic mechanisms have been developed to attach ceramic brackets to the adhesive. The first method is mechanical retention, which is achieved by creating indentations or recesses in the bracket base, much like the mesh on the base of metal brackets. These indentations provide a mechanical interlocking with the resin adhesive and thus facilitate debonding. The second method is by coating an intermediate layer of glass on the ceramic bracket base and then using a silane coupler to obtain a chemical bond between the bracket and the adhesive. The silane molecule is a bifunctional molecule; that is, one end is a reactive silanol group that can bind tenaciously to glass, while the other end of the molecule reacts with other acrylic resins and polymerizes, producing a cohesive bond with the resin material.[12]

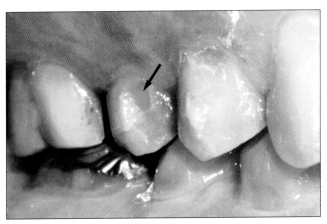

Fig 3-20 Enamel tearout *(arrow)* following debonding of a ceramic bracket.

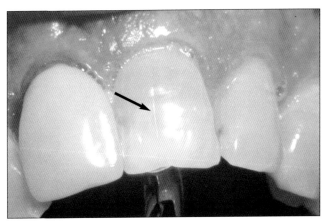

Fig 3-21 Enamel crack *(arrow)* made visible via fiberoptic trans-illumination.

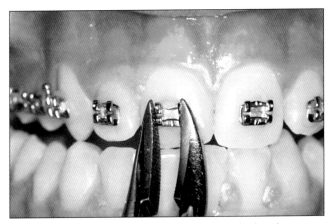

Fig 3-22 Debonding of bracket by squeezing the bracket wings with a Weingart pliers.

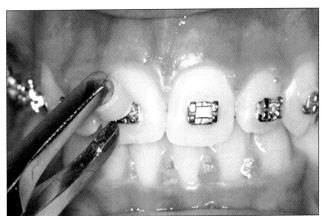

Fig 3-23 Debonding of bracket by squeezing one bracket wing with a band remover.

Bond strength of ceramic brackets depends on *(a)* the type of retention of the ceramic bracket (eg, chemical versus mechanical bond or combinations); *(b)* the conditioning method used (eg, phosphoric acid versus polyacrylic acid); and/or *(c)* the bonding material used (eg, filled versus unfilled adhesives). Usually, ceramic brackets that rely on mechanical retention debond easier than chemically retained ceramic brackets. Nevertheless, the adhesion between the resin and the ceramic bracket base has increased to a point where the most common site of bond fracture during debonding has shifted from the bracket base–adhesive interface to the enamel-adhesive interface. This shift has led to an increased incidence of bond failures within the enamel surface.[12]

Although the tensile strength of ceramics is greater than that of stainless steel, less energy is required to cause fracture of ceramic brackets than of conventional stainless-steel brackets. This phenomenon is related to "fracture toughness," or the ability of a material to resist fracture. During loading, stainless steel will elongate approximately 20% of its original length before failing, while sapphire will elongate less than 1% before failing. Thus, ceramics are more likely to fracture than metals under the same conditions during debonding (Fig 3-24). Another factor related to the fracture of ceramic brackets is the condition of the surface of the ceramic. A shallow scratch on the surface or a microscopic crack will drastically reduce the load required for fracture of ceramic brackets, whereas

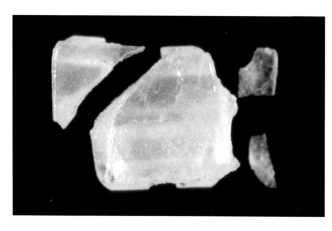

Fig 3-24 Ceramic bracket fractured during debonding.

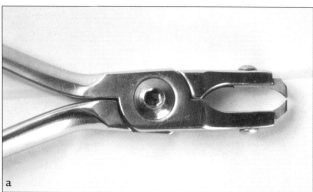

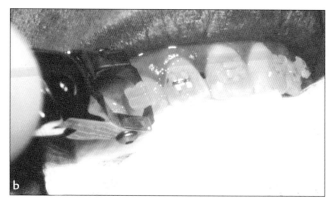

Fig 3-25 Debonding of ceramic bracket using a sharp-edged pliers (a) with the blades at the enamel-adhesive interface (b).

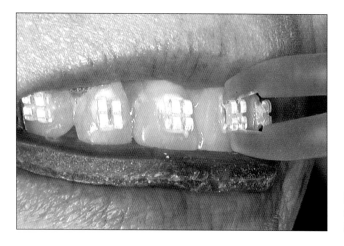

Fig 3-26 Special pliers (Inspire) for debonding the single crystal sapphire brackets. (Courtesy of Dr Michael L. Swartz, Encino, CA.)

the same scratch or crack on a metal surface will have little effect on fracture under load.[12]

As noted earlier, the optimal method for removing orthodontic metal brackets is to apply a force that peels the bracket base away from the tooth. Because of the nature of ceramic brackets, debonding methods that employ a shear force often result in fracture. As a result, manufacturers have developed four different types of debonding techniques specifically designed for ceramic brackets: mechanical, ultrasonic, electrothermal, and laser.

Mechanical debonding The most widely accepted mechanical debonding technique for ceramic brackets is to use a sharp-edged pliers and place the blades at the enamel-adhesive interface (Fig 3-25). A slow, gradual

Fig 3-27 Series showing how to debond ceramic brackets with a vertical scribe using a Howes or Weingart pliers. (Courtesy of 3M Unitek.)

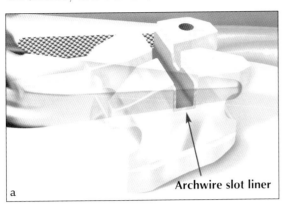

Archwire slot liner

a

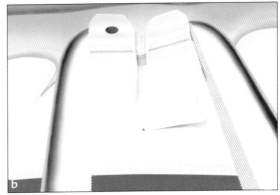

b

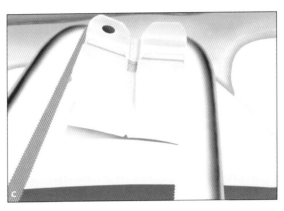

c

Fig 3-27a Position the tips of the pliers over the mesial or distal sides of the metal archwire.

Figs 3-27b and 3-27c Squeeze gently with the hand instrument until the bracket collapses. Do not place the instrument tips below the bottom of the archwire slot liner. Removal of adhesive flash prior to debonding is recommended to reduce the risk of bracket breakage.

squeezing force is applied until the bracket fails. This method depends either on the deformation of the bracket to break the bond at the bracket-adhesive interface or on stressing the adhesive to the point of causing cohesive failure within the resin composite. Some debonding pliers have narrow (2.0 mm) or wide (3.0 mm) blades. The narrow-bladed pliers are recommended because they are as effective as the wide blades but transmit debonding forces that are significantly (approximately 25%) less than those transmitted by the wide blades.[12]

Recently, a specially designed plastic pliers was introduced (Fig 3-26) to address the special needs of debonding a ceramic bracket. Because ceramics are rigid, they cannot be distorted to create a peel type of force. By crushing it mesiodistally, the bracket will fracture (see Fig 3-24), often leaving the ceramic base

still attached to the enamel and making it very difficult to remove safely. The plastic pliers is designed to grasp the bracket firmly without fracturing it. The bracket is then removed by rotating the pliers slowly, either gingivally or toward the incisal/occlusal. The bracket comes off in one piece, leaving the bonding resin to be removed and the enamel polished. The important part of the debonding technique is to compress the handles of the pliers together until they touch to gain a very firm grip on the bracket. The tips of the pliers quickly become worn and distorted and should be discarded after a single patient use (personal communication, Dr Michael L. Swartz, Encino, CA).

Some ceramic brackets have a vertical scribe line that will easily split when the bracket is squeezed (Fig 3-27). However, part of the bracket may break and remain on the enamel surface following debonding,

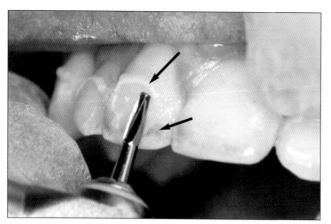

Fig 3-28a Adhesive remnants removed with a tungsten carbide bur. Note the excess adhesive material and discoloration *(arrows)*.

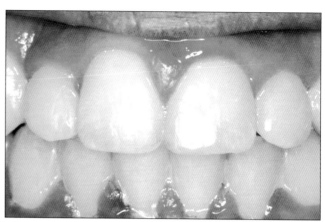

Fig 3-28b The enamel surface after clean-up.

and the remnants have to be removed carefully with a bur. Ceramic brackets should certainly not be bonded to teeth that have cracks or other signs of physical defects.

Ultrasonic bracket removal Despite longer debonding time (30 to 60 seconds per bracket), effective bracket removal can be achieved by means of the ultrasonic technique. The advantages of this approach include potentially less enamel damage and a decreased likelihood of bracket failure. In addition, adhesive removal after debonding can be accomplished with the same ultrasonic tip. Some of the disadvantages associated with the ultrasonic technique include increased debonding time, excessive wear of the expensive ultrasonic tip, the need to apply some force and water spray to reduce the heat buildup and minimize any possibility of pulpal damage, and the potential for soft tissue injury. Although the method requires further testing and is not yet recommended for clinical use, ultrasonic debonding may be effective when a ceramic bracket fractures with conventional methods and part of it remains attached to the tooth.[12]

Electrothermal debonding The advantages of electrothermal debonding include a reduced incidence of bracket failure and a relatively short debonding time. The reduced incidence of bracket failure is attributable to the small amount of force required to break the bond after the heat-induced tip has promoted bond

failure by softening the adhesive. The main disadvantage of this method is the potential for pulp damage and mucosal burns, although recent studies have not indicated any such iatrogenic effects.[131,132]

Laser debonding Both carbon dioxide and YAG (yttrium-aluminum-garnet) lasers have been tested and work on the same principle as electrothermal debonding through heat generation to soften the adhesive. When combining mechanical debonding of ceramics with laser in vitro, the debonding forces on the incisors have been lowered by a factor of 16. The laser approach, although still experimental, is more precise than other techniques in terms of time and the amount of heat application required, but a major disadvantage is the high cost of the instrument.[12]

Removal of residual bonding material

Safe debonding techniques aim to break the bond between the bracket base and the adhesive rather than that between the adhesive and the enamel surface. Accordingly, most of the adhesive remains on the surface after debonding (see Fig 3-27). This material must certainly be removed and the enamel surface polished to avoid discoloration and plaque buildup. Conditioning the enamel surface with phosphoric acid prior to bonding the attachment induces irreversible changes to the enamel structure. Furthermore, enamel color alterations may occur as a result of the irreversible penetration of resin tags into the enamel structure at depths reaching 30 to 50 μm or more (see Fig 3-5).[133,134] Only limited research has been done on the long-term effects of leaving residual adhesive on the enamel surface after debonding, although clinical experience indicates no significant detrimental effects. A recent in vitro study indicated that the debonding cleaning process involving adhesive grinding was more important for enamel color alterations than whether the surface had been etched or not.[134]

To remove residual material, tungsten carbide burs (Fig 3-28) are preferable to other methods, such as diamond burs, sandpaper disks, or rubber wheels. Water cooling is recommended when bulk material is removed at high speeds (>30,000 rpm) to avoid pulpal damage. When remnants of the adhesive are removed at lower speeds, better contrast between the adhesive and enamel is obtained without water cooling. However, conventional carbide burs may be aggressive and produce irreversible changes in the enamel surface due to their shape and the sharpness of their blades. Recently, a carbide-finishing bur with a larger wedge angle and oblique ground chamfer has been shown to produce less damage to the enamel surface than conventional carbide burs.[135] The enamel surface is often polished with pumice or a paste after the adhesive has been removed even if some (5 to 10 μm) of the enamel surface is lost.[136]

Clinical Guidelines

The bonding and debonding of attachments to the enamel surface and treatment with fixed appliances are based on techniques and principles developed over time and based on clinical experience and research. Some enamel is inevitably lost when conventional bonding and debonding procedures are followed; other adverse effects include decalcification during treatment and the development of enamel cracks and fractures during debonding of ceramic brackets.

Acid penetrates to a depth of about 50 μm following acid etching of the enamel surface with 30% phosphoric acid; consequently, resin tags may also reach this depth. During bracket debonding and "clean up," varying amounts of enamel are lost, ranging from 1 or 2 μm to more than 20 μm. Therefore, there is a risk that resin tags may still remain in the

enamel surface following debonding, and these may later discolor. Clearly, the use of self-etching primers or conditioning of the enamel surface with polyacrylic acid prior to bonding will reduce the damage to the enamel surface as well as the risk of leaving residual adhesive.

Following is a summary of the major conclusions and recommendations of this chapter.

Bonding attachment to the enamel

Conditioning
Pumicing prior to etching is not required. Most plaque is removed by the patient during brushing. Poor oral hygiene is a contraindication for orthodontic treatment with fixed appliances. The concentration of phosphoric acid for conditioning of the enamel surface must not exceed 37%, and etching should not exceed 30 seconds. There is a reduced loss of the enamel surface with the use of self-etching primers. The use of resin-reinforced glass ionomers eliminates the need for phosphoric acid etching since conditioning with polyacrylic acid is recommended, but the initial bond strength is reduced.

Unfilled sealants
Unfilled sealants penetrate more easily than bonding material into the micropores of the etched enamel, although bonding without sealants may not influence bond strength. The potential for a caries-preventive effect of sealants has not been established.

Bonding material
The choice of bonding material depends on clinician preference. The cariostatic effect of fluoride-containing composites is low. More fluoride is released from glass ionomers with a possible cariostatic potential. In vitro measurements have consistently shown initial lower bond strength of resin-reinforced glass ionomers than composite adhesives. A slight excess of material is needed on the attachment base to avoid voids and fill out irregular surfaces.

Excess materials should be removed during and after bonding to avoid plaque buildup. This can be accomplished either by a scaler prior to curing or with tungsten carbide burs after curing. The use of tungsten carbide burs for removing excess material induces less damage to the enamel surface than any other procedure.

Preventive measures during treatment

It is essential for the clinician to understand that the cariostatic effect of fluoride is limited when the pH in plaque is very low. Such situations appear frequently in association with orthodontic appliances, especially on the maxillary anterior teeth. This induces an environment that reduces the efficiency of fluoride. Good oral hygiene during treatment is thus essential to obtain an optimal cariostatic effect of fluoride.

Patients should be instructed to brush twice daily with a fluoride dentifrice (≥0.1% F) and to rinse every evening after brushing with a fluoride mouthrinse. Predictors of caries risk include poor oral hygiene, past caries experience, failure to brush regularly with a fluoride dentifrice, and regular consumption of sucrose between meals in the form of snacks and soft drinks. Carbonated soft drinks have a very low pH, and frequent consumption may induce erosion of the enamel in spite of good oral hygiene.

Oral hygiene must be monitored during treatment.[137,138] The best indicator of poor oral hygiene is gingival bleeding. There is a positive association between oral hygiene and caries incidence in orthodontic patients. Fluoride and good oral hygiene have a synergistic effect. Complex appliances that complicate plaque removal should be avoided on the maxillary anterior teeth. Plaque pH may drop rapidly in this area, reducing the cariostatic effect of fluoride.

Topical fluoride solutions, gels, or varnishes should be applied at regular intervals to decrease caries risk. The clinical effect of these fluoride products and procedures is more or less similar. The method of choice depends on cost, convenience, patient acceptance, and safety.

Preventive measures after debonding

Anterior teeth
White spot lesions found on the maxillary anterior teeth should not be treated with topical fluoride during the first few weeks after orthodontic therapy is completed. There is no risk that lesions will progress in this area following debonding. Fluoride increases redeposition of fluorhydroxyapatite and seals the surface. This prevents further remineralization, although it will not reduce the optical appearance of the white spot. Surface abrasion by toothbrushing will most often reduce the extent of white spots after debonding. At present there are no simple methods to "treat" unesthetic lesions persisting on the anterior teeth.

Posterior teeth
There is risk that carious lesions in posterior teeth may progress even after debonding due to plaque accumulation. Optimal oral hygiene and some fluoride therapy are recommended in these locations.

Debonding attachments

The bracket retention mechanism, the method of debonding, the composition of the adhesive, and the method of enamel conditioning influence bond strength and the force applied during debonding.

When using conventional debonding methods, the force applied must not exceed 13 MPa to prevent enamel cracks, flaking, or fracture. Care must be exercised when debonding attachments from compromised teeth.

Several optional methods to remove metal brackets can be used to avoid damaging the enamel surface of normal teeth.

A safe, simple, and efficient method for removing ceramic brackets has yet to be designed. Conventional ceramics are most gently removed using pliers to apply a squeezing force to the bracket with the blades of the pliers at the enamel surface and within the adhesive. Ceramic brackets that have a vertical scribe line and metal slots are preferred since they allow the side of the brackets to collapse when it is squeezed. Alternative methods for debonding ceramic brackets (ultrasonic, electrothermal, laser) are available, but more research is needed before definite clinical recommendations can be made. After debonding, residual adhesive should be removed using tungsten carbide burs followed by polishing with pumice or a paste.

References

1. Fejerskov O, Thylstrup A. Dental enamel. In: Mjør IA, Fejerskov O (eds). Human Oral Embryology and Histology. Copenhagen: Munksgaard, 1985:50–89.

2. Risnes S. Circumferential continuity of perikymata in human dental enamel investigated by scanning electron microscopy. Scand J Dent Res 1985;93:185–191.

3. Arends J, Jongebloed W, Øgaard B, Rølla G. SEM and microradiographic investigation of initial enamel caries. Scand J Dent Res 1987;95:193–201.

4. Newman GV. Epoxy adhesives for orthodontic attachments: Progress report. Am J Orthod 1965;51:901–912.

5. Buonocore MG. A simple method of increasing the adhesion of acrylic filling materials to enamel surface. J Dent Res 1955;34:849.

6. Swift EJ. Bonding systems for restorative materials—A comprehensive review. Pediatr Dent 1998;20:80–84.

7. Smith DC, Cartz L. Crystalline interface formed by polyacrylic acid and tooth enamel. J Dent Res 1973;52:1155.

8. Årtun J, Bergland S. Clinical trials with crystal growth conditioning as an alternative to acid-etch enamel pretreatment. Am J Orthod 1984;85:333–340.

9. Maijer R, Smith DC. Crystal growth on the outer enamel surface—An alternative to acid etching. Am J Orthod Dentofacial Orthop 1986;89:183–193.

10. Farquhar RB. Direct bonding comparing a polyacrylic acid and a phosphoric acid. Am J Orthod Dentofacial Orthop 1986;90:187–194.

11. Knox J, Jones ML. Crystal bonding—An adhesive system with a future? Brit J Orthod 1995;22:309–317.

12. Bishara SE, Dale EF. Ceramic brackets: Something old, something new, a review. Semin Orthod 1997;3:178–188.

13. Fuhrman R, Gutknecht N, Magunski A, Lampert F, Diedrich P. Conditioning of enamel with Nd:YAG and CO_2 dental laser systems and with phosphoric acid. J Orofacial Orthop 2001;62:375–386.

14. Zachrisson BU. Bonding in orthodontics. In: Graber TM, Vanarsdall RL (eds). Orthodontics, Current Principles and Techniques, ed 3. St. Louis: Mosby, 2000:557–645.

15. Zachrisson BU, Brobakken BO. Clinical comparison of direct versus indirect bonding with different bracket types and adhesives. Am J Orthod 1978;74:62–78.

16. Chan DCN, Swift EJ, Bishara SE. In vitro evaluation of a fluoride-releasing orthodontic resin. J Dent Res 1990;69:1576–1579.

17. Bishara SE, Swift EJ Jr, Chan DC. Evaluation of fluoride release from an orthodontic bonding system. Am J Orthod Dentofacial Orthop 1991;100:106–109.

18. Eliades T, Viazis AD, Eliades G. Enamel fluoride uptake from an experimental fluoride-releasing orthodontic adhesive. Am J Orthod Dentofacial Orthop 1992;101:420–424.

19. Aasrum E, Ng'ang'a PM, Dahm S, Øgaard B. Tensile bond strength of orthodontic brackets bonded with a fluoride-releasing light-curing adhesive. An in vitro comparative study. Am J Orthod Dentofacial Orthop 1993;104:48–50.

20. Trimpeneers LM, Dermaut R. A clinical evaluation of the effectiveness of a fluoride-releasing visible light-activated bonding system to reduce demineralization around orthodontic brackets. Am J Orthod Dentofacial Orthop 1996;110:18–22.

21. Rock WP, Abdulla MS. Shear bond strength produced by composite and compomer light cured orthodontic adhesives. J Dent 1997;25:243–249.

22. Millett DT, Cattanach D, McFadzean R, Pattison J, McColl J. Laboratory evaluation of a compomer and a resin-modified glass ionomer cement for orthodontic bonding. Angle Orthod 1999;69:58–63.

23. Millett DT, McCluskey LA, McAuley F, Creanor SL, Newell J, Love J. A comparative clinical trial of a compomer and a resin adhesive for orthodontic bonding. Angle Orthod 2000;70:233–240.

24. Büyükyilmaz T, Øgaard B. Caries-preventive effects of fluoride-releasing materials. Adv Dent Res 1995;9:377–383.

25. Steckel SE, Rueggeberg FA, Whitford GM. Effect of cure mode and fluoride content on bracket debonding. Angle Orthod 1999;69:282–287.

26. Kvam E, Broch J, Nissen-Meyer IH. Comparison between a zinc phosphate cement and a glass ionomer cement for cementation of orthodontic bands. Eur J Orthod 1983;5:307–334.

27. Rezk-Lega F, Øgaard B, Rølla G. Availability of fluoride from glass-ionomer luting cements in human saliva. Scand J Dent Res 1991;99:60–63.

28. Seppä L, Forss H, Øgaard B. The effect of fluoride application on fluoride release and the antibacterial action of glass-ionomer. J Dent Res 1993;72;1310–1314.

29. Forsten L. Resin-modified glass ionomer cements: Fluoride release and uptake. Acta Odontol Scand 1995;53:222–225.

30. Øgaard B. Oral microbiological changes, long-term enamel alterations due to decalcification, and caries prophylactic aspects. In: Brantley WA, Eliades T. Orthodontic Materials: Scientific and Clinical Aspects. Stuttgart: Thieme, 2001:123–142.

31. Klockowski R, Davis EL, Joynt RB, Wieczkowski G, McDonald A. Bond strength and durability of glass-ionomer cements used as bonding agents in the placement of orthodontic brackets. Am J Orthod Dentofacial Orthop 1989;96:60–64.

32. Fajen VB, Duncanson MG, Nanda RS, Currier GF, Angolkar PV. An in vitro evaluation of bond strength of three glass-ionomer cements. Am J Orthod Dentofacial Orthop 1990;97:316–322.

33. Oen JO, Gjerdet NR, Wisth PJ. Glass ionomer cements used as bonding materials for metal orthodontic brackets: An in vitro study. Eur J Orthod 1991;13:187–191.

34. Rezk-Lega F, Øgaard B. Tensile bond force of glass-ionomer cements in direct bonding of orthodontic brackets: An in vitro comparative study. Am J Orthod Dentofacial Orthop 1991;100:357–361.

35. Rezk-Lega F, Øgaard B, Arends J. An in vivo study on the merits of two glass ionomers for the cementation of orthodontic bands. Am J Orthod Dentofacial Orthop 1991;99:162–167.

36. Evans R, Oliver R. Orthodontic bonding using glass-ionomer cements: An in vitro study. Eur J Orthod 1991;13: 493–500.

37. Compton AM, Meyers CE, Hondrum SO, Lorton L. Comparison of the shear bond strength of a light-cured glass ionomer and a chemically cured glass ionomer for use as an orthodontic bonding agent. Am J Orthod Dentofacial Orthop 1992;101:138–144.

38. Fricker JP. A 12-month clinical evaluation of a light-activated glass polyalkenoate (ionomer) cement for the direct bonding of orthodontic brackets. Am J Orthod Dentofacial Orthop 1994;105:502–505.

39. Wiltshire WA. Shear bond strengths of a glass ionomer for direct bonding in orthodontics. Am J Orthod Dentofacial Orthop 1994;106:127–130.

40. Miguel JA, Almeida MA, Chevitarese O. Clinical comparison between a glass ionomer cement and a composite for direct bonding of orthodontic brackets. Am J Orthod Dentofacial Orthop 1995;107:484–487.

41. Silverman E, Cohen M, Demke RS, Silverman M. A new light-cured glass ionomer cement that bonds brackets to the teeth without etching in the presence of saliva. Am J Orthod Dentofacial Orthop 1995;108:231–236.

42. Miller JR, Mancl L, Arbuckle G, Baldwin J, Phillips RW. A three-year clinical trial using a glass ionomer cement for the bonding of orthodontic brackets. Angle Orthod 1996; 66:309–312.

43. Norevall LI, Marcusson A, Persson M. A clinical evaluation of a glass ionomer cement as an orthodontic bonding adhesive compared with an acrylic resin. Eur J Orthod 1996; 18:373–384.

44. Bourke AM, Walls AW, McCabe JF. Light-activated glass polyalkenoate (ionomer) cements: The setting reaction. J Dent Res 1992;20:115–120.

45. Komori A, Ishikawa H. Evaluation of a resin-reinforced glass ionomer cement for use as an orthodontic bonding agent. Angle Orthod 1997;67:189–196.

46. Czochrowska E, Øgaard B, Duschner H, Ruben J, Arends J. Cariostatic effect of a light-cured, resin reinforced glass-ionomer for bonding orthodontic brackets in vivo. A combined microradiography and confocal laser scanning microscopy study. J Orofacial Orthop 1998;59:265–273.

47. Czochrowska E, Burzykowski T, Buyukyilmaz T, Øgaard B. The effect of long-term water storage on the tensile strength of orthodontic brackets bonded with resin-modified glass-ionomer cements. J Orofacial Orthop 1999;60:361–370.

48. Rix D, Foley TF, Mamandras A. Comparison of bond strength of three adhesives: Composite resin, hybrid GIC, and glass-filled GIC. Am J Orthod Dentofacial Orthop 2001;119:36–42.

49. Kirovski I, Madzarova S. Tensile bond strength of a light-cured ionomer cement when used for bracket bonding under different conditions: An in vitro study. Eur J Orthod 2000;22:719–723.

50. Flores AR, Saez EG, Barcelo F. Metallic bracket to enamel bonding with a photopolymerizable resin-reinforced glass ionomer. Am J Orthod Dentofacial Orthop 1999;116: 514–517.

51. Shammaa I, Ngan P, Kim H, Kao E, Gladwin M, Gunel E, Brown C. Comparison of bracket debonding force between two conventional resin adhesives and a resin-reinforced glass ionomer cement: An in vitro and in vivo study. Angle Orthod 1999;69:463–469.

52. Bishara SE, VonWald L, Laffoon JF, Jakobsen JR. Effect of changing enamel conditioner concentration on the shear bond strength of a resin-modified glass ionomer adhesive. Am J Orthod Dentofacial Orthop 2000;118:311–316.

53. Larmour CJ, Stirrups DR. An ex vivo assessment of a resin-modified glass ionomer cement in relation to bonding technique. J Orthod 2001;28:207–210.

54. Powers JM, Messersmith ML. Enamel etching and bond strength. In: Brantley WA, Eliades T. Orthodontic Materials: Scientific and Clinical Aspects. Stuttgart: Thieme, 2001:105–122.

55. Reynolds IR. A review of direct orthodontic bonding. Br J Orthod 1979;2:171–182.

56. Adolfsson U, Larsson E, Øgaard B. Bond failure of a no-mix adhesive during orthodontic treatment. Am J Orthod Dentofacial Orthop 2002;122:277–281.

57. Zachrisson B. A posttreatment evaluation of direct bonding in orthodontics. Am J Orthod 1977;71:173–189.

58. Mizrahi E. Success and failure of banding and bonding. A clinical study. Angle Orthod 1982;52:113–117.

59. Millett DT. A 5-year clinical review of bond failure with a no-mix adhesive (Right on). Eur J Orthod 1994;16:203–211.

60. Miguel JAM. Clinical comparison between a glass ionomer cement and a composite for direct bonding of orthodontic brackets. Am J Orthod Dentofacial Orthop 1995;197: 484–487.

61. Norevall LI, Marcusson A, Persson M. A clinical evaluation of a glass ionomer cement as an orthodontic bonding adhesive compared with an acrylic resin. Eur J Orthod 1996;18:373–384.

62. Trimpeneers LM, Dermaut LR. A clinical trial comparing the failure rates of two orthodontic bonding systems. Am J Orthod Dentofacial Orthop 1996;110:547–550.

63. Frost T, Norevall LI, Persson M. Bond strength and clinical efficiency for two light guide sizes in orthodontic bracket bonding. Brit J Orthod 1997;24:35–40.

64. Sunna S, Rock WP. Clinical performance of orthodontic brackets and adhesive systems: A randomized clinical trial. Br J Orthod 1998;25:283–287.

65. Millett DT. A 5-year clinical review of bond failure with a light cured resin adhesive. Angle Orthod 1998;68:351–356.

66. Armas Galindo HR, Sadowsky PL, Vlachos C, Jacobson A, Wallace D. An in vivo comparison between a visible light-cured bonding system and a chemically cured bonding system. Am J Orthod Dentofacial Orthop 1998;113: 271–275.

67. Mattick CR, Hobson RS. A comparative micro-topographic study of the buccal enamel of different tooth types. J Orthod 2000;27:143–148.

68. Linklater RA, Gordon PH. An ex vivo study to investigate bond strength of different tooth types. J Orthod 2001;28: 59–65.

69. Smith RS, Spinelli JA, Tartakow DJ. Phosphoric acid penetration during direct bonding. Am J Orthod 1976;70: 543–550.

70. Legler LR, Retief DH, Bradley EL. Effects of phosphoric acid concentration and etch duration on enamel depth of etch: An in vitro study. Am J Orthod Dentofacial Orthop 1990;98:154–160.

71. Zentner A, Duschner H. Structural changes of acid etched enamel examined under confocal laser scanning microscope. J Orofacial Orthop 1996;57:202–209.

72. Webster M, Nanda R, Duncanson M, Khajotia S, Sinha P. The effect of saliva on shear bond strengths of hydrophilic bonding systems. Am J Orthod Dentofacial Orthop 2001;119:54–58.

73. Grandhi RK, Combe EC, Speidel TM. Shear bond strength of stainless steel orthodontic brackets with a moisture insensitive primer. Am J Orthod Dentofacial Orthop 2001;119:251–255.

74. Zachrisson BU, Heimgard E, Ruyter IE, Mjör IA. Problems with sealants for bracket bonding. Am J Orthod 1979; 75:641–649.

75. Tang ATH, Björkman L, Lindbäck KF, Andlin-Sobocki A, Ekstrand J. Retrospective study of orthodontic bonding without liquid resin. Am J Orthod Dentofacial Orthop 2000;118:300–306.

76. Cinader D. Chemical processes and performance comparisons of Transbond Plus self etching primer. Orthod Perspec 2001;7:8–9.

77. Bishara SE, VonWald L, Laffoon JF, Warren JJ. Effect of a self-etch primer/adhesive on the shear bond strength of orthodontic brackets. Am J Orthod Dentofacial Orthop 2001;119:621–624.

78. Buyukyilmaz T, Usumez S, Karaman AI. Effect of self-etching primers on bond strength—Are they reliable? Angle Orthod 2003;73:64–70.

79. Zachrisson BU, Zachrisson S. Caries incidence and orthodontic treatment with fixed appliances. Scand J Dent Res 1971;79:183–192.

80. Gorelick L, Geiger AM, Gwinnett AJ. Incidence of white spot formation after bonding and banding. Am J Orthod 1982;81:93–98.

81. Mizrahi E. Surface distribution of enamel opacities following orthodontic treatment. Am J Orthod Dentofacial Orthop 1983;84:323–331.

82. Årtun J, Brobakken BO. Prevalence of carious white spots after orthodontic treatment with multibonded appliances. Eur J Orthod 1986;8:229–234.

83. Øgaard B. Incidence of filled surfaces from 10-18 years of age in an orthodontically treated and untreated group in Norway. Eur J Orthod 1989;11:116–119.

84. Øgaard B. Prevalence of white spot lesions in 19-year olds: A study on untreated and orthodontically treated persons 5 years after treatment. Am J Orthod Dentofacial Orthop 1989;96:423–427.

85. Chatterjee R, Kleinberg I. Effect of orthodontic band placement on the chemical composition of human incisor plaque. Arch Oral Biol 1979;24:97–100.

86. Gwinnett JA, Ceen F. Plaque distribution on bonded brackets. Am J Orthod 1979;75:667–677.

87. Zachrisson BU, Zachrisson S. Caries incidence and oral hygiene during orthodontic treatment. Scand J Dent Res 1971;79:394–401.

88. Løe H, Theilade E, Jensen SB. Experimental gingivitis in man. J Periodontol 1965;36:177–188.

89. Scheie AA, Arneberg P, Krogstad O. Effect of orthodontic treatment on prevalence of Streptococcus mutans in plaque and saliva. Scand J Dent Res 1984;92:211–217.

90. Fournier A, Payant L, Bouclin R. Adherence of Streptococcus mutans to orthodontic brackets. Am J Orthod Dentofacial Orthop 1998;14:414–417.

91. Øgaard B, Larsson E, Bishara SE, Birkhed D. Effects of a combined application of antimicrobial and fluoride varnishes in orthodontic patients. Am J Orthod Dentofacial Orthop 2001;120:28–35.

92. Hausen H, Seppä L, Fejerskov O. Can caries be predicted? In: Thylstrup A, Fejerskov O (eds). Textbook of Clinical Cariology. Copenhagen: Munksgaard, 1994:393–411.

93. Bach EN. Incidence of caries during orthodontic treatment. Am J Orthod 1953;39:756–778.

94. Ingervall B. The influence of orthodontic appliances on caries frequency. Odontol Rev 1962;13:175–190.

95. Wisth PJ, Nord A. Caries experience in orthodontically treated individuals. Angle Orthod 1977;47:59–64.

96. Hollender L, Rönnerman A. Proximal caries progression in connection with orthodontic treatment. Swed Dent J 1978;2:153–160.

97. Southard MS, Cohen ME, Ralls SA, Rouse LA. Effects of fixed appliance orthodontic treatment on DMF indices. Am J Orthod Dentofacial Orthop 1986;81:93–98.

98. O'Reilly MM, Featherstone JDB. Demineralization and remineralization around orthodontic appliances: An in vivo study. Am J Orthod Dentofacial Orthop 1987;92:33–40.

99. Øgaard B, Rölla G, Arends J. Orthodontic appliances and enamel demineralization. Part 1. Lesion development. Am J Orthod Dentofacial Orthop 1988;94:68–73.

100. Arneberg P, Giertsen E, Emberland H, Øgaard B. Intra-oral variations in total plaque fluoride related to plaque pH. A study in orthodontic patients. Caries Res 1997;31:451–456.

101. Fejerskov O, Thylstrup A, Larsen MJ. Rational use of fluoride in caries prevention. A concept based on the possible cariostatic mechanisms. Acta Odontol Scand 1981;39:241–249.

102. König KG. Role of fluoride toothpastes in a caries-preventive strategy. Caries Res 1993;27(suppl 1):23–28.

103. Øgaard B, Rölla G, Cruz R. Fluoride dentifrices a possible cariostatic mechanism. In: Embery G, Rölla G (eds). Clinical and Biological Aspects of Dentifrices. Oxford, UK: Oxford Univ Press, 1992:305–312.

104. Øgaard B, Gjermo P, Rölla G. Plaque-inhibiting effect in orthodontic patients of a dentifrice containing stannous fluoride. Am J Orthod 1980;78:266–272.

105. Boyd RL, Chun YS. Eighteen-month evaluation of the effects of a 0.4% stannous fluoride gel on gingivitis in orthodontic patients. Am J Orthod Dentofacial Orthop 1994;105:35–41.

106. Herlofson BB, Barkvoll P. The effect of two toothpaste detergents on the frequency of recurrent aphthous ulcers. Acta Odontol Scand 1996;54:150–153.

107. Barkvoll P, Rølla G. Triclosan reduces the clinical symptoms of the allergic patch test reaction (APR) elicited with 1% nickel sulphate in sensitized patients. J Clin Periodontol 1995;22:485–487.

108. Kjærheim V, Barkvoll P, Waaler SM, Rølla G. Triclosan inhibits histamine-induced inflammation in human skin. J Clin Periodontol 1995;22:423–426.

109. Geiger AM, Gorelick L, Gwinnett AJ, Benson BJ. Reducing white spot lesions in orthodontic populations with fluoride rinsing. Am J Orthod Dentofacial Orthop 1992;101:403–407.

110. Geiger AM, Gorelick L, Gwinnett AJ, Griswold PG. The effect of a fluoride program on white spot formation during orthodontic treatment. Am J Orthod Dentofacial Orthop 1988;93:29–37.

111. Øgaard B, Seppä L, Rølla G. Professional topical fluoride applications—Clinical efficacy and mechanism of action. Adv Dent Res 1994;8:190–201.

112. Øgaard B, Rølla G, Arends J, ten Cate JM. Orthodontic appliances and enamel demineralization. Part 2. Prevention and treatment of lesions. Am J Orthod Dentofacial Orthop 1988;94:123–128.

113. Büyükyilmaz T, Tangugsorn V, Øgaard B, Arends J, Ruben J, Rølla G. The cariostatic effect of titanium tetrafluoride (TiF$_4$) application around orthodontic brackets in vivo. Am J Orthod Dentofacial Orthop 1994;105:293–296.

114. Millett DT, Nunn JH, Welbury RR, Gordon PH. Decalcification in relation to brackets bonded with glass ionomer cement and resin adhesive. Angle Orthod 1999;69: 65–70.

115. Wenderoth CJ, Weinstein M, Borislow AJ. Effectiveness of a fluoride-releasing sealant in reducing decalcification during orthodontic treatment. Am J Orthod Dentofacial Orthop 1999;116:629–634.

116. Mattick CR, Mitchell L, Chadwick SM, Wright J. Fluoride-releasing elastomeric modules reduce decalcification: A randomized controlled trial. J Orthod 2001;28:217–219.

117. Øgaard B. Effects of fluoride on caries development and progression in vivo. J Dent Res 1990;69(special issue): 813–819.

118. Øgaard B, ten Bosch JJ. Regression of white spot enamel lesions. A new optical method for quantitative longitudinal evaluation in vivo. Am J Orthod Dentofacial Orthop 1994;106:238–242.

119. Al-Khateeb S, Forsberg CM, de Josselin de Jong E, Angmar-Månsson B. A longitudinal laser fluorescence study of white spot lesions in orthodontic patients. Am J Orthod Dentofacial Orthop 1998:113:595–602.

120. Årtun J, Thylstrup A. Clinical and scanning electron microscopic study of surface changes of incipient enamel caries lesions after debonding. Scand J Dent Res 1986; 94:193–210.

121. Kapila S, Currier F. Hydrochloric acid-pumice treatment for post-orthodontic localized decalcification. Am J Dent 1988;1:15–19.

122. Bishara SE, Denehy GE, Goepferd SJ. A conservative postorthodontic treatment of enamel stains. Am J Orthod Dentofacial Orthop 1987;92:2–7.

123. Al-Khateeb S, Exterkate R, Angmar-Månsson B, ten Cate B. Effect of acid-etching on remineralization of enamel white spot lesions. Acta Odontol Scand 2000;58:31–36.

124. Årtun J, Spadafora AT, Shapiro PA, McNeill RW, Chapko MK. Hygiene status associated with different types of bonded, orthodontic canine-to-canine retainers. A clinical trial. J Clin Periodontol 1987;14:89–94.

125. Årtun J, Spadafora AT, Shapiro PA. A 3-year follow-up study of various types of orthodontic canine-to-canine retainers. Eur J Orthod 1997;19:501–509.

126. Gwinnett AJ, Gorelick L. Microscopic evaluation of enamel after debonding: Clinical application. Am J Orthod 1977;71:651–665.

127. Zachrisson BU, Årtun J. Enamel surface appearance after various debonding techniques. Am J Orthod 1979;75: 121–127.

128. Bishara SE, Trulove TS. Comparisons of different debonding techniques for ceramic brackets: An in vitro study. Parts I and II. Am J Orthod Dentofacial Orthop 1990;98: 145–153, 263–273.

129. Campbell PM. Enamel surfaces after orthodontic bracket debonding. Angle Orthod 1995;65:103–110.

130. Hong YH, Lew KK. Quantitative and qualitative assessment of enamel surface following five composite removal methods after bracket debonding. Eur J Orthod 1995;17: 121–128.

131. Jost-Brinkmann PG, Radlanski RJ, Årtun J, Loidl H. Risk of pulp damage due to temperature increase during thermodebonding of ceramic brackets. Eur J Orthod 1997; 19:623–628.

132. Dovgan JS, Walton RE, Bishara SE. Electrothermal debracketing: Patient acceptance and effects on the dental pulp. Am J Orthod Dentofacial Orthop 1995;108: 249–255.

133. Ceen RF, Gwinnett AJ. Indelible iatrogenic staining of enamel following debonding. J Clin Orthod 1980;14: 713–715.

134. Eliades T, Kakaboura A, Eliades G, Bradley TG. Comparison of enamel colour changes associated with orthodontic bonding using two different adhesives. Eur J Orthod 2001;23:85–90.

135. Radlanski RJ. A new carbide finishing bur for bracket debonding. J Orofacial Orthop 2001;62:296–304.

136. Pus MD, Way DC. Enamel loss due to orthodontic bonding with filled and unfilled resins using various clean-up techniques. Am J Orthod 1980;77:269–283.

137. Lundström F, Hamp SE. Effect of oral hygiene education on children with and without subsequent orthodontic treatment. Scand J Dent Res 1980;88:53–59.

138. Lundström F, Hamp SE, Nyman S. Systematic plaque control in children undergoing long-term orthodontic treatment. Eur J Orthod 1980;2:27–39.

CHAPTER 4

Metabolic Profile of Orthodontic Patients Exhibiting Root Resorption:

An Assessment of the Biologic Predisposition Hypothesis

Stavros Papaconstantinou

The issue of root resorption has attracted the interest of investigators because of the alarming clinical and legal implications associated with its occurrence. In this chapter, an exhaustive search of the literature is presented along with evidence supporting a biologic predisposition to this iatrogenic effect.

Historic Perspectives of Root Resorption

The earliest reports of root resorption in permanent teeth, as cited by Ketcham,[1] were made by Bates in 1856, Chase in 1875, and Harding in 1878; the first study of apical root resorption associated with orthodontic procedures was reported by Ottolengui in 1914.[1] However, it was a report on apical root resorption presented by Ketcham in 1927,[1,2] followed by a second report in 1929,[3] that finally drew the concern of the orthodontic profession. Initially, Ketcham reported that the incidence of root resorption in nor-

mal individuals ranged from 1%[1,4] to 5%,[6] whereas in orthodontic patients the incidence of root resorption rose to 21%.[2–5] Ketcham stated that "apical root loss was so startling, so potent in danger to the orthodontic patient, so prolific of recrimination to the orthodontist himself," that he "made bold" to present his findings to the orthodontic world. Ketcham's[1] dramatic assertions acted as a catalyst, challenging every orthodontist to review practices. All of these early investigators showed remarkable unanimity in their findings. However, Rudolf[6,7] found that at the end of the first year of treatment, 49% of the patients showed root resorption; at the end of two years of treatment, the percentage rose to 75%.

In 1951, Henry and Weinman[8] reported the results of a histologic study of the morphologic and physiologic characteristics of the cementum in terms of number, size, distribution, and types of resorption areas in the permanent teeth of 15 cadavers. Their findings disclosed that over 90% of the teeth showed evidence that root resorption had occurred and often subsequently resolved. The resorption areas were observed more often in the apical third of the roots (76.8%) than in the middle (19%) or gingival third (4%). There were also more instances of resorption on the mesial and buccal surface, indicating that resorption occurred more readily on surfaces that face the direction of physiologic drift. The potential for repair of the cementum after root resorption, first shown by Henry and Weinman, has been confirmed by other researchers.[9–11]

In 1954, Massler and Malone[12] studied 708 sets of radiographs of the complete dentitions of normal individuals aged 12 to 49 years and compared them to 81 sets of radiographs of patients aged 12 to 19 years who had undergone orthodontic treatment. They found that over 80% of the untreated group exhibited root resorption compared to 93.3% of the orthodontic group. However, the frequency of moderate degrees of root resorption rose from 9.2% in the untreated group to 31.4% in the treated group. The frequency of severe root resorption rose from 0.3% to 10.8% and of very severe resorption from 0.11% to 3.4%. The percentage of teeth exhibiting slight root resorption decreased from 71% to 54.7%.

There seems to be few disagreements among epidemiologic studies concerning the frequency and susceptibility of different teeth to root resorption after orthodontic treatment.[5,12,13] Overall, there is agreement that the teeth most susceptible to root resorption are the maxillary and mandibular incisors followed by the maxillary first molars, maxillary first and second premolars, and maxillary canines, while the mandibular canines, first and second premolars, and first molars show less susceptibility. There is also evidence[13] supporting a similarity in the teeth that are most and least susceptible between the treated and untreated populations; the only difference is the severity of root resorption displayed. Gender was not found to be a variable related to root resorption.[4,14–17]

Some controversy exists concerning the influence of the age of the patients who underwent orthodontic treatment as well as the length of the treatment. Several researchers[6–8,15] found a significant increase in root resorption among older patients, while others[16–18] did not find any relationship between them. Similarly, some found a mild relationship[14,16] between the length of treatment and root resorption, while others found no such relationship.[15,18–20] The amount of

tooth movement was related to root resorption by some[13,21] and refuted by others.[18,20] No association was found between initial malocclusion and root resorption.[20]

The use of rectangular archwires did not increase the incidence of root resorption,[20] while Begg appliances increased the incidence of root resorption by 2 to 3 times when compared to cases treated with edgewise appliances.[21]

Mechanisms of Root Resorption

Numerous studies have attempted to elucidate the mechanism behind root resorption and account for changes in supporting structures of the teeth as they relate to orthodontic tooth movements. Present knowledge on that subject is based on experiments on dogs,[22–26] monkeys,[27–46] and humans.[47–53] However, the most accurate portrayal of the situation is obtained by several electron microscopy studies.[30,31,41,42,49,53–55]

The principle findings of these studies indicate that the initial response to the application of force is the dilation of blood vessels and packing of erythrocytes along with the interspersing of platelets and follicular material between the cellular elements. The vessel walls appear to be intact at this stage, and, although the erythrocytes have been pressed against each other, an open lumen remains in these vessels.[41] During the next stage, part of the endothelial walls disappears along with the basement lamina, thus allowing communication between the lumen of the blood vessels and the perivascular space.[41]

Crystallization of the erythrocytes develops in the periodontal ligament (PDL), indicating a local degradation of the erythrocytes as a result of pressure and hemostasis.[42] Cementoblasts, fibroblasts, and osteoblasts show no difference in cellular reaction to the orthodontic force.[55] They all exhibit various stages of disintegration characterized by intracellular swelling, advanced dilation of the endoplasmic reticulum, moderate swelling of the mitochondria, rupture of the cell membrane followed by separation of the nucleus from the cytoplasm, and decomposition of the nucleus. This process indicates that cell death occurs in the cytoplasm, while the nucleus disintegrates later. Furthermore, it demonstrates that the previous assumption, which held that the death of a cell is more prominent in the nucleus than in the cytoplasm due to the appearance of a pyknotic nucleus, was incorrect. This process would continue until complete hyalinization of the PDL at the pressure sites is achieved. Multinuclear giant cells then appear near the cementum surface at some distance from the hyalinized tissues; these cells resorb tooth substance. The resorption of the cementum appears under the electron microscope as a resorption from the rear.[53] Once the cementum is resorbed, there is an indication that the resorption continues in the dentin at a greater rate. In other words, the cementum acts as a barrier so that resorption of the entire root of the tooth does not take place. The PDL adjacent to the cementum being resorbed from the rear is rich in blood vessels and cells.[53] Hyalinized structures disappeared concomitantly with an invasion of cells and blood vessels from the neighboring PDL. These findings are common both in animal and human material[31,49,52] and indicate that the formation of hyalinized zones on the PDL due to force application lead to root resorption during the invasion of new cells from the healthy periodontium and the bone marrow.

It might be concluded that the mechanism by which root resorption occurs is presently clear. However, although it has been well-established[2,3,6,7,12–16,18] that orthodontic treatment can significantly increase both the number of teeth that exhibit this defect and its severity, the literature does not contribute substantially to our understanding of why individuals respond to orthodontic treatment with varying degrees of root resorption.

Factors Influencing Root Resorption

Cementum

Cementum is a tissue that has morphologic characteristics similar to those of bone. That is, it is produced by cementoblast cells that are very similar to osteoblasts, and it is calcified in the same manner as bone and resorbed by large multinucleate cells that remove first the minerals and then the organic matrix. Never-

theless it has some distinct differences from bone that help to explain why cementum is much more resistant to resorption as well as why resorption can occur.

There are four primary reasons why cementum is more resistant to resorption than bone: (1) Cementum has a higher fluoride content then bone; (2) bony tissue has an ample blood supply whereas cementum is completely devoid of vascular tissue; (3) cementum is surrounded by older and more mature collagen, which is more resistant to the actual chemical changes than bone[12]; and (4) cementum is covered by a layer of nonmineralized precementum, called the *cementoid*, which, like the osteoid, is considered a resorption-resistant coating.[22,52] It is reasonable to consider that any variations in these four factors can greatly influence the capacity of cementum to resist resorption, particularly when a local stimulus changes the equilibrium of the PDL.

Since cementum is considered to be very closely related to bone, it would be logical to speculate that the mechanisms that induce cellular activity to form or resorb bone would also influence cellular activity to form or resorb cementum.

Many studies have shown that bone is formed from cells that proliferate from the vascular endothelium of thin-walled sinusoid vessels.[56,57] Cells that originate from these vessels are often called *osteogenic precursor cells* (and sometimes *undifferentiated mesenchymal cells*). A variety of factors operate to influence the proliferation of these cells, some of them common to all connective tissue cells and some specific to bone.

Common to all cells is the need for an adequate supply of energy before cell division can take place.[58] Since energy production is brought about by means of oxidation of certain cellular high-energy products, a plentiful supply of oxygen is needed for cell proliferation and activity.

In the PDL, the undifferentiated mesenchymal cells become osteoblasts, which lay down the bone matrix. If a decreased oxygen supply occurs, the amount of osteoid matrix produced is decreased or ceases altogether. Equally important for cell division is the local concentration of carbon dioxide. Concentrations of carbon dioxide that are too high or too low inhibit cell proliferation. Since local concentrations of oxygen and carbon dioxide are partly regulated by the rate of blood flow, the latter should be an important practical consideration. When the rate of blood flow diminishes, as on the pressure side of the PDL, the available oxygen is decreased and, at the same time, the rate of carbon dioxide removal is decreased. With a diminished blood flow, therefore, fewer osteoblasts and less osseous tissue are formed, while at the same time the osteoclasts that are formed from the undifferentiated mesenchymal cells are also reduced in number. However, it has been demonstrated[59] that as the rate of the flow of blood through bone is reduced, macrophages increase in size and coalesce to form phagocytic osteoclasts. This mode of osteoclastic activity and bone removal is therefore enhanced.

Hormones

Another regulating mechanism of cell division and intercellular matrix production is the balance of anabolic and catabolic hormones.[59] There are two types of osteoclasts. Both are multinucleated cells and secrete enzymes that hydrolyze and degrade bone tissue and thus are able to resorb bone.

One type of osteoclast is formed by the coalescence of undifferentiated mesenchymal cells in the presence of excess cortisol or corticosteroids.[60] Although they show considerable cytoplasmic activity, osteoclasts formed in this manner remain in one place, still attached to neighboring cells.

The second type of osteoclast is freely moving and is formed from macrophages. These cells are formed in the bone marrow and have phagocytic capability. Before the macrophages can coalesce, the cells enlarge. This is prevented by cortisol or corticosteroids[61] so that these catabolic agents inhibit the production of the freely moving osteoclasts. The presence of parathyroid hormone (PTH) is required before macrophages can coalesce to form osteoclasts.[62] With an excessive amount of PTH present, these osteoclasts display a correspondingly exuberant activity. The presence of thyroid hormones seems to be necessary for parathyroid hormone activity.[59]

Different hormones regulate bone metabolism to maintain a constant level of extracellular calcium.[63,64] Calcium is an important substance required (1) in the form of calcium phosphate and calcium carbonate to form the principal chemical constituents of bone,

cementum, and enamel; (2) for the coagulation of blood (clotting formation); and (3) for the regulation of neural function by keeping the excitability of nerve endings at a normal level. It is believed[63] that the maintenance of a constant extracellular calcium concentration depends mainly on the dual reciprocal control of bone resorption by PTH and calcitonin (CT). Other important factors controlling calcium homeostasis and bone resorption are the level of extracellular phosphorus (PO_4), the presence of vitamin D, the thyroid hormones (T_3, T_4), and the corticosteroids. Secondary factors include sucrose, fatty acids, heparin, serum proteins, male and female hormones, etc.[63]

PTH has both a regulatory and a permissive role in bone resorption. The overall resorption rate is maintained by continuous secretion of PTH, which can be increased or decreased in response to calcium concentration.[62,63] The hormone must also be present for changes in bone resorption to occur locally in response to immobilization.[62] PTH raises the calcium blood level by causing osteoclastic resorption of bone and by increasing the excretion of PO_4 from the kidneys, causing inhibition of reabsorption of PO_4 from the tubules and by inhibiting calcification of newly formed bone.

Two types of hyperparathyroidism are distinguished. The primary form of hyperparathyroidism is usually caused by a tumor of the parathyroid gland, while the secondary form can be caused by calcium-deficient diets, vitamin D deficiency, and kidney insufficiency.

Experimentally, it was reported[63] that repeated injections of phosphates could lead to one type of secondary hyperparathyroidism, as the organism tries to increase the excretion of phosphates through the kidneys. Weinman and Sisher[64] state that latent hyperparathyroidism, which is developed through moderate renal insufficiency, causes sometimes localized and minute bone changes in areas that have suffered a mechanical or infectious injury. They hypothesized that these localized changes were the response of the sensitized skeleton to a localized injury.

Vitamin D deficiency primarily causes reduced absorption of calcium and secondarily the reduced absorption of PO_4 from the intestinal tract.[64] This occurs because calcium in the gastrointestinal lumen combines with the PO_4 to form insoluble $Ca_3(PO_4)_2$, resulting in a secondary hyperparathyroidism in order to maintain a normal blood level of calcium. The PO_4 deficiency is increased by the hyperactivity of the parathyroid.

Vitamin D is found to be permissive for PTH stimulated bone resorption.[63] They are considered to be physiologic synergists that act not at the same receptor site in bone-resorbing cells but at separate sites linked so that the effects of one can enhance the response of the other. When lacking in vitamin D, experimental animals become unresponsive to all but extraordinarily large doses of PTH, while large doses of vitamin D have hypercalcemic effects.[65] CT together with the PO_4 blood concentration are considered to be the two physiologic synergists for inhibiting bone resorption.[66] CT mainly causes inhibition of mineral resorption in vivo, while PO_4 concentration primarily causes inhibition of matrix resorption by increasing the deposition of mineral on collagen and therefore blocking its resorption. Another way by which PO_4 can inhibit bone resorption is by enhancing increased deposition of calcium minerals on bone surfaces that are less mineralized.[67] In contrast to PTH, which causes bone resorption along with release of calcium by stimulating collagenolytic and proteolytic enzymatic activity, the CT and PO_4 block calcium release without inhibiting enzyme release.[68] This indicates that while PTH acts directly on the cells, the CT does not.

Thyroid hormones regulate calcium homeostasis by controlling the renal secretion of calcium and phosphates. Consequently, the changes in bones are expected to be a response to depletion of calcium. Reduced bone apposition and increased bone resorption in cases of hyperthyroidism are to be understood as an attempt by the organism to mobilize enough calcium and PO_4 to compensate for the increased loss of these elements.[52] In addition, thyroid hormones seem to be necessary so that PTH can act on the cells.[49]

The complicated interplay of hormones, which can be influenced by local or generalized factors (primary endocrine malfunction, diet, renal insufficiency, gastrointestinal problems, etc), influences the cellular activity in forming or resorbing bone. Based on the similarity of cementum and bone, it has been assumed[5,34,69–77] that these factors should influence the resorption of the cementum.

The Hormonal Implication

Orthodontists have speculated for a number of years about hormonal and dietetic influences on root resorption, and several researchers have attempted to study these relationships.

Early experiments on monkeys[24,73–75] showed that absorption occurred on either the lateral or apical aspect of the root under conditions where unusual force was applied, independent of the type of appliance used. This process seemed to develop more rapidly and proceed farther when the diets of the experimental animals were deficient in vitamin A. Furthermore, when experimental animals maintained diets adequate in protein, vitamins, mineral salts, fats, and carbohydrates, new tissue was always found in the areas where slight absorption had previously occurred, thus restoring the original contour.

When diets with normal salt mixtures and those with low calcium salt mixtures, both devoid of cod liver oil (vitamin D), were given to a series of 25 dogs for a period of 7 to 12 months, atrophic and dystrophic bone changes were observed in the active skeleton. These changes were accompanied by marked root resorption.[69]

In a subsequent study,[5] 100 individuals with root resorption underwent complete physical examination, urinalysis, differential blood count, dietary survey, clinical and roentgenographic examination of the teeth and jaws, determination of basal metabolic rate, and determination of the serum and saliva calcium and PO_4. It was reported that 60% of the orthodontic group and 40% of the nonorthodontic group exhibited a definite hypothyroidism. Hypothyroidism together with other endocrinopathies accounted for another 20% in the orthodontic group and 26% in the nonorthodontic group. Hyperpituitarism was also noted in this study and correlated with root resorption as well as intestinal problems, the latter causing disturbances in mineral metabolism and therefore leading to pathologic bone formation.

In 1951, Tager[77] searched for medical evidence of endocrine and metabolic disease in 100 children who presented with special orthodontic problems, among them root resorption. Basal metabolic rate, calcium and PO_4 serum concentration, sugar tolerance, protein-bound iodine (PBI), and serum cholesterol were measured. It was concluded that only 10% of the children revealed a "frank endocrinopathy." One case presented hypopituitarism, and the other 9 cases were hypothyroid. The greatest proportion of these cases revealed neither specific endocrine disease nor congenital anomalies. What did appear significant was evidence that certain types of orthodontic defects, more specifically root resorption and architectural abnormalities of the bone, repeated themselves in a particular type of accelerated growth pattern connected with puberty. This observation led to the notion of a "relative metabolic insufficiency," that is, insufficiency of a hormone or nutrients in the bone not in an absolute sense but with respect for the greater demands made by the accelerated growth pattern.

In 1975, Newman[78] screened 47 orthodontic patients, each of whom exhibited moderate to severe root resorption on a minimum of three teeth, in terms of their genetic make-up, endocrine status, and nutritional health. He concluded that no definite relationship could be drawn, and that concerning the genetic aspect, the metabolic aspect was not at all related to root resorption.

Two patients with low serum PO_4[79] and one case with high PTH[72] exhibited extensive root resorption.

Secondary hyperparathyroidism was not found to increase the incidence of root resorption,[80] while thyroxin administration was found to decrease it.[81]

Concerning the effect of corticosteroid treatment on root resorption, one study showed that administration of hydrocortisone increased the potential for root resorption in monkeys,[76] while another researcher showed that prednisolone administration significantly reduces the degree of root resorption.[82]

Root resorption was shown to take place during high alveolar bone turnover due to hypercalcemia induction in cats.[70,71] The situation was markedly improved during subsequent induced low alveolar bone turnover due to bisphosphonate treatment.

Interaction of Biologic Parameters

In 1981, the present author[83] selected 12 individuals, ages 17 to 22 years, who were undergoing orthodontic treatment to participate in a study. Six of the individuals displayed moderate to severe generalized root resorption. The resorption constituted a source of concern to both the orthodontist and the patient. The prognosis in these cases, for both the orthodontic treatment and the future health of the dentition, was poor. The other six individuals, who did not exhibit any radiographic evidence of root resorption, were used as controls. Of the patients who exhibited root resorption, three were male and three female, while four of the control patients were male and two were female. All subjects appeared to be healthy and had negative medical histories. In an attempt to exclude patients whose root resorption could be readily attributed to excessive and prolonged trauma of the supporting tissues of the dentition, one principal criterion of selection was that patients exhibiting root resorption had to be in treatment for less than 18 months; the control patients could be in treatment for a longer time. Gender was not a criterion of case selection.

The sample was carefully selected to allow for comparisons between two extreme situations. The percentage of orthodontic patients exhibiting generalized idiopathic root resorption is less than 10%, while the large majority of orthodontic patients exhibit only a minor degree of root resorption.

Blood specimens and 24-hour urine specimens were collected from every patient for the determination of the following clinical values:

1. Serum calcium
2. Serum phosphorus level
3. 24-hour urine calcium
4. 24-hour urine phosphorus
5. Tubular resorption of phosphorus (TRP)
6. Blood level of alkaline phosphatase
7. Blood level of thyroid hormone T_3
8. Blood level of thyroid hormone T_4
9. Blood level of cortisol
10. Blood level of parathyroid hormone (PTH)

Table 4-1 Means, standard deviations, *t* values, and level of significance for between-group comparisons of each variable

Variables	Control group		Root resorption group		*t* value	*P*
	Mean	SD	Mean	SD		
Serum PO$_4$	3.05	0.64	3.28	0.16	0.854	.10
Serum Ca	9.4	0.19	9.48	0.43	0.417	.10*
24 h urine Ca	154.3	77.8	185.5	93.9	0.627	.10
24 h urine PO$_4$	1	0.17	1.04	0.45	0.204	.10
TRP	77.8%	6.9	77.7%	4.7	0.029	.10
Alk phosphatase	77.3	24.5	71	26.1	0.431	.10
T$_3$	118	9.6	130.5	23.8	1.117	.10
T$_4$	7.7	0.9	7.9	2.1	0.214	.10
Cortisol	18.8	5.1	18.8	10.5	0	.10
PTH	782	123	981	501	0.945	.10

*At $P = 0.1$, the difference between the groups is not significant.

An attempt to statistically relate individual metabolic variables to root resorption failed (Table 4-1), though some greater variability among the values of some metabolic factors can be observed. Also, occasional values outside their normal ranges could be seen in the root resorption group. These preliminary conclusions were similar to those of Newman,[78] who examined the relationship of thyroid hormone T$_4$, protein-bound iodine, serum calcium, serum phosphorus, and alkaline phosphatase to tooth resorption and found them to be unrelated.

Use of the SAS[84] direct discriminant analysis (SAS Institute, Raleigh, NC) (Table 4-2), which allowed each patient's measurements to be taken as a biochemical unit, demonstrated that the control and root resorption patients were classified in two separate groups with a certainty ranging from 93 to 100%, with the exception of one control patient who was classified as a root resorption case. This divergent datum indicates that, in addition to the selected variables, other variables influence root resorption. Some of these additional variables could be related to the anatomy of the root and periodontal ligament and to the chemical composition of the cementum. Another possible explanation for divergence could be that the chemical analyses provide a metabolic fingerprint only at a particular time. Perhaps that patient would have been classified as a control in this analysis if the tests had been performed earlier. It is also possible that the patient will develop root resorption as treatment progresses.

Becks'[5] study of 100 patients with root resorption concluded that 66% of the orthodontic patients and 86% of the nonorthodontic patients exhibited definite hyperthyroidism. These findings were based mainly on readings of patients' basal metabolic rate. The present study, using more precise methods for determining thyroid function, does not support this finding. On the contrary, it showed that in the root resorption group, there was one patient exhibiting a high value of T$_3$ and also that the mean values for T$_3$ and T$_4$ were greater, though when compared to the mean values exhibited in the control group, these findings were not statistically significant.

Table 4-2 Probability of membership by patient according to the SAS discriminant analysis

Patient	Actual group	Group 1 (control)*	Group 2 (root resorption)*
F.D.	1	0.928	0.9072
F.S.	1	0.9998	0.0002
L.D.	1	0.9994	0.0006
F.G.	1	1.0000	0.0000
H.M.	1	0.9996	0.0004
K.J.	1	0.9999	0.0001
W.R.	2	0.0620	0.9380
M.R.	2	0.0002	0.9998
S.K.	2	0.0038	0.9962
V.L.	2	0.0005	0.9995
M.M.	2	0.0001	0.9999
D.M.	2	0.0003	0.9997

*Placement according to statistical analysis

The results of Tager[77] could not be evaluated and compared to this study because his study sample included patients with several problems, including delayed tooth eruption, tooth deformities, and root resorption.

The SPSS stepwise discriminant analysis[85] (SPSS, McGraw-Hill, New York, NY) shows that the single most important separating variable is the hormone T_3, while the factor that best enhances the separating action of T_3 is T_4 (Fig 4-1). This result indicates that thyroid function is closely related to tooth resorption. Nevertheless, it is apparent that the separation of the sample into two groups is insignificant, and only after five variables are included in the discriminant analysis can one observe the sample separation. The sequence by which the variables were included one after another in the stepwise analysis is based on the potential of each variable to increase the separating action of the previously added variables and does not necessarily imply any biologic mechanism, nor does the sequence follow any biologic pertinence. An impression was given that the sequence by which the variables were included in the stepwise discriminant analysis does not express a particular pattern or syndrome not detectable in the graphical two-dimensional representation of each case. On the contrary, it is tempting to speculate that, based on the small difference between the mean values and the large standard deviations shown in Table 4-1, there could be several biologic mechanisms involved. Some of these may possibly be related to nutritional status, as Marshall and Becks have shown; some may be related to renal function, as Marshall and Becks have shown; some of them may be related to renal and gastrointestinal problems, as Sisher and Weinman suggested; and some of them may be related to primary endocrine problems.

This study clearly described a definite relationship between the metabolic picture of the patients, as given by the tests that were selected, and generalized root resorption. Furthermore, it is suggested that the

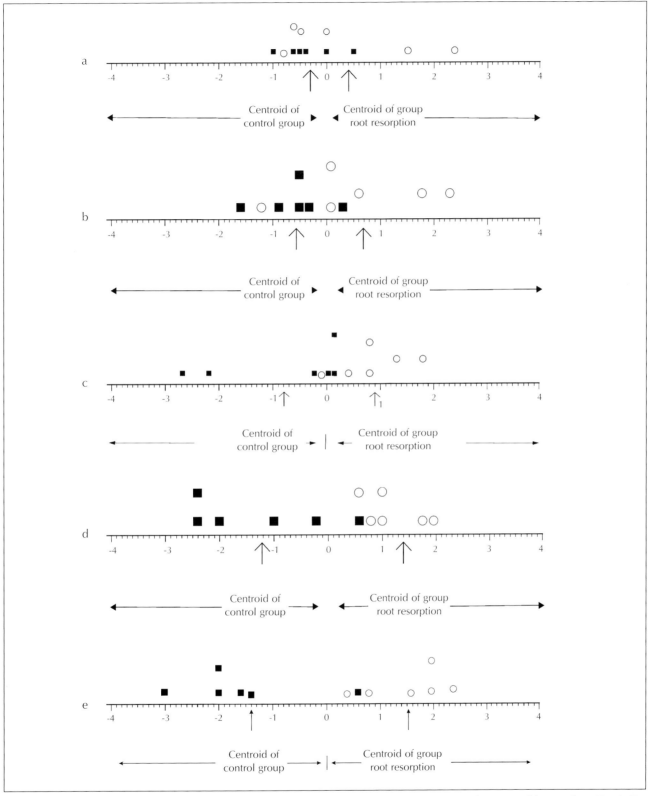

Fig 4-1 Histograms of classification of the sample in two groups by the SPSS discriminant analysis. Variables used: *(a)* T_3; *(b)* T_3, T_4; *(c)* T_3, T_4, 24-hour urine Ca; *(d)* T_3, T_4, 24-hour urine Ca, serum PO_4; *(e)* T_3, T_4, 24-hour urine Ca, serum PO_4, TRP.

(cont)

○ Represents one root resorption patient selected according to root condition.
■ Represents one control patient selected according to root condition.

Fig 4-1 *(f)* T$_3$, T$_4$, 24-hour urine Ca, serum PO$_4$, TRP, serum Ca; *(g)* T$_3$, T$_4$, 24-hour urine Ca, serum PO$_4$, TRP, serum Ca, alkaline phosphatase; *(h)* T$_3$, T$_4$, 24-hour urine Ca, serum PO$_4$, TRP, serum Ca, alkaline phosphatase, 24-hour urine PO$_4$; *(i)* T$_3$, T$_4$, 24-hour urine Ca, serum PO$_4$, TRP, serum Ca, alkaline phosphatase, 24-hour urine PO$_4$, PTH; *(j)* T$_3$, T$_4$, 24-hour urine Ca, serum PO$_4$, TRP, serum Ca, alkaline phosphatase, 24-hour urine PO$_4$, PTH, cortisol.

○ Represents one root resorption patient selected according to root condition.
■ Represents one control patient selected according to root condition.

procedure applied in this study could be used prospectively as a prediction test concerning the behavior of the roots of the dentition of future orthodontic patients.

Based on this review of the literature on root resorption, the following statements can be made:

1. Root resorption can occur in individuals whether they undergo orthodontic treatment or not.
2. During orthodontic treatment, both the sequence and the severity of root resorption increases.
3. Root resorption does undergo a certain degree of repair.
4. Whether age, time, and extent of orthodontic movement can increase the amount of root resorption remains controversial.
5. There has been some speculation regarding the influence of metabolic factors on the development of root resorption.
6. What really concerns the orthodontic profession is the small percentage of patients who exhibit moderate to severe generalized root resorption.
7. It has been shown that there should be a metabolic picture of healthy individuals under which the occurrence of moderate to severe generalized root resorption can increase.

References

1. Ketcham A. A preliminary report of an investigation of root resorption of permanent teeth. Int J Orthod Oral Surg Oral Radiol 1927;13:97–127.
2. Ketcham A. A radiographic study of orthodontic tooth movement: A preliminary report. JADA 1927;14:577–598.
3. Ketcham A. Progress report of an investigation of root resorption of permanent teeth. Int J Orthod Oral Surg Oral Radiol 1929;15:310–328.
4. Hemley S. The aetiology of root resorption of vital permanent teeth. Bull NY State Dent Soc 1938;5:7–18.
5. Becks H. Root resorption and their relation to pathologic bone formation. Int J Orthod 1936;22:455–478.
6. Rudolf CE. A comparative study in root resorption in permanent teeth. JADA 1936;23:822–826.
7. Rudolf CE. An evaluation of root resorption occurring during orthodontic treatment. J Dent Res 1940;19:367–371.
8. Henry JL, Weinman JP. The pattern or resorption and repair of human cementum. JADA 1951;42:170–280.
9. Langford SR, Sims MR. Root surface resorption, repair and periodontal attachment following rapid maxillary expansion in man. Am J Orthod 1982;81:108–115.
10. Vardimon AD, Graber TM, Voss LR, Lenke J. Determinants controlling iatrogenic external root resorption and repair during and after palatal expansion. Angle Orthod 1991; 61:113–124.
11. Vardimon AD, Graber TM, Pitaru S. Repair process of external root resorption, subsequent to palatal expansion treatment. Am J Orthod 1993;103:120–130.
12. Massler M, Malone A. Root resorption in human permanent teeth. Am J Orthod 1954;40:619–633.
13. Hemley S. The incidence of root resorption of vital permanent teeth. J Dent Res 1941;20:133–141.
14. DeShields RW. A study of root resorption in treated class II, division 2 malocclusions. Angle Orthod 1969;39: 231–245.
15. Linge B, Linge L. Apical root resorption in upper anterior teeth. Eur J Orthod 1983;5:173–183.
16. McFalden WM, Engstrom C, Engstrom H, Anholm JM. A study of the relationship between incisor intrusion and root shortening. Am J Orthod 1989;96:390–395.
17. Sjolien T, Sachrisson BU. Periodontal bone support and tooth length in orthodontically treated and untreated persons. Am J Orthod 1973;64:28–37.
18. Phillips JR. Apical root resorption under orthodontic treatment. Angle Orthod 1955;25:1–22.
19. Otto RL, Anholm JM, Engel GA. A comparative analysis of intrusion of incisor teeth achieved in adults and children according to facial type. Am J Orthod 1980;77:437–446.
20. Mirabella AD, Artun J. Risk factors for apical root resorption of maxillary anterior teeth in adult orthodontic patients. Am J Orthod 1995;108:48–55.
21. McNab S, Battistuta D, Taverne A, Symons AL. External root resorption following orthodontic treatment. Angle Orthod 2000;70:227–232.
22. Gottlieb B, Orban B. Die Veranderungen der Gewebe bein ubernassiger Beanspruchung der Zabue. Leipzig: Thieme, 1931.
23. Reitan K, Skiellen WG. Tissue changes following the rotation of teeth in the dog. Angle Orthod 1940;10:140–147.
24. Sandstedt C. Einige Beitrage zur Theorie der Zahnregulering Nord. Tandl Tidsska 1904;236–256.
25. Sandstedt C. Einige Beitrage zur Theorie der Zahnregulering Nord. Tandl Tidsska 1905;6:1–25.
26. Schwarz A. Tissue changes incident to tooth movement. Int J Orthod 1932;18:331–352.
27. Baumrind S, Buck DL. Rate changes in cell replication and protein synthesis in the periodontal ligament incident to tooth movement. Am J Orthod 1970;57:109–131.
28. Crumley PJ. Collagen formation in the normal and stressed periodontium. Periodontics 1964;2:53–61.
29. Johnson AL, Appleton JLT, Rittershafer LS. Tissue changes involved in tooth movement. Int J Orthod Oral Surg 1926; 12:889–898.
30. Kwan E. Tissue Changes Incident to Movement of Rat Molars [thesis]. Oslo: Universitetsforloget, 1957.
31. Kwan E. A study of cell-free zone following experimental tooth movment in the rat. Trans Europ Orthod Soc 1969; 419–435.

32. Lilja E, Lindskog S, Hammarstrom L. Histochemistry of enzymes associated with tissue degradation incident to orthodontic tooth movement. Am J Orthod 1983;83: 62–75.

33. Macapanpan LC, Weinman JP, Prodie AG. Early tissue changes following tooth movement in rats. Angle Orthod 1954;24:79–95.

34. Marshall JA. Deficient diets and experimental malocclusions considered from the clinical aspect. Int J Orthod 1932;18:438–442.

35. Oppenheim A. Tissue changes particularly of bone, incident to tooth movment. Am J Orthod Oct 1911;Jan 1912.

36. Oppenheim A. The crisis in orthodontia. Int J Orthod 1933; 19:1201–1213.

37. Oppenheim A. The crisis in orthodontia. Int J Orthod 1934; 20:18–24, 137–144, 331–336, 461–466, 542–554, 639–644, 759–769.

38. Oppenheim A. The crisis in orthodontia. Int J Orthod 1935; 21:50–55, 153–156, 243–247.

39. Oppenheim A. Biologic orthodontic therapy and reality. Angle Orthod 1935;5:159–211, 233–270; 1935;6:5–38, 69–116.

40. Oppenheim A. Possibility for orthodontic physiologic movement. Am J Orthod Oral Surg 1944;30:277–328, 345–368.

41. Rygh P. Ultrastructural cellular reactions in pressure zones of rat molar periodontium incident to orthodontic tooth movement. Acta Odontol Scand 1972;80:575–593.

42. Rygh P, Selvig AKV. Erythrocytic crystallisation in rat molar periodontium incident to tooth movement. Scand J Dent Res 1973;81:62–73.

43. Waldo CM, Rothblatt JM. Histologic response to tooth movement in the laboratory rat, procedure and preliminary observations. J Dent Res 1954;33:481–486.

44. Wesselink RR, Beertsen W, Everts V. Resorption of the mouse incisor after application of cold to the periodontal attachment apparatus. Calcif Tissue Int 1986;39:11–21.

45. Wesselink PR, Beertsen W. Initiating factors in dental root resorption. In: The Biological Mechanisms of Tooth Eruption and Root Resorption. Birmingham, AL: EBSCO Media, 1988:329–334.

46. Zaki AE, Heysen G. Histology of the periodontium following tooth movement. J Dent Res 1963;42:1373–1379.

47. Boyde A, Lester KS. Electron microscopy of resorbing surfaces of dental hard tissues. Z Zellforsch Mikrosk Anat 1967;83:538–548.

48. Herzberg B. Bone changes incident to orthodontic tooth movement in men. JADA 1932;19:1777.

49. Kwan E. Scanning electron microscopy of tissue changes on the pressure surface of human premolars following tooth movement. Scand J Dent Res 1972;80:357–368.

50. Reitan K. The initial tissue reaction incident to orthodontic tooth movement. Acta Odontol Scand 1951;(suppl 6).

51. Reitan K, Kwan E. Comparative behavior of human and animal tissue during experimental tooth movement. Angle Orthod 1971;41:1–14.

52. Reitan K. Initial tissue behavior during apical root resorption. Angle Orthod 1974;44:63–82.

53. Rygh PV. Orthodontic root resorption studied by electron microscopy. Angle Orthod 1977;47:1–16.

54. Barber AF, Sims M. Rapid maxillary expansion and external root resorption in man: An SEM study. Am J Orthod 1981;79:630–652.

55. Rygh P. Ultrastructural vascular changes in pressure zones of rat molar periodontium incident to orthodontic tooth movement. Scand J Dent Res 1972;80:307–321.

56. Trueta J, Amato VP. The vascular contribution to osteogenesis changes in the growth cartilage caused by experimentally induced ischemia. J Bone Joint Surg 1960;428: 571–587.

57. Trueta J. A theory of bone formation. Acta Orthop Scand 1962;32:190–198.

58. Bullough WS. The energy relations of mitotic activity. Biol Rev 1952;27:133–168.

59. Little K. Osteoporotic mechanisms. Int Med Res 1973;1: 509–529.

60. Little K, Valderama JA. Some mechanisms involved in the osteoporotic process. Gerontologia 1968;14:109.

61. Dougherty TF. Effect of hormones on lymphotic tissue. Physiol Rev 1952;32:379–401.

62. Burkhart JM, Jowey J. Parathyroid and thyroid hormones in the development of immobilisation of osteoporosis. Endocrinol 1967;81:1053–1062.

63. Raisz L. Physiologic and pharmacologic regulation of bone resorption. Seminars in Medicine of the Beth Israel Hospital, Boston 1970;282:909–916.

64. Weinman JP, Sisher H. Bone and Bones. Fundamentals of Bone Biology. St Louis: Mosby, 1955.

65. Blunt JW, Tanaka Y, Deluca HF. The biologic activity of 25-HC, a metabolite of vitamin D. Proc Natl Acad Sci USA 1968;61:1503–1506.

66. Hirsch PF, Munson PL. Thyrocalcitonin. Physiol Rev 1969; 49:548–622.

67. Feinblatt J, Balanger LF, Rasmussen H. The effect of phosphate infusion upon bone metabolism and PTH action. Am J Physiol 1970;218:1624–1631.

68. Vaas G. Lysosomes and the cellular physiology of bone resorption. In: Dingle JT, Fell HB (eds). Frontiers of Biology. Amsterdam: Holland Publishing, 1969:217–253.

69. Becks H, Weber M. The influence of diet on the bone system with special reference to the alveolar process and the labyrinthine capsule. JADA 1931;18:197–264.

70. Engstrom C. Odontoblast metabolism in rats deficient in vitamin D and calcium. IV: Lysosomal and energy metabolic enzymes. J Oral Pathol 1980;9:246–254.

71. Engstrom C, Thilander B. Effect of orthodontic force on periodontal tissue metabolism. Am J Orthod 1988;93: 486–495.

72. Goultchin J, Kaufman E. Resorption of cementum in renal dystrophy. J Oral Med 1982;37:84–86.

73. Marshall JA. The relation of malnutrition to dental pathology. Int J Orthod Oral Surg Oral Radiol 1931;17:527–551.

74. Marshall JA. The classification, etiology, diagnosis, prognosis and treatment of radicular resorption of teeth. Int J Orthod 1934;20:731–746.

75. Marshall JA. A study of bone and tissue changes incident to experimental tooth movement and its application to orthodontic practice. Int J Orthod 1933;19:1–17.

76. Pinsker LJ. Root resorption under orthodontic appliances as affected by corticosteroids in the rhesus monkey. Int J Orthod 1962;48:4–12.

77. Tager BB. Endocrine problems in orthodontics. Am J Orthod 1951;37:867–875.

78. Newman WG. Possible etiologic factors in external root resorption. Am J Orthod 1975;67:522–538.

79. Olson A, Matsson L, Blomquist HK, Larson A, Sjiodin B. Hypophosphatasia affecting the permanent dentition. J Oral Pathol Med 1996;25:343–347.

80. Goldie SR, King JG. Root resorption and tooth movement in orthodontically treated calcium deficient and lactating rats. Am J Orthod 1984;85:424–433.

81. Shirazi M, Dehpour AR, Jafari F. The effect of thyroid hormone on orthodontic tooth movement in rats. J Clin Pediatr Dent 1999;23:259–264.

82. Ong CK, Walsh LJ, Harbrow D, Taverne AA, Symons AL. Orthodontic tooth movement in the prednisolone treated rat. Angle Orthod 2000;70:118–125.

83. Papaconstantinou S. Characterisation of healthy orthodontic patients on the basis of metabolic tests, as a function of the presence or absence of moderate to severe generalised root resorption [thesis]. Chicago: Loyola Univ, 1981.

84. SAS. Statistical Analysis System. Raleigh, North Carolina: SAS Institute, 1979.

85. SPSS. Statistical Package for the Social Sciences. McGraw-Hill, 1979.

Minimizing Orthodontically Induced Root Resorption

Olle Malmgren and Eva Levander

High frequencies of orthodontically induced apical root resorption have been reported in histologic studies, and the tissue reactions are well documented. In clinical radiographic studies, the reported frequency varies. Phillips[1] found apical resorption exceeding one fourth of the original root length in 1.5% of maxillary central incisors and in 2.2% of lateral incisors. Linge and Linge[2] reported apical root resorption of 3 mm or more in 4% of investigated maxillary incisors. Individual variations between patients and between different teeth in the same person have also been reported.[3] Because extensive root resorption might have untoward sequelae such as tooth mobility and loss of supporting bone,[4] a strategy to minimize resorption must be considered and a plan for follow-up should be established before orthodontic treatment. The strategy includes evaluation of the risk of root resorption before treatment and at a predetermined stage early in the treatment.[5] Resorption detected early should be followed up and documented at the end of treatment.

Pretreatment

Because the individual response is unknown, all systemic and local factors must be considered before the start of treatment. Assessment of the risk of root resorption starts with the patient's medical history to evaluate the hypothetical influence of systemic factors. The history should include:

1. Hereditary factors[6]: The outcome of any orthodontic treatment received by parents, siblings, or other relatives (Fig 5-1)
2. Systemic factors[7]: Diabetes, allergic reactions, or other systemic diseases (Fig 5-2)
3. Local factors[8,9]: Nail biting and other oral habits
4. Trauma[10]: Earlier trauma, type, and follow-up, including dental records from the trauma event, if available (Fig 5-3)

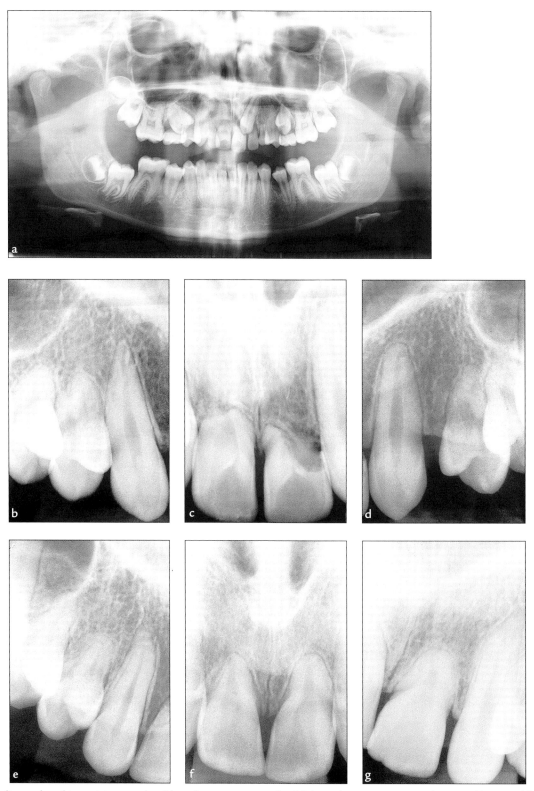

Fig 5-1 Radiographs of two sisters, each with a short root anomaly. *(a)* An orthopantomogram shows a 13-year-old girl with a short root anomaly of the maxillary anterior teeth and premolars. The left central and lateral incisors are severely resorbed during eruption of the canine. *(b–d)* Radiographs of the same patient 1 year later. The premolars have a plump form and the left central incisor is severely resorbed. The left canine was moved in a distal direction with a removable appliance. Both lateral incisors were extracted. *(e–g)* Radiographs of the sister at 18 years of age also showing a short root anomaly.

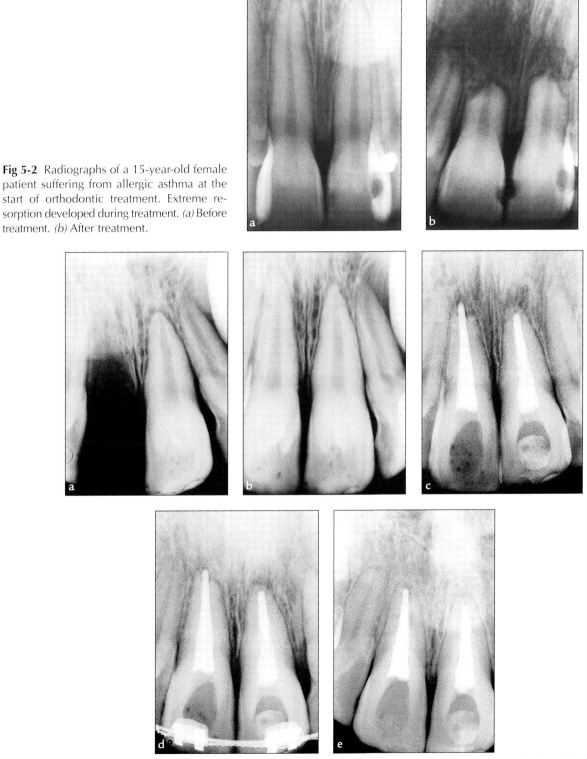

Fig 5-2 Radiographs of a 15-year-old female patient suffering from allergic asthma at the start of orthodontic treatment. Extreme resorption developed during treatment. *(a)* Before treatment. *(b)* After treatment.

Fig 5-3 A 9.7-year-old girl suffered a fall during gymnastics. The maxillary right central incisor was avulsed, and the left central was laterally luxated. *(a)* After the trauma, the right incisor was kept first in the mouth in saliva and then in saline. *(b)* After 85 minutes, 11 was replanted and 21 repositioned. Both teeth were endodontically treated with an interim dressing of Calasept (Nordiska Dental) and filled with gutta-percha. *(c)* At 13.8 years of age, the orthodontic diagnosis was normal occlusion, severe crowding of the maxillary and mandibular anteriors, and a deep overbite. A moderate apical root resorption on the maxillary central incisors (index score 2) can be seen. Orthodontic treatment comprised extraction of the four first premolars and fixed appliance therapy for 1.7 years. No further root resorption developed. *(d)* Radiograph at the end of orthodontic treatment. *(e)* Follow-up 2 years later.

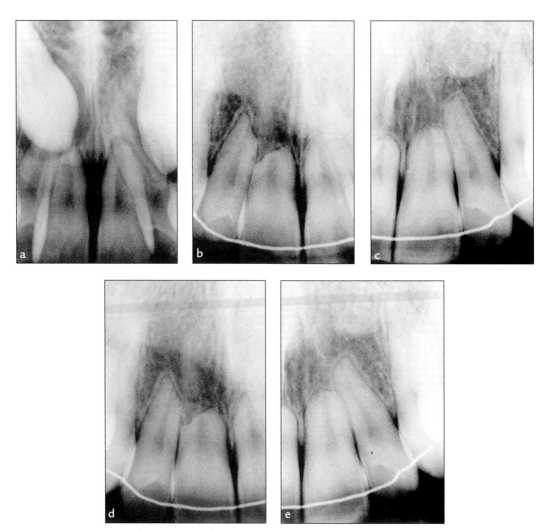

Fig 5-4 Radiographs of a patient with severe apical root resorption due to eruption disturbances. Follow-up period: 7 years. *(a)* Before treatment. *(b,c)* After treatment. Severe apical root resorption of all maxillary incisors. *(d,e)* At the follow-up control. Total root lengths: the right lateral, left central, and left lateral incisors were greater than 9 mm; the right central incisor was less than 9 mm and showed increased mobility. (Reprinted from Levander and Malmgren[4] with permission.)

A clinical examination, including standardized peri-apical radiographs taken with a film holder, should be performed to assess the potential contribution of local factors. Periodontal conditions should be registered. Based on the radiographic findings, the following important factors should be evaluated: existing root resorption, including that due to disturbances of eruption[11,12] (Fig 5-4); apical root form[13,14] (Fig 5-5a); invagination[15] (Fig 5-5b); agenesis[16] (Fig 5-6); and short root anomalies[17–19] (see Fig 5-1).

Treatment planning primarily involves evaluation of the type and extent of tooth movement needed to correct the deviations, the duration of treatment, and the need for extraction. In patients with several predisposing factors, the individual treatment plan should be modified to make allowance for the risk of root resorption—for example, shorter treatment time, less force, and a limited goal.

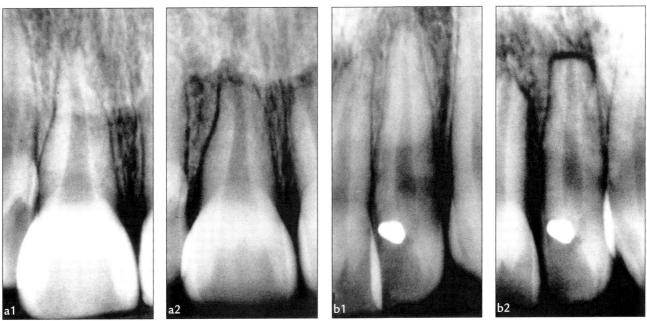

Fig 5-5 Typical effect of root resorption. A pipette-shaped root *(a1)* before and *(a2)* after treatment. Tooth crown with invagination *(b1)* before and *(b2)* after treatment. (Reprinted from Levander and Malmgren[5] with permission.)

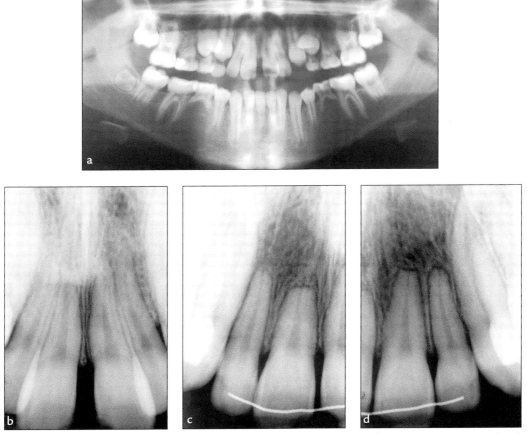

Fig 5-6 Radiographs of a girl with agenesis of four premolars. *(a)* Orthopantomogram before treatment. Periapical radiographs of maxillary incisors *(b)* before and *(c,d)* after treatment. Severe resorption is evident after treatment. (Reprinted from Levander et al[16] with permission.)

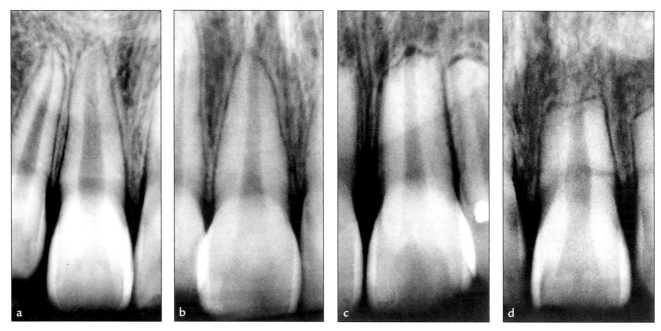

Fig 5-7 An index for evaluation of root resorption. *(a)* Irregular root contour. *(b)* Apical root resorption of less than 2 mm (minor resorption). *(c)* Apical root resorption from 2 mm to one third the original root length (severe resorption). *(d)* Root resorption of greater than one third the original root length (extreme resorption). (Reprinted from Levander and Malmgren[5] with permission.)

Treatment

Once treatment has begun, an initial follow-up is recommended at 6 months[5] and should include periapical radiographs of all maxillary and mandibular incisors, since these are the teeth most susceptible to root resorption.[20] It is important that the root apices can be viewed on at least two radiographs taken from different directions. In order to standardize the assessment of root resorption, a four-point index can be applied (Fig 5-7).[5]

If there are no radiographic signs of root resorption at this stage of treatment, the risk of severe resorption at the end of treatment is minimal (Fig 5-8a). Resorption at 6 months of treatment indicates a risk of progressive resorption as treatment proceeds (Fig 5-8b).[5] This risk may be reduced by temporary suspension of active treatment for 2 to 3 months (Figs 5-9a and 5-9b).[21] In teeth showing progressive resorption, further radiographic follow-up every 3 months is recommended.

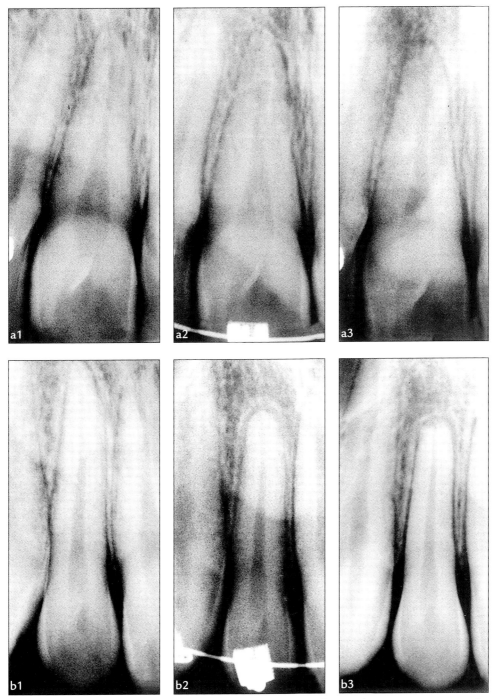

Fig 5-8 Root resorption: post-treatment outcome in relation to degree of resorption 6 to 9 months after the start of treatment. Before treatment *(a1)*; no resorption after 6 to 9 months *(a2)*; minor resorption after treatment *(a3)*. Before treatment *(b1)*; minor resorption after 6 to 9 months *(b2)*; severe resorption after treatment *(b3)*. (Reprinted from Levander and Malmgren[5] with permission.)

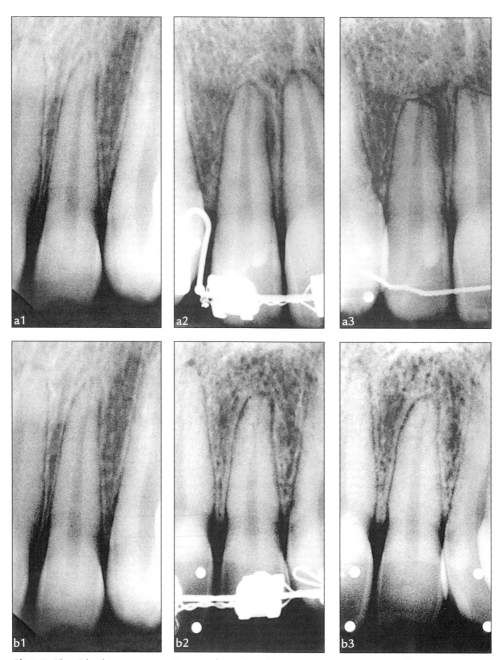

Fig 5-9 The risk of severe resorption may be reduced by temporary suspension of active treatment for 2 to 3 months. Uninterrupted treatment before treatment *(a1)* and at registration of initial apical root resorption *(a2)*. Severe resorption after treatment *(a3)*. Interrupted treatment before treatment *(b1)* and at registration of initial resorption *(b2)*. Minimal further resorption after treatment *(b3)*. (Reprinted from Levander et al[21] with permission.)

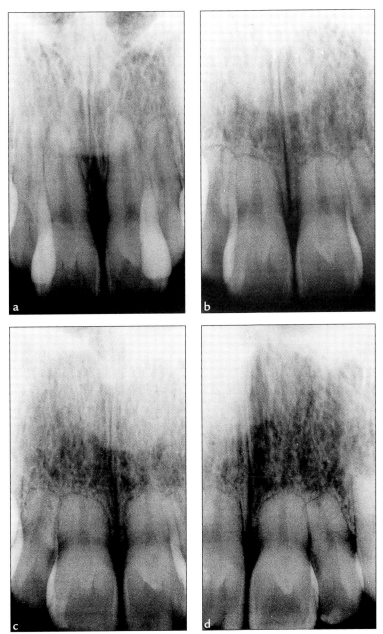

Fig 5-10 Radiographs of a 31-year-old patient with severe apical root resorption. Follow-up period was 15 years. *(a)* Before treatment. *(b)* After treatment. Severe apical root resorption of maxillary incisors. *(c,d)* At follow-up 15 years later. Total root length of each of the four incisors was less than 9 mm. Increased mobility was found in all four incisors. (Reprinted from Levander and Malmgren[4] with permission.)

Post-treatment

After treatment, a radiographic examination is mandatory, and the patient and referring dentist should be informed if a root resorption has occurred. If it is mild or moderate, no further action is indicated. If it is severe and the foreshortened root remaining is no longer than the tooth crown, there is a risk of tooth mobility (Fig 5-10).[4] In such a case, further follow-up and instructions to the patient are necessary.

Evidence Based on Clinical Studies

There is no definitive evidence in the literature of the importance of the interaction between biologic and mechanical factors during treatment.[22,23] However, these factors must be taken into account in assessing the risk of root resorption and should be included in the treatment plan.

Familial susceptibility to root resorption during orthodontic treatment was found in a study of a large number of full siblings, indicating a heritable component.[6] A correlation between gender and apical root resorption has been reported.[18,24–26] Linge and Linge[2] reported that females are more susceptible than males. Other studies[27–29] failed to verify this finding.

Davidovitch et al[7] have proposed that individuals with pre-existing inflammatory conditions, such as periodontitis, diabetes, and allergy, are at high risk for orthodontic root resorption. Furthermore, Kjaer[15] demonstrated a relationship between some dental anomalies, particularly ectopia and agenesis of teeth, and a tendency to root resorption during orthodontic treatment. This observation was verified by an investigation designed to analyze the risk of root resorption associated with agenesis.[16] In patients with multiple agenesis, the risk of root resorption must be considered carefully because the teeth are often intended to serve as prosthetic abutments. Two variables—treatment with rectangular archwires plus intermaxillary elastics and duration of treatment—were significantly related to the severity of root resorption. This may reflect the difficulty of controlling the force applied when few teeth are available for anchorage.[16]

Some morphologic characteristics of root anatomy can be diagnosed in pretreatment intraoral radiographs. Oppenheim[30] alleged that incisors with deviant root forms are especially at risk. Lind[17] and Newman[18] claimed that the condition "short root anomaly" predisposes to root resorption during orthodontic treatment. The roots are abnormal from an early stage of development, and the final shape is not due to resorption. The anomaly always affects both central incisors almost symmetrically: As a rule, these roots are characteristically plump. Premolars and canines are less frequently involved. No clear evidence of the

risk for root resorption in these teeth has been shown. However, even minor resorption might jeopardize their long-term prognosis.

In a study by Malmgren et al,[31] root resorption after orthodontic treatment of traumatized teeth was analyzed. The study comprised 55 luxated incisors and their noninjured antimeres. At the time of injury, all teeth had been carefully examined by experienced pedodontists following standardized procedures. The extent of resorption was the same in the traumatized as in the contralateral noninjured control teeth. However, a few teeth exhibiting resorption before orthodontic treatment became severely resorbed during treatment.

In an ongoing study by Morin et al, 17 patients with 27 severely injured teeth with complete records from the trauma episode and follow-up after the trauma were treated with fixed appliances and followed up. The conclusions were that in cases of severe trauma, teeth with severe periodontal damage, particularly exarticulated and replanted teeth and teeth with intrusive luxations, should be extracted if the follow-up period after trauma showed that the teeth had a poor prognosis. Successfully treated injured teeth, which show normal periodontal ligaments after an adequate post-trauma observation period, may be subjected to orthodontic movement without increased risk of root resorption. Furthermore, a tooth with a root fracture, healed with bone or connective tissue, is looked upon as a tooth with a short root. If the fracture line is located in the middle third of the root, there is a risk of further shortening of the short coronal fragment during orthodontic movement.[10]

The importance of forces has been discussed for years. Most authors consider only heavy forces to be responsible for root resorption, but intensity and duration are also of great importance. The conclusions in the literature, however, are conflicting. Kvam,[32] Harry and Sims,[33] and Vardimon et al[34] found an association between severity of resorption and the magnitude of force, while Owman-Moll[3] concluded that root resorption did not seem to be very force-sensitive. It is often stated that forces causing jiggling of teeth, intrusion, and/or torquing of roots increase the risk of root resorption.[2,28] A correlation between resorption and the duration of active treatment has been shown in some studies[35,36] but has not been shown in others.[37,38]

A recent study of root resorption associated with standard and straight edgewise techniques disclosed significantly more resorption of central incisors in patients treated with the standard edgewise technique.[39] In another recent study, a technique using heat-activated and superelastic wires resulted in less resorption than either standard or straight-wire edgewise techniques where stainless-steel archwires had been used.[20]

It has been shown that movement into labial and cortical bone can initiate root resorption. It is thus important to establish the borders of the cortical bone, based on profile radiographs, prior to treatment.[10] If the alveolar crest is narrow, resorption can easily occur during retraction of maxillary incisors. The maxillary incisors are often protrusive and require palatal root torque during retraction; this root movement should be made in the roomier cancellous bone area, preferably using an approach that intrudes the anterior teeth at the onset of treatment.

Owman-Moll[3] found great variability in tissue response regardless of the magnitude of the applied force. In some patients, substantial resorption was detected after a short period of treatment, although light forces were used. It may be concluded that treatment duration, mechanical factors, and individual variations are all of importance.

A major consideration is the management of apical root resorption detected early during active orthodontic treatment. Reitan[40] recommended temporary suspension of treatment in cases showing a strong tendency to root resorption. Rygh[41] goes even further by proposing the scheduling of periods of treatment suspension throughout the course of orthodontic therapy.

There is consensus that root resorption usually ceases after orthodontic treatment, when applied forces are discontinued.[37,42,43] Histologic studies have shown that repair of resorption cavities will take place after force removal. Brudvik and Rygh[44] studied the reparative process in animal experiments in rats and observed new mineralized cementum on the resorbed root surface 21 days after the forces were discontinued. In human experiments, Owman-Moll[3] found various degrees of repair after 8 weeks, and Odenrick et al[45] reported deposition of hard tissue in resorption lacunae after 53 to 90 days. In a study of patients in whom active treatment of initially resorbed teeth had

been suspended for 2 to 3 months, there was significantly less post-treatment resorption than in cases where treatment proceeded without interruption.[21]

Little is known of the long-term prognosis of teeth with severely or extremely resorbed roots. In concurrence with an earlier study by VonderAhe,[37] Remington et al[43] reported that even teeth with severe orthodontically induced resorption seemed to function reasonably well clinically several years post-treatment. In a case report of a patient with extremely foreshortened maxillary central incisor roots examined 33 years after treatment, radiographic, visual, and tactile examination revealed that the resorbed teeth functioned well.[46] It has been claimed that resorption of as much as one third the original root length does not result in decreased stability[47] because the highest percentage of periodontal attachment is in the crestal two thirds of the root.[48] If there is considerable foreshortening of the original root, the longevity of the tooth might be compromised; such a tooth might not resist normal functional load.[49] A further risk is that in the event of crestal alveolar bone loss, a critical stage for the residual periodontal attachment may be reached prematurely in teeth with pronounced apical root resorption.[47]

The clinical sequelae to severe root resorption are of major concern. Wainwright[50] concluded that resorption could lead to mobility and even to exfoliation of the tooth. Of 57 teeth with postorthodontic root resorption, VonderAhe[37] reported only one mobile tooth. Sharpe et al[36] investigated orthodontic relapses and reported a higher prevalence of root resorption in the relapse group than in the control group. In a study by Levander and Malmgren,[4] increased mobility was found in incisors with a total root length of less than 9 mm. There was no difference between central and lateral incisors. Loss of root length moves the center of resistance coronally; thus, the same amount of force will have a greater impact than on an intact root. The results of the study indicate enhanced risk of tooth mobility associated with a crown-root ratio greater than 1:1.

It has been claimed that alveolar bone loss increases with age. Albandar and Abbas[51] found little loss in subjects up to 32 years of age and a loss of 0.2 mm per year in those from age 33 to 45 years. This implies that the stability of incisors with less resorption also may decrease. Ericsson and Lindhe[52] reported that experimentally induced tooth mobility in dogs with a healthy but markedly reduced periodontium did not cause attachment loss. Enhanced mobility may function as a codestructive factor, however, in the presence of ongoing plaque-induced destruction of the periodontal tissue.[53] The increased mobility of teeth with short roots should therefore be regarded as a long-term risk factor. Such teeth should be carefully monitored.

Summary

Radiographic follow-up is indicated after 6 to 9 months of orthodontic treatment with fixed appliances. There is a significant correlation between initial and post-treatment apical root resorption. If no radiographic sign of resorption is found at the 6- to 9-month control, there is little risk of severe resorption by the end of treatment. Minor resorption early in treatment indicates a risk of progressive resorption as treatment continues. The risk of severe resorption may be reduced by temporary suspension of active treatment for 2 to 3 months by means of an inactive archwire. There is an increased risk of apical root resorption in maxillary incisors with roots having a deviating root form, particularly with pipette-shaped roots. Treatment planning for patients with multiple agenesis of teeth should take into consideration the risk of excessive apical root resorption during orthodontic therapy. If orthodontic treatment leads to severe root resorption and a crown-root ratio of less than or equal to 1:1, there is a risk of tooth mobility.

References

1. Phillips JR. Apical root resorption under orthodontic therapy. Angle Orthod 1955;25:1–22.
2. Linge BO, Linge L. Apical root resorption in upper anterior teeth. Eur J Orthod 1983;5:173–183.
3. Owman-Moll P. Orthodontic Tooth Movement and Root Resorption with Special Reference to Force Magnitude and Duration. A Clinical and Histological Investigation in Adolescents [thesis]. Gothenburg: Univ of Gothenburg, 1995.
4. Levander E, Malmgren O. Long-term follow-up of maxillary incisors with severe apical root resorption. Eur J Orthod 2000;22:85–92.
5. Levander E, Malmgren O. Evaluation of the risk of root resorption during orthodontic treatment: A study of upper incisors. Eur J Orthod 1988;10:30–38.
6. Harris EF, Kineret SE, Tolley EA. A heritable component for external apical root resorption in patients treated orthodontically. Am J Orthod Dentofacial Orthop 1997; 111:301–309.
7. Davidovitch Z, Godwin SL, Part YG, Taverne AA, Dobeck JM, Lilly CM, et al. The etiology of root resorption. In: Orthodontic Treatment: Management of Unfavourable Sequelae. Proceedings of the Twenty-Second Annual Moyers Symposium, Ann Arbor, MI. Craniofacial Growth Series 1995;31:93–117.
8. Odenrick L, Brattstrom V. The effect of nailbiting on root resorption during orthodontic treatment. Eur J Orthod 1983;5:185–188.
9. Odenrick L, Brattstrom V. Nailbiting: Frequency and association with root resorption during orthodontic treatment. Br J Orthod 1985;12:78–81.
10. Malmgren O, Malmgren B, Goldson L. Orthodontic management of the traumatized dentition. In: Andreasen JO, Andreasen FM (eds). Textbook and Color Atlas of Traumatic Injuries to the Teeth. Copenhagen: Munksgaard, 1994:587–633.
11. Ericson S, Kurol J. Resorption of maxillary lateral incisors caused by ectopic eruption of the canines. A clinical and radiographic analysis of predisposing factors. Am J Orthod Dentofacial Orthop 1988;94:503–513.
12. Brin I, Becker A, Zilberman Y. Resorbed lateral incisors adjacent to impacted canines have normal crown size. Am J Orthod Dentofacial Orthop 1993;104:60–66.
13. Mirabella AD, Artun J. Risk factors for apical root resorption of maxillary anterior teeth in adult orthodontic patients. Am J Orthod Dentofacial Orthop 1995;108: 48–55.
14. Sameshima GT, Sinclair PM. Predicting and preventing root resorption: Part II. Treatment factors. Am J Orthod Dentofacial Orthop 2001;119:511–515.
15. Kjaer I. Morphological characteristics of dentitions developing excessive root resorption during orthodontic treatment. Eur J Orthod 1995;17:25–34.

16. Levander E, Malmgren O, Stenback K. Apical root resorption during orthodontic treatment of patients with multiple aplasia: A study of maxillary incisors. Eur J Orthod 1998;20:427–434.

17. Lind V. Short root anomaly. Scand J Dent Res 1972;80:85–93.

18. Newman WG. Possible etiologic factors in external root resorption. Am J Orthod 1975;67:522–539.

19. Apajalahti S, Holtta P, Turtola L, Pirinen S. Prevalence of short-root anomaly in healthy young adults. Acta Odontol Scand 2002;60:56–59.

20. Janson GR, De Luca Canto G, Martins DR, Henriques JF, De Freitas MR. A radiographic comparison of apical resorption after orthodontic treatment with 3 different fixed appliance techniques. Am J Orthod Dentofacial Orthop 2000;118:262–273.

21. Levander E, Malmgren O, Eliasson S. Evaluation of root resorption in relation to two orthodontic treatment regimes. A clinical experimental study. Eur J Orthod 1994;16:223–228.

22. Brezniak N, Wasserstein A. Orthodontically induced inflammatory root resorption. Part 1. The basic science aspect. Angle Orthod 2002;72:175–179.

23. Brezniak N, Wasserstein A. Orthodontically induced inflammatory root resorption. Part 2. The clinical aspect. Angle Orthod 2002;72:180–184.

24. Massler MM, Perreault JG. Root resorption in the permanent teeth of young adults. J Dent Child 1954;21:158–164.

25. Dougherty HL. The effect of mechanical forces upon the mandibular buccal segments during orthodontic treatment. Am J Orthod 1968;54:83–103.

26. Dougherty HL. The effect of mechanical forces upon the mandibular buccal segments during orthodontic treatment. Am J Orthod 1968;54:29–49.

27. Kennedy DB, Joondeph DR, Osterberg SK, Little RM. The effect of extraction and orthodontic treatment on dentoalveolar support. Am J Orthod 1983;84:183–190.

28. McFadden WM, Engstrom C, Engstrom H, Anholm JM. A study of the relationship between incisor intrusion and root shortening. Am J Orthod Dentofacial Orthop 1989;96:390–396.

29. Goldin B. Labial root torque: Effect on the maxilla and incisor root apex. Am J Orthod Dentofacial Orthop 1989;95:208–219.

30. Oppenheim A. Human tissue response to orthodontic intervention of short and long duration. Am J Orthod Oral Surg 1942;52:263–301.

31. Malmgren O, Goldson L, Hill C, Orwin A, Petrini L, Lundberg M. Root resorption after orthodontic treatment of traumatized teeth. Am J Orthod 1982;82:487–491.

32. Kvam E. Tissue Changes Incident to Tooth Movement of Rat Molars [thesis]. Oslo: Universitetsförlaget, 1967.

33. Harry MR, Sims MR. Root resorption in bicuspid intrusion. A scanning electron microscope study. Angle Orthod 1982;52:235–258.

34. Vardimon AD, Graber TM, Voss LR, Lenke J. Determinants controlling iatrogenic external root resorption and repair during and after palatal expansion. Angle Orthod 1991;61:113–124.

35. Stenvik A, Mjor IA. Pulp and dentine reactions to experimental tooth intrusion. A histologic study of the initial changes. Am J Orthod 1970;57:370–385.

36. Sharpe W, Reed B, Subtelny JD, Polson A. Orthodontic relapse, apical root resorption, and crestal alveolar bone levels. Am J Orthod Dentofacial Orthop 1987;91:252–258.

37. VonderAhe G. Postretention status of maxillary incisors with root-end resorption. Angle Orthod 1973;43:247–255.

38. Dermault LR, De Munck A. Apical root resorption of upper incisors caused by intrusive tooth movement: A radiographic study. Am J Orthod Dentofacial Orthop 1986;90:321–326.

39. Mavragani M, Vergari A, Selliseth NJ, Boe OE, Wisth PL. A radiographic comparison of apical root resorption after orthodontic treatment with a standard edgewise and a straight-wire edgewise technique. Eur J Orthod 2000;22:665–674.

40. Reitan K. Effects of force magnitude and direction of tooth movement on different alveolar bone types. Angle Orthod 1964;34:244–255.

41. Rygh P. Orthodontic root resorption studied by electron microscopy. Angle Orthod 1977;47:1–16.

42. Hollender L, Ronnerman A, Thilander B. Root resorption, marginal bone support and clinical crown length in orthodontically treated patients. Eur J Orthod 1980;2:197–205.

43. Remington DN, Joondeph DR, Artun J, Riedel RA, Chapko MK. Long-term evaluation of root resorption occurring during orthodontic treatment. Am J Orthod Dentofacial Orthop 1989;96:43–46.

44. Brudvik P, Rygh P. Transition and determinants of orthodontic root resorption-repair sequence. Eur J Orthod 1995;17:177–188.

45. Odenrick L, Karlander EL, Pierce A, Kretschmar U. Surface resorption following two forms of rapid maxillary expansion. Eur J Orthod 1991;13:264–270.

46. Parker WS. Root resorption—Long-term outcome. Am J Orthod Dentofacial Orthop 1997;112:119–123.

47. Lupi JE, Handelman CS, Sadowsky C. Prevalence and severity of apical root resorption and alveolar bone loss in orthodontically treated adults. Am J Orthod Dentofacial Orthop 1996;109:28–37.

48. Henry JL, Weinmaan JP. The pattern of resorption and repair of human cementum. J Am Dent Assoc 1951;42:270–290.

49. Jacobson O. Clinical significance of root resorption. Am J Orthod Dentofacial Orthop 1952;38:687–696.

50. Wainwright M. Facial lingual tooth movement. Its influence on the root and cortical plate. Am J Orthod Dentofacial Orthop 1973;64:278–302.

51. Albandar JM, Abbas DK. Radiographic quantification of alveolar bone level changes. Comparison of 3 currently used methods. J Clin Periodontol 1986;9:810–813.

52. Ericsson I, Lindhe J. Lack of effect of trauma from occlusion on the recurrence of experimental periodontitis. J Clin Periodontol 1977;4:115–117.

53. Ericsson I, Lindhe J. Effect of longstanding jiggling on experimental marginal periodontitis in the beagle dog. J Clin Periodontol 1982;9:497–503.

Damage to Tooth-Supporting Tissues in Orthodontics

Birgit Thilander

Orthodontic treatment involves the use and control of forces acting upon the teeth. During tooth movement, the tooth-supporting tissues (ie, gingiva, periodontal ligament, alveolar bone) usually exhibit favorable responses. However, some clinical, radiologic, and histologic investigations have indicated that such forces may cause damage not only to the root substance, but also to the bone-supporting tissues. Food debris and plaque represent a risk factor for gingival inflammation, which can be reduced or eliminated by better oral hygiene and by fluorides. Orthodontic treatment can also have an adverse effect upon the periodontal tissues (eg, gingival recession, marginal bone loss, infrabony pockets) depending on the magnitude, direction, and duration of the force applied and on the age of the treated patient. This chapter discusses the facts and fiction of possible adverse effects on the tooth-supporting tissues associated with orthodontic treatment.

Adverse Effects on Gingival Tissues

In a clinically healthy gingiva, the free gingiva is in close contact with the enamel surface, and its margin is located 0.5 to 2 mm coronal to the cementoenamel junction after the completion of tooth eruption (Fig 6-1). The attached gingiva is firmly attached to the underlying alveolar bone and root cement by connective tissue fibers and is, therefore, comparatively immobile in relation to the underlying tissue.

Bacterial plaque at the gingival margin is the initiating and most significant factor in *gingival inflammation* (Fig 6-2a). Patients undergoing orthodontic treatment have increased retention sites for microbial samples, which may be responsible for gingivitis (Fig 6-2b). It has been shown that patients with fixed appliances have significantly higher total numbers of *Strepto-*

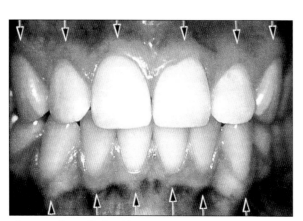
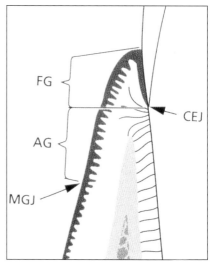

Fig 6-1 Clinically healthy gingiva. Free gingiva (FG), attached gingiva (AG), mucogingival junction (MGJ) *(arrows)*, cementoenamel junction (CEJ), gingival pocket (FG–CEJ).

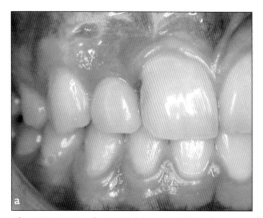
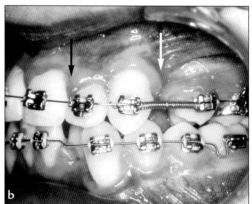

Fig 6-2 *(a)* Simple gingivitis caused by plaque accumulation. *(b)* Hyperplastic gingivitis *(black arrow)* in a young patient with a fixed appliance; interdental fold *(white arrow)*.

coccus mutans and lactobacilli than nonorthodontic subjects.[1,2] Davies et al found a significant reduction in all plaque and gingival indices in children after completion of orthodontic treatment; however, this reduction related more to behavioral factors than to improved tooth alignment, which underscores the importance of plaque control in orthodontic patients.[3]

Higher Plaque Indices, bleeding tendencies and pocket depths have been observed for molars with orthodontic bands than for bonded brackets (Fig 6-3).[4]

Loss of attachment was also more common for molars with orthodontic bands. A likely explanation for these differences is difficulty in plaque removal on the gingival margin of the bands.[5] An alternative explanation for at least part of the attachment loss is the mechanical injury caused by the placement of the bands too deep within the gingival pocket.

Orthodontic closure of extraction sites often results in compressed gingival tissue with an *interdental fold*, most frequently at the buccal aspect of the maxillary

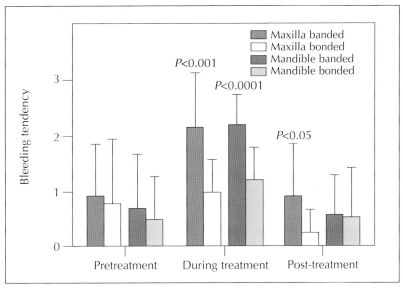

Fig 6-3 Mean bleeding tendency for maxillary and mandibular banded or bonded molars before appliances were placed, during treatment, and 3 months after treatment. (Reprinted from Boyd and Baumrind[5] with permission.)

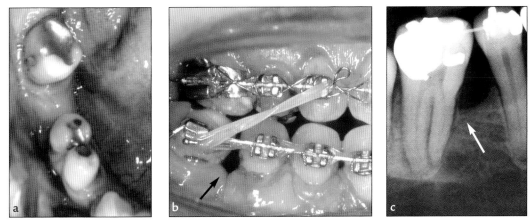

Fig 6-4 *(a)* Orthodontic closure of the mandibular first molar extraction area in an adult patient. *(b)* Interdental fold *(black arrow)*. *(c)* Bone loss after the final closure *(white arrow)*.

first premolar extraction site (see Fig 6-2b) or at the mandibular first molar extraction site (Fig 6-4). Excision of such gingival tissue showed a long-lasting epithelial fold, or invagination, with loss of collagen in the surrounding connective tissue and an increased amount of glucose aminoglycans in the intercellular substance of the connective tissue (Fig 6-5).[6]

Orthodontic forces, especially heavy ones, thus may cause sublethal damage and stimulate a hyperplastic tendency in the tissue components. In some extraction areas, a slight bone loss has been observed after the final closure of the extraction sites (see Fig 6-4c). Moreover, the increased amount of glucose aminoglycans will act as an elastic tissue, which,

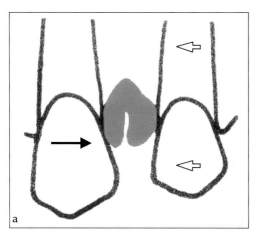
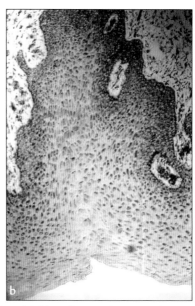
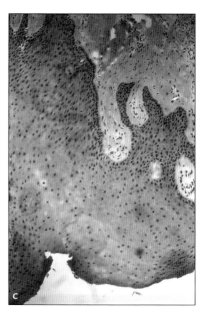

Fig 6-5 *(a)* Hyperplastic gingival tissue with interdental fold *(red area)*. *(b,c)* Histologic sections from this area showing deep proliferation of oral epithelium and increased amount of glucose aminoglycans. (Adapted from Rönnerman et al[6] with permission.)

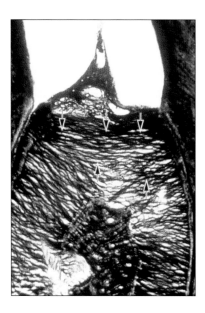

Fig 6-6 Histologic section of the supra-alveolar portion of the interdental area, illustrating the orientation of the transseptal fiber bundles *(arrows)*.

together with the compression of the transseptal fibers and their general toughness and resistance (Fig 6-6), may be responsible for relapse after closure of the extraction gap.

In summary, a proper oral hygiene regimen in patients with fixed orthodontic appliances (especially around molar bands) prevents plaque accumulation, bleeding tendency, and loss of attachment. Furthermore, the use of light forces in closing extraction sites will minimize compression of gingival tissue with interdental folds, which may be responsible for relapse after closure of the gap.

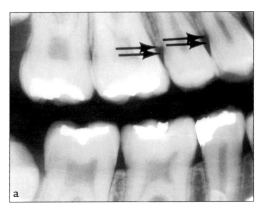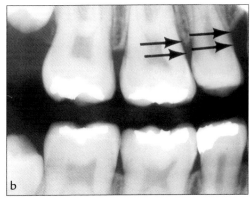

Fig 6-7 Radiographs showing the marginal bone support at the mesial surfaces of the maxillary first molar and second premolar *(a)* before and *(b)* after orthodontic treatment. *Arrows* indicate CEJ and alveolar crest. (Adapted from Hollender et al[8] with permission.)

Loss of Marginal Bone Support

Some studies have shown that orthodontic appliances have the potential to damage the periodontal support of the treated teeth.[7,8] These clinical studies have demonstrated that treated subjects showed larger mean values than controls (nontreated subjects) for the distance between the cementoenamel junction and the alveolar crest, although the differences were small. However, many factors influence the alveolar bone height besides the orthodontic treatment, including systematic differences existing prior to orthodontic treatment between groups. The incidence and degree of changes in marginal bone support in treated maxillae compared to untreated mandibles registered in bitewing radiographs showed a statistically significant *reduction of the marginal bone* for the treated maxilla but not for the untreated mandible (Fig 6-7).[8] The majority of the orthodontic patients presented little or no damage, in contrast to a small number who showed considerably more damage, especially those who had difficulties with the oral hygiene regimen during the treatment.

This observation indicates that orthodontic treatment can aggravate a pre-existing plaque-induced gingival lesion, which may cause loss of alveolar bone and periodontal attachment. In fact, experimental studies in the beagle dog could verify that it is possible by orthodontic tipping forces to shift plaque from a supragingival to a subgingival position, resulting in the formation of *infrabony pockets* (Fig 6-8).[9]

These findings deserve attention in patients with *periodontal disease,* especially for intruding and tipping tooth movements. For *intruding displacements,* deepened gingival pockets must be eliminated before the start of orthodontic treatment to prevent a plaque-induced lesion from being displaced into an infrabony position (Fig 6-9a), since the risk of additional loss of attachment is evident when a tooth is moved into such an area. After the completion of orthodontic treatment, additional surgical pocket elimination may be performed if necessary (Fig 6-9c).

General spacing in the maxillary anterior region, often combined with proclined incisors, is a common characteristic among patients with periodontal disease (Figs 6-10a to 6-10c). Orthodontic alignment of the dental arch involves *palatal tipping* of the incisors. On the pressure zone, a landmark (indicating the CEJ in Fig 6-10d) will be displaced, not only in a palatal but also in an apical direction. When orthodontic forces direct incisors that harbor bacterial plaque into such an "intruded" position, even the plaque-induced lesion will be shifted from a suprabony to an infrabony level—that is, into an area in which orthodontic forces have an injurious effect on the periodontium.

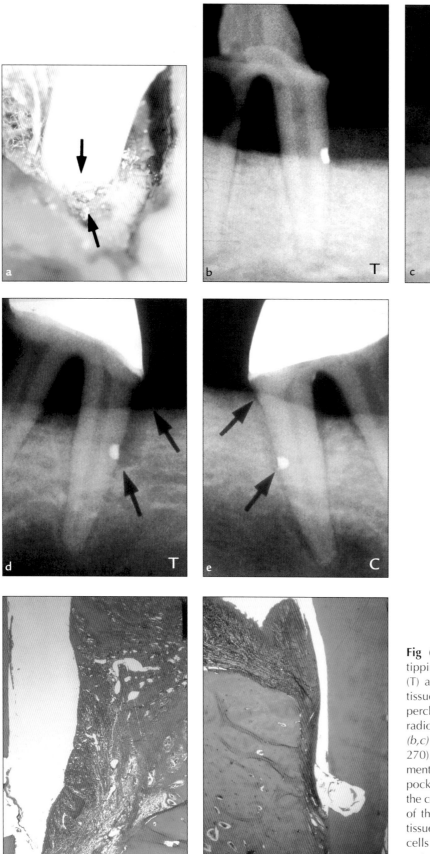

Fig 6-8 The effect of orthodontic tipping force in a dog with infected (T) and noninfected (C) periodontal tissues. *(a)* A cavity filled with gutta-percha served later as a landmark in radiographs and histologic sections. *(b,c)* At the start of the tipping (day 270). *(d)* At the end of the experiment (day 450), showing an infrabony pocket on the test tooth *(e)* but not on the control tooth. *(f)* Histologic section of the test area shows a connective tissue heavily infiltrated by round cells *(g)* in contrast to the noninflammatory control area. (Adapted from Ericsson et al[9] with permission.)

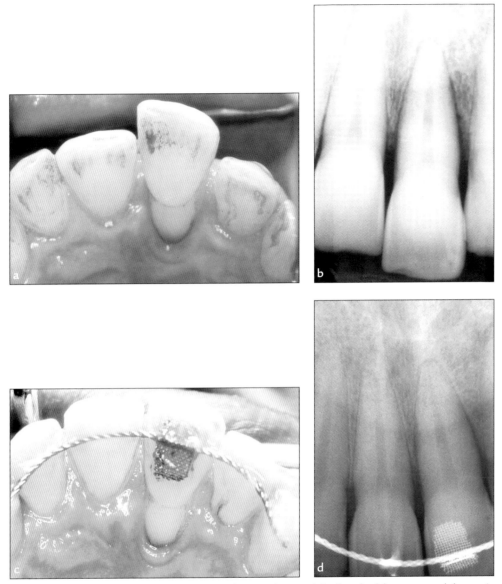

Fig 6-9 *(a,b)* A 42-year-old man with an elongated central incisor had been treated for periodontal disease. After surgical pocket elimination, the tooth was repositioned in the dental arch by very light orthodontic forces. *(c,d)* Retention was performed 10 months later with a bonded lingual retainer strengthened with a net. Additional surgical pocket elimination had to be carried out to allow proper plaque control.

Thus, surgical pocket elimination palatal to the incisors should be considered before the start of orthodontic treatment.

In summary, clinical and experimental studies have demonstrated that in the absence of plaque, orthodontic forces and tooth movements fail to induce gingivitis. In the presence of plaque, however, similar forces may cause marginal bone loss. Furthermore, tipping and intruding movements are capable of shifting a supragingival plaque into a subgingival position; consequently, a gingival inflammation is converted into a lesion associated with attachment loss and infrabony pockets. In patients who have been treated for periodontal disease, surgical pocket elimination should be performed if the patient has deficient capacity for proper oral hygiene. Such a procedure should be performed *before* any orthodontic treatment is started.

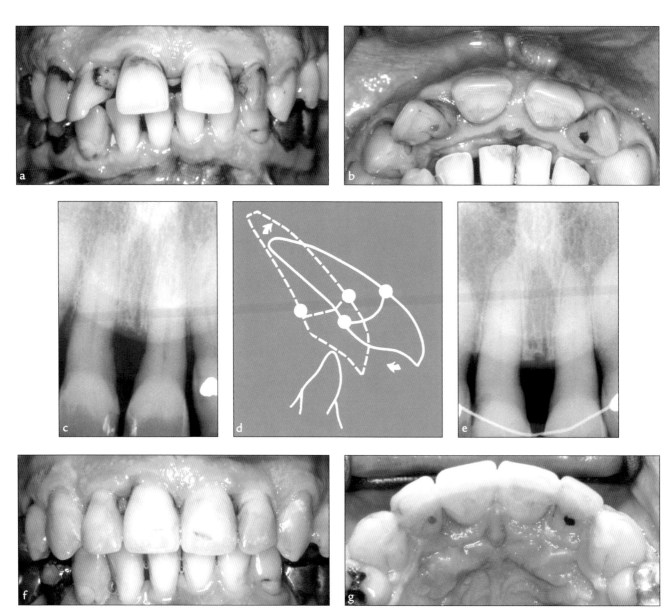

Fig 6-10 *(a–c)* A 50-year-old man with general spacing in the maxillary incisor region and excessive overjet had been treated for periodontal disease. *(d)* Fixed appliances were used for orthodontic alignment, including palatal tilting of the incisors. *(f,g)* Retention 12 months later with a bonded lingual retainer in an enamel groove. *(e)* Note the improvement of the gingival conditions and absence of evidence of further loss of alveolar bone. No need for surgical pocket elimination due to the patient's capacity for proper oral hygiene.

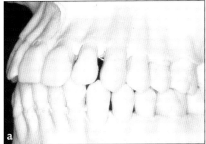
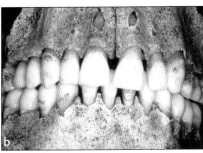
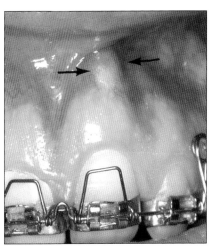

Fig 6-11 *(a)* Thickness of the cortical bone plate in different locations of the alveolar process as shown in skull material. *(b)* Note the thin bone plate at the labial aspect of the maxillary incisors, resulting in fenestrations.

Fig 6-12 Bone fenestration *(arrows)* after torque movement.

Adverse Effects of Labial/Buccal Tooth Movements

The alveolar process, which forms and supports the sockets of the teeth, consists of dense outer cortical bone plates separated by varying amounts of spongy cancellous bone. The thickness of the cortical laminae varies in different locations (Fig 6-11). In the incisor and canine region, for example, the cortical bone plate at the labial aspect of the teeth is considerably thinner than at the lingual aspect. The same is true for the maxillary premolars and molars, and exposed root surfaces (*fenestration* and *dehiscence* defects) are common in skull materials. The type of bone through which the tooth is moved must be taken into consideration in the orthodontic treatment plan. Tooth movements in the mesial or distal direction displace the roots within the spongiosa with rapid bone remodeling. Conversely, labial and buccal tooth movements displace the roots toward, and sometimes (unintentionally) through, the thin cortical plate. Thus, for example, with an orthodontic *torque* movement the apex of the root is tipped slightly in a labial direction. If more torque is incorporated into the archwire, the magnitude of force is increased and the apex may

be displaced through the cortical bone, resulting in a *fenestration* (Fig 6-12).

Contrary to a bone fenestration, which is localized in the apical part of the root, a bone *dehiscence* involves marginal bone loss at the labial/buccal aspect of the root (Fig 6-13a). An experimental study in the beagle dog demonstrated that bone dehiscences can be produced in the buccal alveolar bone by moving the teeth in a facial direction and are not necessarily accompanied by loss of connective tissue attachment (Fig 6-13b).[10] Retention of the displaced tooth in this position for a period of 5 months demonstrated no signs of bone formation of the dehiscence (Figs 6-13e and 6-13h). Such a lack of bone regeneration was speculated to be a result of degradation of both the organic and inorganic components of the bone, including osteogenic cells, as a result of the orthodontic forces. The most striking observation in this study was a complete regeneration of the alveolar bone when the teeth were moved back to their original position (Figs 6-13c, 6-13f, and 6-13i). The mechanism of this reversal of bone loss is not known, but it seems logical to assume that cells with the capacity to form bone may have invaded the area of bone dehiscence on the labial/buccal aspect of the teeth during their movement back to their original position. These

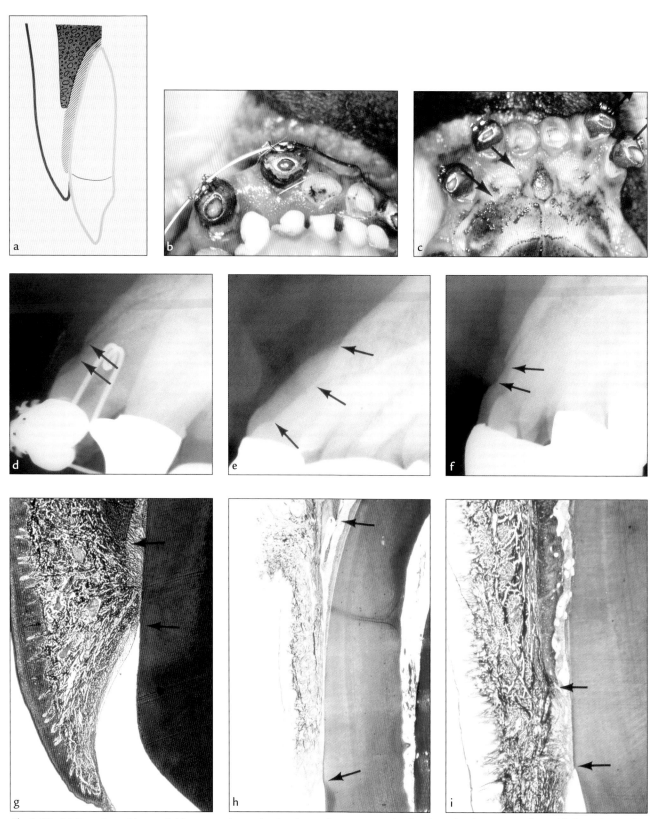

Fig 6-13 *(a)* Drawing of bone dehiscence after orthodontic tooth movement in the dog. *(b)* The incisors ²I and ³I have been displaced through the alveolar bone plate. *(c)* They had then been moved back to their original position; I² and I³ were simultaneously displaced labially. *(d,g)* Radiographs and histologic sections show the alveolar crest and cementoenamel junction *(arrows)* before and *(e,h)* after the anterior displacement. *(f, i)* Note the completely reestablished bone height for the tooth that had been moved back to its original position. (Adapted from Thilander et al¹⁰ with permission.)

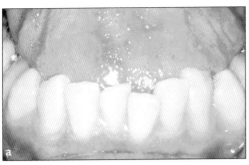
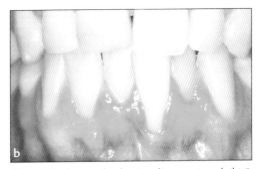

Fig 6-14 A 24-year-old woman with anterior crowding *(a)* before orthodontic alignment and *(b)* 8 years postretention, showing marginal bone recession.

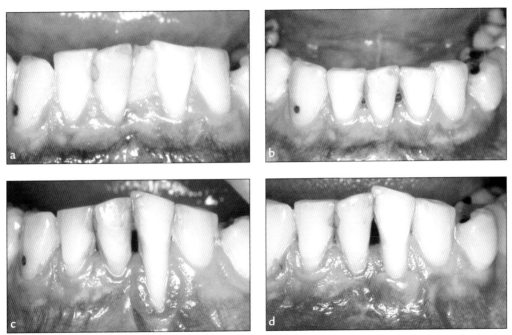

Fig 6-15 *(a)* A 22-year-old man with anterior crowding and hyperplastic gingivitis. *(b)* Orthodontic alignment after extraction of the left central incisor. *(c)* Marginal bone recession with a plaque-induced inflammatory lesion was observed 12 years later. *(d)* After root coverage with a soft tissue flap.

results might indicate that bone will re-form in the area of a dehiscence, unfortunately formed during orthodontic treatment, when the tooth is retracted toward a proper positioning of the root within the alveolar process.

Marginal bone recession, ie, displacement of the soft tissue margin apical to the cementoenamel junction with exposure of the root surface, is a common feature in individuals who have not undergone orthodontic treatment. However, such recessions are also observed in association with orthodontic therapy, for example, after alignment of crowded teeth (Fig 6-14). This type of recession may be associated with localized plaque-induced inflammatory lesions (Fig 6-15).

The presence of an alveolar bone dehiscence is a prerequisite for the development of a marginal reces-

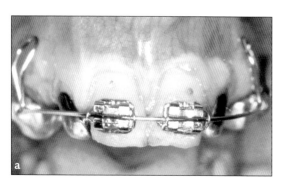
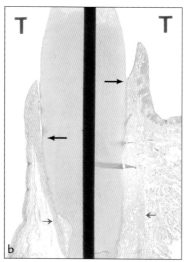
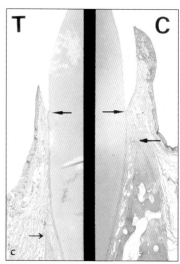

Fig 6-16 *(a)* Anterior movement of incisors in the monkey. The volume of the attached gingiva had been surgically reduced to different degrees on left and right sides of the incisors. *(b,c)* Histologic sections show reduced alveolar bone height and soft tissue margin at three test teeth (T) compared to the normal height in a control tooth (C). (Adapted from Wennström et al[11] with permission.)

sion, but it has also been suggested that recessions may occur during orthodontic treatment involving areas with an inadequate zone of keratinized gingiva. An experimental study in the monkey in which teeth were moved in a labial direction into areas with varying thickness and quality of marginal soft tissue could demonstrate a small apical displacement of the soft tissue margin and a reduced alveolar height (Fig 6-16).[11] In other words, the apical displacement of the gingival margin was a result of the reduced soft tissue thickness and the reduced height of the free gingiva, which in turn may be related to "stretching" in the soft tissues during the anterior tooth movement. These findings suggest that the thickness (volume) of the marginal soft tissue, rather than the apicocoronal width of the keratinized and attached gingiva, is the determining factor in the development of gingival recession and attachment loss during orthodontic tooth movement.

In summary, as long as a tooth can be moved within the envelope of the alveolar process, risk of the development of harmful side effects in the marginal tissue is minimal regardless of the dimensions and quality of the soft tissue. If, however, the tooth movement results in an alveolar bone dehiscence, it must be stressed

that no bone regeneration will occur, even after a long period of retention. Furthermore, the volume (thickness) of the soft tissue cover should be considered as a factor that may cause a soft tissue recession to develop during or after active orthodontic therapy.

RME Treatment in Posterior Skeletal Crossbite

There are two distinct types of posterior crossbite: the *dentoalveolar crossbite* (palatally inclined maxillary teeth) and the *skeletal crossbite* (narrower dimension in the maxilla than in the mandible). Treatment of the dentoalveolar crossbite is aimed at tipping the maxillary teeth into a vertical position (Fig 6-17a). In the skeletal crossbite, buccal tipping of the premolars and molars may result in *bone dehiscence* and *gingival recession*; therefore, rapid maxillary expansion (RME) is required (Fig 6-17b). RME broadens the maxilla, and eruption of the teeth further widens the maxillary dental arch (Fig 6-17c). RME also widens the nasal cavity, which is beneficial for patients with airway problems. It is important to note that such an expan-

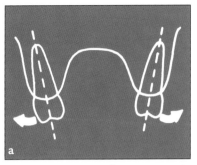
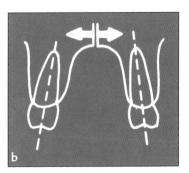
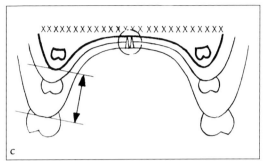

Fig 6-17 Drawings illustrating *(a)* dentoalveolar and *(b)* skeletal crossbites. *(c)* Effect of RME and further widening of the dental arch due to tooth eruption.

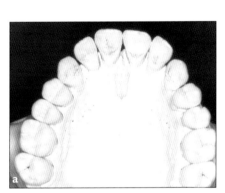
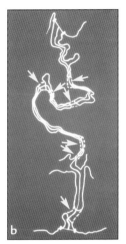
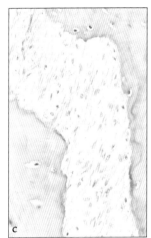
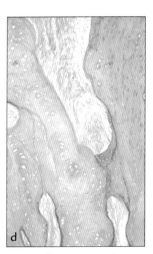

Fig 6-18 *(a)* Maxilla showing the palatal sutures. *(b)* Tracing of a section in the frontal plane of the intermaxillary suture of a 31-year-old man. Bony bridges occur at the *arrows*. *(c)* Photomicrographs from the same suture of a 14-year-old girl *(d)* and of the 31-year-old man. (Adapted from Persson and Thilander[12] with permission.)

sion also affects the total circummaxillary suture system, by which all craniofacial bones of the maxilla are adjoined.

An RME treatment can hardly be performed when the sutures are closed (unless there is surgical assistance). Histologic studies on facial sutures from humans (15 to 35 years old) have shown large individual variations in palatal suture closure with regard to start of closure and advance of closure with age.[12] According to an obliteration index, signs of bone bridging were observed as early as the adolescent period (Fig 6-18). The most favorable outcome of RME

is achieved at young ages, as illustrated in Fig 6-19. Recovery of the expanded suture is demonstrated by the radiograph (Fig 6-19f). Traction generated by orthopedic forces has long been purported to stimulate sutural growth; thus, bone deposition following the expansion/traction will allow the suture to recover a normal histologic picture, as verified in postexpansion photographs of the intermaxillary suture in the rat (Fig 6-20).[13]

RME treatment in patients with fully or partially closed sutures will result in tipping or tilting of the premolars and molars toward the cortical bone plate

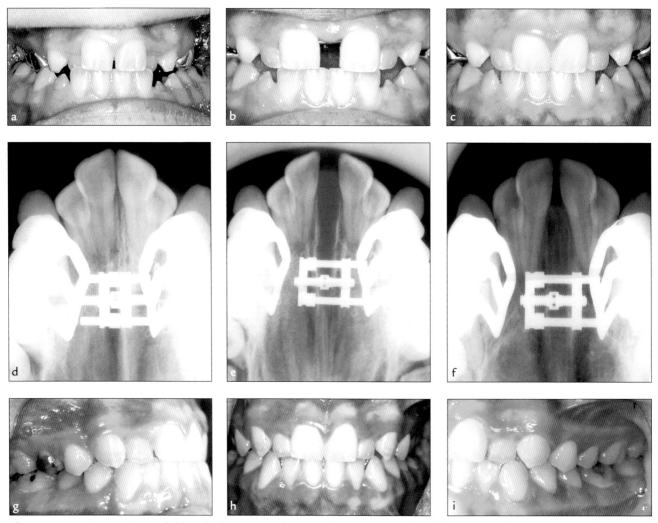

Fig 6-19 RME treatment in a child in the late-mixed dentition. *(a,d)* The expansion plate cemented at the start, *(b,e)* at the end of the RME (day 21), *(c,f)* and at the end of retention (day 60). *(g–i)* Five years postretention.

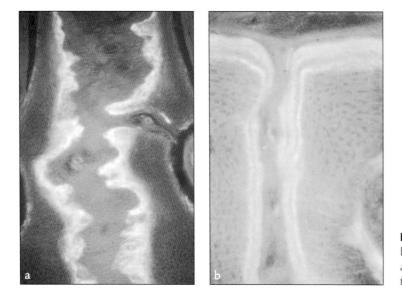

Fig 6-20 Photomicrographs of the intermaxillary suture in the rat. *(a)* After RME for 7 days and *(b)* spontaneous closure at day 28. (Adapted from Engström and Thilander[13] with permission.)

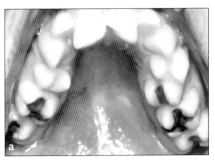
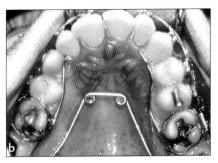
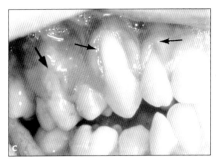

Fig 6-21 RME treatment in a 15-year-old boy. *(a)* Before and *(b)* after the expansion with quad-helix and alignment of the dental arch with a fixed appliance. *(c)* Note the marginal recession *(arrows)*.

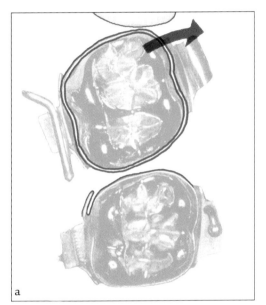
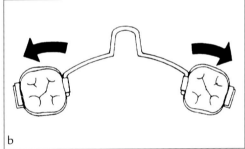

Fig 6-22 Drawings illustrating *(a)* rotation of a maxillary molar with *(b)* a transpalatal bar. A heavy force may result in overrotation of the mesiobuccal root and marginal recession, as shown in Fig 6-21c.

and may lead to marginal bone recession (Fig 6-21). This is most likely when the quad-helix type of expansion device (anchorage) is used instead of tissue-borne appliances, as shown in Fig 6-19. Such adverse effects may also result from the use of transpalatal bars for distalization or rotation of maxillary molars (Fig 6-22). An activation force above the recommended value (1.0 to 1.5 mm per activation) will result in overrotation of the mesiobuccal root, which may cause marginal reces-

sion similar to that shown in Fig 6-21c. Finally, it must be stressed that marginal recession caused by RME can be exposed many years after treatment has been completed and generally requires a soft tissue graft for root coverage (Fig 6-23). The primary indications for root coverage procedures are esthetic demands, root hypersensitivity, and management of shallow root caries lesions and cervical abrasions.

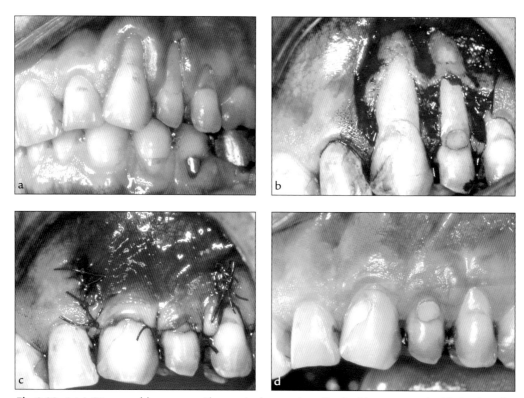

Fig 6-23 *(a)* A 35-year-old woman with marginal recession. She had been treated with RME at the age of 16 years. *(b)* The extension of the dehiscences is seen before root coverage. *(c)* The soft tissue flap sutured. *(d)* The 1-year postoperative healing result.

In summary, RME treatment is indicated in patients with airway problems and severe crowding in a narrow maxillary dental arch. The rigidity of the expansion device is important not only for long-term stability, but especially to avoid tipping of the molars and premolars, which can damage the periodontal tissues. Thus, maximal anchorage is a must in the individual case. RME can be used as long as the sutures are not obliterated. Treatment success is high in the mixed and early permanent dentition, decreases with age, and is questionable in adults for whom surgical expansion must be considered. The wise, tissue-conscious clinician avoids excessive RME and instead aims at providing ultimate stable, healthy teeth and tooth-supporting tissues.

Potential Problems with Implants in Adolescent Patients

A 10-year follow-up study of the use of single-tooth implants in adolescents has shown that they are a good treatment option for replacing missing teeth provided that the subject's dental and skeletal development is complete (Fig 6-24).[14] However, in the maxillary incisor area, slight continuous eruption of teeth may result in an *infra-occluded implant-supported crown,* with high individual variations (Figs 6-25 to 6-27). The mean change in this infra-occluded position of the incisor gradually increased 0.1 mm per year throughout the observation period. Besides differences

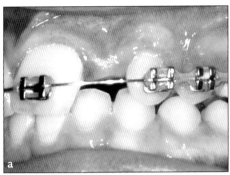
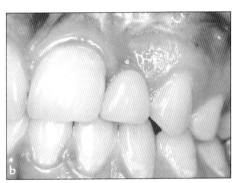
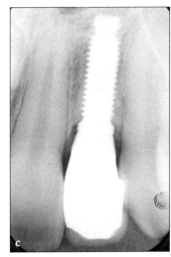

Fig 6-24 A boy with a congenitally missing lateral incisor. *(a)* After space-gaining treatment, an implant was placed at the age of 16 years, 4 months, skeletal stage R-IJ. *(b)* The final control (at age 26 years, 11 months) showed a good long-term result, ie, inter-incisal stability, no infra-occluded implant-supported crown, and *(c)* no marginal bone loss. (Adapted from Thilander et al[14] with permission.)

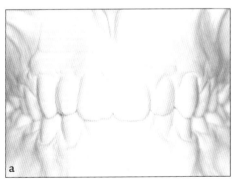
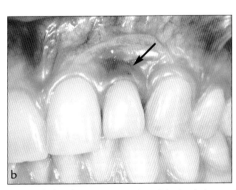
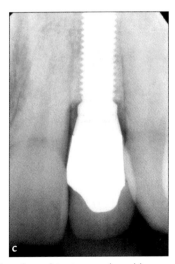

Fig 6-25 *(a)* Study casts of a girl (16 years, 2 months, skeletal stage MP3-G) with the left maxillary lateral incisor replaced by an implant-supported crown. *(b)* At the latest control (25 years, 2 months), an infra-occlusion (0.8 mm) and discolored gingiva *(arrow)* were observed. *(c)* The periapical radiograph showed no bone loss at the implant, but note the loss of supporting bone at the adjacent central incisor (4.8 mm). The increase in body height during the entire observation period was 4.5 cm. (Adapted from Thilander et al[14] with permission.)

in the level of the incisor edges (range 0.1 to 2.2 mm), an apical shift of the soft tissue margin of the implant-supported crown also could be seen in a few cases. Of note is that infra-occlusion also may occur in patients who had received single implants in the incisor region at adult ages (Fig 6-28).[15]

Throughout the follow-up period, minor *loss of marginal bone at implant sites* was also observed. Radiographic assessments (Fig 6-29) showed that most bone loss occurred between abutment connection and crown placement (mean 0.5 mm; SD 0.99 mm), with additional loss of approximately 0.3 mm at the

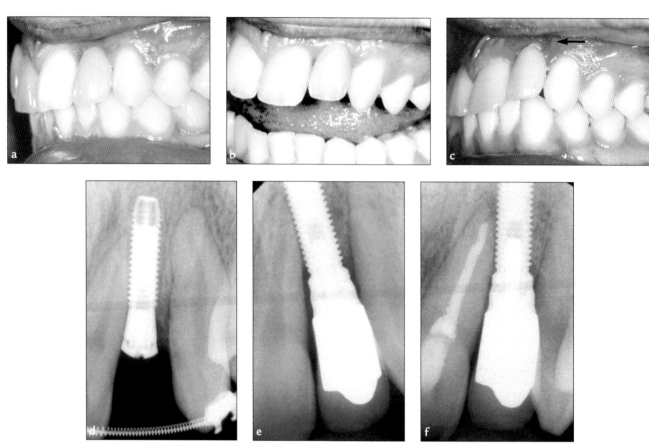

Fig 6-26 *(a)* A boy with a congenitally missing lateral incisor, which was replaced by an implant-supported crown at the age of 15 years, 5 months (skeletal stage MP3-FG). *(b)* At the 3-year control, an infra-occlusion of 1.6 mm was registered; the increase in body height during this period was 18 cm. *(c)* At the latest observation (25 years, 2 months), no further increase in body height was found, but the infra-occlusion had increased to 2.2 mm. The shift in the gingival margin and the marginal bone loss at the buccal aspect *(arrow)* resulted in an unesthetic appearance. Periapical radiographs from these three different observations show bone loss at the adjacent incisor *(d)* as early as crown placement and *(e,f)* further loss with age. At the latest observation, even loss of bone at the implant was registered (1.2 mm). (Adapted from Thilander et al[14] with permission.)

most recent examinations (although with individual variations) (mean 0.75 mm; SD 0.44 mm). The soft tissue also became discolored, indicating loss of marginal bone support at the buccal aspect of the implant that was further verified by gingival retraction (see Figs 6-26c and 6-27a,b).

Reduction of the marginal bone level at the teeth adjacent to the lateral incisor was observed in some patients (see Figs 6-25c and 6-26d to 6-26f). The largest reduction occurred during the interval between preoperative examination and crown placement, although additional changes were observed throughout the study. Altogether, a mean of 4.3 mm mesial and 2.2 mm distal to the incisor implant was registered (although with

large individual variations). The data indicated that the shorter the distance between the implant and the adjoining tooth surface, the larger the reduction of marginal bone level.

In *orthodontic-prosthodontic treatment*, implants serve as orthodontic anchorage units and then as abutments for prosthetic reconstructions of missing teeth in adults.[16] In *regular orthodontic treatment*, the anchorage units must be placed in regions other than the alveolar bone, such as the palate. Because of the thin bone height in the palate, an endosseous implant must have small dimensions, especially in length, so as not to perforate the nasal cavity. Another disadvantage of palatal implants is that they must be removed

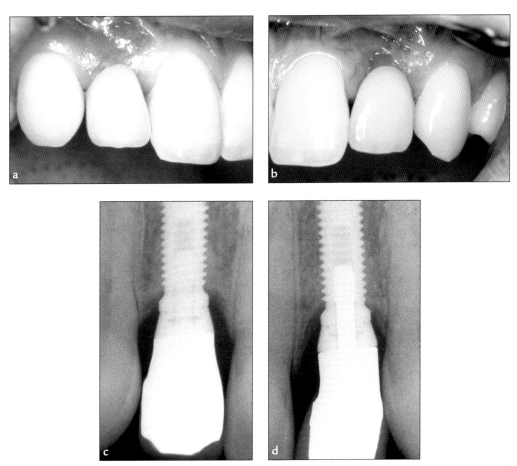

Fig 6-27 (a,b) Clinical photographs and (c,d) periapical radiographs of the two maxillary lateral incisors in a 25-year-old woman, 10 years after placement of implant-supported crowns. Note infra-occlusion (1.6 mm), (a) discolored gingiva, and (b) gingival retraction with bone loss. No bone loss took place at the adjacent teeth, but only at the implants (c,d) (0.5 and 1.0 mm, respectively). (Adapted from Thilander et al[14] with permission.)

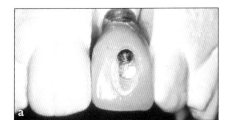
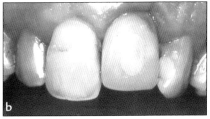
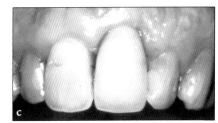

Fig 6-28 (a) Study cast with an implant-supported crown as replacement for a missing maxillary central incisor in a 34-year-old woman. (b) Control 12 years later with an infra-occlusion of 2.1 mm due to eruption of the adjacent teeth. (c) Replacement of the implant-supported crown. (Adapted from Thilander et al[15] with permission.)

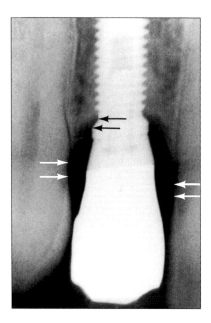

Fig 6-29 Periapical radiograph showing the reference points used for analyzing the marginal bone level changes at the implant (distance between a fixed reference point at the implant and marginal bone level: *black arrows*) and at adjacent teeth (distance between CEJ and marginal bone level: *white arrows*). (Adapted from Thilander et al[14] with permission.)

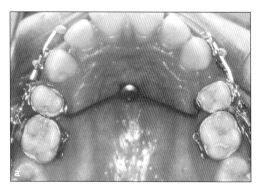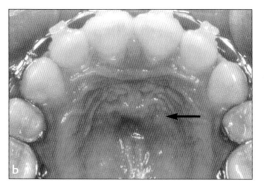

Fig 6-30 *(a)* A dental implant used as orthodontic anchorage and *(b)* 9 months after removal of the implant. Note the incomplete healing *(arrow)*.

after the completion of orthodontic treatment with the risk of bony defects or soft tissue damage (Fig 6-30). Onplants may be an alternate choice.

In summary, single dental implants are a good treatment option for replacing missing teeth in adolescents. However, disadvantages may be related to the maxillary incisor region, due to a slight continuous eruption of adjacent teeth. In addition, periodontal problems may arise with marginal bone loss around the adjacent teeth and marginal bone recession buccal to the implants.

Dental implants resist tooth movements and are excellent orthodontic anchorage units in orthodontic-prosthodontic adult patients. In regular orthodontic patients, however, there is need for further research in developing new implants and components to avoid possible tissue damage.

Conclusions

This chapter is based on experimental studies whose results have been tested in the orthodontic clinic. The long-term outcomes observed in these patients verify that the following facts deserve attention in the orthodontic patient to avoid/minimize damage to tooth-supporting tissues in orthodontics:

1. A proper oral hygiene regimen during the total treatment period is required to prevent plaque accumulation and thus minimize the risk for *gingivitis, attachment loss, infrabony pockets* (of special importance in patients who had been treated for periodontal disease), and *loss of marginal alveolar bone.*

2. The use of light orthodontic forces in closure of extraction sites will minimize formation of *interdental folds,* whose increased amount of glucose aminoglycans may cause *relapse* after closure of the extraction gap.

3. Labial and buccal tooth movements should be preceded by careful examination of the tissues covering the labial/buccal aspects of those teeth. During such movements, the roots are displaced toward and sometimes even through the thin cortical bone plate, which may result in *fenestrations* and *dehiscences. Torquing* tooth movements and *rapid maxillary expansion* (in patients with partially or totally obliterated sutures) heightens the risk of such complications. A thin soft tissue covering the cortical bone plate may serve as a locus minoris resistente, even causing *marginal bone recessions.*

4. The use of dental implants in adolescents appears to be a good option provided that the patient's dental and skeletal development are complete. However, disadvantages may be associated with the maxillary incisors due to *slight continuous eruption of adjacent teeth* post-adolescence. Periodontal problems may arise with *marginal bone loss* around the adjoining teeth and buccal to the implant.

References

1. Lundström F, Krasse B. *Streptococcus mutans* and lactobacilli frequency in orthodontic patients: The effect of chlorhexidine treatment. Eur J Orthod 1987;9:109–116.
2. Rosenblom RG, Tinanoff N. Salivary *Streptococcus mutans* levels in patients before, during and after orthodontic treatment. Am J Orthod Dentofacial Orthop 1991;100:35–37.
3. Davies TM, Shaw WC, Worthington HV, Addy M, Dummer P, Kingdom A. The effect of orthodontic treatment on plaque and gingivitis. Am J Orthod Dentofacial Orthop 1991;99:155–162.
4. Boyd R, Baumrind S. Periodontal considerations in the use of bonds or bands on molars in adolescents and adults. Angle Orthod 1992;62:117–126.
5. Alexander SA. Effects of orthodontic attachments on the gingival health of permanent second molars. Am J Orthod Dentofacial Orthop 1991;100:337–340.
6. Rönnerman A, Thilander B, Heyden G. Gingival tissue reactions to orthodontic closure of extraction sites. Histologic and histochemical studies. Am J Orthod 1980;77:620–625.
7. Alstad S, Zachrisson BU. Longitudinal study of periodontal condition associated with orthodontic treatment in adolescents. Am J Orthod 1979;76:277–286.
8. Hollender L, Rönnerman A, Thilander B. Root resorption, marginal bone support, and clinical crown length in orthodontically treated patients. Eur J Orthod 1980;3:197–205.
9. Ericsson I, Thilander B, Lindhe J, Okamoto H. The effect of orthodontic tilting movements on the periodontal tissues of infected and non-infected dentitions in dogs. J Clin Periodontol 1977;4:278–293.
10. Thilander B, Nyman S, Karring T, Magnusson I. Bone regeneration in alveolar bone dehiscences related to orthodontic tooth movements. Eur J Orthod 1983;5:105–114.
11. Wennström J, Lindhe J, Sinclair F, Thilander B. Some periodontal tissue reactions to orthodontic movement in monkeys. J Clin Periodontol 1987;14:121–129.
12. Persson M, Thilander B. Palatal suture closure in man from 15 to 35 years of age. Am J Orthod 1977;72:42–52.
13. Engström C, Thilander B. Premature synostosis: The influence of biomechanical factors in normal and hypocalcemic young rats. Eur J Orthod 1985;7:35–47.
14. Thilander B, Ödman J, Lekholm U. Orthodontic aspects of the use of oral implants in adolescents: A 10-year follow-up study. Eur J Orthod 2001;23:715–731.
15. Thilander B, Ödman J, Jemt T. Single implants in the upper incisor region and their relationship to the adjacent teeth. Clin Oral Implants Res 1999;10:346–355.
16. Thilander B. Implant anchorage in orthodontic treatment. In: Higuchi K (ed). Orthodontic Applications of Osseointegrated Implants. Chicago: Quintessence, 2000:71–88.

Release of Wear and Corrosion Products from Orthodontic Alloys:

A Review of Mechanisms and Biologic Properties

Theodore Eliades, George Eliades,
William A. Brantley, Athanasios E. Athanasiou

The use of various alloys in orthodontics is an integral part of the standard procedures performed by the clinician, and the application of a wide array of utilities and auxiliaries may impose a risk for the adjacent and distant tissues.[1]

In general, research on the biologic properties of orthodontic alloys is limited. Most of the evidence available is derived from two types of publications: case reports presenting various conditions or adverse reactions induced by the application of materials, and reports describing efforts to simulate the clinical situation through ex vivo experimental configurations. However, the approaches used in the relevant literature (discussed later in this chapter) are flawed by fundamental errors in structuring the analogue of the clinical conditions, by basic inconsistencies concerning the method to study release kinetics, and by the introduction of assumptions pertinent to parameters of alloy aging that find no support in the relevant materials science literature.[2] Thus, most of these

research efforts have not contributed unambiguous evidence to the issue, and the qualitative and quantitative aspects of ionic leaching from alloys remain vague. Concurrently, demands for safety on behalf of the patients and operators have been strongly expressed by various legislations[1] because of the potential side effects arising from the proven action of various metals to induce allergic, mutagenic, and carcinogenic reactions at the cell, tissue, and organ levels, as illustrated in the biomedical literature.[3]

In this chapter, we first explore the composition and structure of the alloys currently used in orthodontic applications. The need to avoid exposure to corrosion products and ions, along with a review of the methods employed for investigation of metal ion levels in biologic fluids, is also considered. Last, a critique of the in vitro, in vivo, and ex vivo protocols used to investigate the hypotheses in published articles is presented.

Structure and Composition of Orthodontic Alloys

The vast majority of the metallic orthodontic appliances and utilities involve stainless-steel and nickel-titanium alloys, whereas beta-titanium wires and cobalt–chromium–molybdenum (Co-Cr-Mo) wires (Elgiloy, Elgin, IL) are used less frequently. Table 7-1 lists the wide range of nickel-containing appliances.[2]

Stainless-steel alloys

Stainless steels are iron-based alloys that contain chromium to provide excellent corrosion resistance from a thin, adherent, passive surface oxide layer.[4,5] These alloys may be divided into five families based on the predominant phase(s) in their microstructure: austenitic, martensitic, ferritic, duplex austenitic plus ferritic, and precipitation-hardened stainless steels with more complex microstructures. The austenitic stainless steels, which generally offer the greatest corrosion resistance, contain nickel as the primary austenite-stabilizing element and are designated as AISI (American Iron and Steel Institute) series 200 and 300 alloys. The 316L type (the "L" denotes a low carbon content) is the most commonly used stainless steel for implantation applications. The presence of nickel in stainless steels increases the resistance to corrosion in neutral chloride solutions and in acids that have low oxidizing capacity; the addition of molybdenum to these alloys also improves the resistance to corrosion in neutral chloride solutions, including seawater.[5] The nickel atoms are not strongly bonded to form some intermetallic compound, increasing the likelihood of in vivo slow nickel ion release from the alloy surface.[6]

The corrosion potential and nickel release feature of the AISI type 316L austenitic stainless-steel alloy currently used for orthodontic brackets has led to the consideration of alternative stainless steels.[7] For example, 2205 stainless-steel alloy, which contains half the amount of nickel found in the 316L alloy, has been proposed for manufacturing of orthodontic brackets.[8,9] This stainless steel has a duplex microstructure consisting of austenitic and delta-ferritic phases and is harder than the 316L alloy. Moreover, the 2205 alloy demonstrated substantially less crevice corrosion than the 316L alloy when coupled with nickel titanium, beta-titanium, or stainless-steel archwires in vitro.[7,8]

The chromium oxide surface film on stainless steels spontaneously forms (passivation) and reforms (repassivation) in air and under most tissue fluid conditions.[10] Oxygen is necessary for the formation of the film, whereas a low pH and the presence of chloride ions can be particularly detrimental to its stability. Increasing the content of chromium reduces the passive current density, increases the potential for breakdown and pitting, and lowers the critical current density and potential necessary for passivation.[11] Nickel decreases the critical current density, whereas molybdenum not only lowers the critical current density but also raises the pitting potential.[4]

Studies have shown that the surface film formed by chromium also contains iron, nickel, and molybdenum. In an aqueous environment, this film consists of an inner oxide layer and an outer hydroxide layer.[5] The chromium oxide passive films on stainless steels are not as stable as their titanium oxide counterparts on titanium and its alloys, contributing to the inferior corrosion resistance of stainless steels relative to titanium and its alloys.[6]

Nickel-titanium alloys

The nickel-titanium wires contain approximately equiatomic proportions of nickel and titanium and are based on the intermetallic compound NiTi.[6] Examination of the binary phase diagram reveals that there can be some deviation from stoichiometry for NiTi. There are two major NiTi phases in the nickel-titanium orthodontic wires: an austenitic phase, which has an ordered body-centered cubic (CsCl-type) structure that occurs at high temperatures and low stresses; and a martensitic phase, which has been reported to have a distorted monoclinic, triclinic, or hexagonal structure and forms at low temperatures and high stresses.[6]

The corrosion resistance of NiTi wires is primarily due to the large amount (48% to 54%) of titanium in the alloy composition. Titanium forms several oxides

Table 7-1 Nickel-containing orthodontic materials and corresponding nickel-free substitutes*

Category	Material	Ni-free substitute and modifications
Standard appliances	Brackets	Ni-free stainless-steel, ceramic, plastic, Ti, and gold-plated brackets
	Bands	Gold-plated bands
Treatment utilities	Stainless-steel archwires	No alternative currently available; development of polymeric wires in progress
	Ni-Ti archwires	β-Ti archwires; nitride- or epoxy-coated Ni-Ti archwires
		β-Ti archwires
	Co-Cr-Ni archwires (Elgiloy)	No alternative currently available
Mechanics auxiliaries	Sliding yokes, transpalatal and lingual arches	β-Ti, plastic, or inert metal (Au) coating of wire segments
Miscellaneous auxiliaries	Stainless-steel ligatures	Teflon-coated ligatures
	Kobayashi hooks	Ni-free brackets with hooks
	Coil springs	Elastomeric ligatures
Fixed expansion appliances	Stainless-steel appliances (quad-helix, rapid palatal expander)	β-Ti wires for quad-helix
	Stainless-steel headgear	Teflon-coated stainless-steel facebow
	Ni-Ti spring screws	No alternative currently available
Removable appliances	Stainless-steel components of Hawley appliance and variations	Plastic or elastic retainers; elastic positioners or acrylic splints
Complex therapeutic interventions	Orthognathic surgery lag screws and plates	Resorbable polylactic–polyglycolic lag screws and plates
	Distraction osteogenesis apparatus	No alternative currently available

*Reprinted from Eliades and Athanasiou[2] with permission.

(TiO_2, TiO, Ti_2O_5), of which titanium dioxide is the most common and stable. This oxide has three crystalline forms: tetragonal anatase and rutile, and orthorhombic brookite. The composition of the titanium oxide surface layer has not been clearly defined, and, because it is unlikely to be stoichiometric, TiO_x more accurately describes this oxide.[12] The rapid, spontaneous formation of TiO_2 in air is due to the substantial negative free energy ($\Delta G = -203.8$ kcal/mol) for oxidation, which makes this reaction energetically highly favorable:

$$Ti + O_2 \rightarrow TiO_2$$

However, considerable dispute exists concerning the pattern, kinetics, and direction of oxide growth.

Although some reports suggest that the oxide thickness increases as a logarithmic function of immersion time in electrolytes, a different relationship for growth and steady-state levels of the TiO_2 has also been observed.[13]

Upon exposure of Ti to water, TiO_2 is expected to form according to the reaction

$$Ti + 2H_2O \rightarrow TiO_2 + 2H_2$$

with $\Delta G = -82.9$ kcal/mol. In electrolyte solutions, anions adsorbed on the oxide surface generate a sufficiently high electric field to facilitate migration of metal (oxide) anions through the film to the oxide-electrolyte interface. During this reaction H^+ ions are produced, increasing the pH. The resulting OH^- anions are adsorbed on the surface, where they create an electric field for ion migration and subsequent oxide growth.[12]

For a thorough analysis of orthodontic wire alloys from both metallurgical and clinical perspectives, the reader is referred to Brantley.[6]

Intraoral Aging of Orthodontic Alloys: Material Alterations

Some corrosion of orthodontic alloys, regardless of their metallurgical structure, occurs in the oral environment; the inevitable surface defects from wire manufacturing are assumed to accelerate this process. Apart from the various types of corrosion found in other applications of materials,[14] intraoral aging of orthodontic alloys is subject to a unique set of parameters arising from environmental factors.[2]

In general, corrosion of orthodontic alloys during the intraoral service of appliances and utilities includes a broad spectrum of corrosion types and a wide array of mechanisms. Thus, *pitting* corrosion has been identified in brackets and wires, while *crevice* corrosion occurs in confined spaces that are exposed to corrosive environments, often through the application of elastomeric ligatures on a bracket, and arises from differences in metal ion or oxygen concentration between the crevice and its vicinity.[11,15] In clinically derived material, the depth of the crevice can reach 2 to 5 mm, perforating the base in one-piece brackets, and the amount of metal dissolved can reach high levels (Fig 7-1).[16] The attack may be attributed to the lack of oxygen associated with plaque formation and the byproducts of microbial flora, which deplete the oxygen and disturb the regeneration of the passive layer of chromium oxides. Also, *fretting* corrosion developed during sliding of a metallic wire on the slot of the bracket, with the underlying mechanism involving cold welding at the interfaces under pressure, results in rupturing of the contact points (wear oxidation). In addition, *enzymatic activity* and microbial attack on material surfaces has been identified in dental applications of materials.[17]

The action of microbiota colonization is two-fold. Certain species can uptake and metabolize metals from alloys, while microbial byproducts and metabolic processes may alter the conditions of the microenvironment (eg, decreasing pH, thereby contributing to initiation of the corrosion process). The metal uptake capacity of microbia has long been known and applied to the problem of metal waste management. Other species, including *Bacteroides corrodens*; *Thiobacillum ferroxidans*; or the acid-producing *Streptococcus mutans*, which plays a major role in dental caries, may adversely affect the surface structure of dental alloys.[11] Bacterial metabolism has been reported as having a role in the surface alteration of dental alloys,[2] with particular emphasis being placed on sulfate- and nitrate-reducing bacteria.[17] These species are aggressive and inflammatory to the host tissues while affecting the corrosion processes of various alloys.

A study of retrieved NiTi orthodontic wires revealed that the used samples were characterized by the formation of a proteinaceous biofilm, the organic constituents of which are mainly alcohol, amides, and carbonate.[15] The irreversible formation of precipitates and the development of microcrystalline sodium chloride, potassium chloride, and calcium phosphorus deposits substantially alter the surface composition and topography of the wire alloy (Fig 7-2). In addition, delamination, pitting, and crevice corrosion defects, as well as an apparent reduction in the alloy grain size, were identified in retrieved NiTi wires (Fig 7-3). These alterations may arise from a

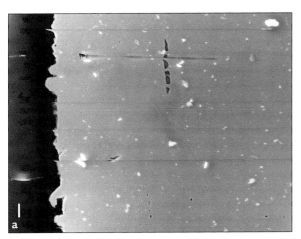
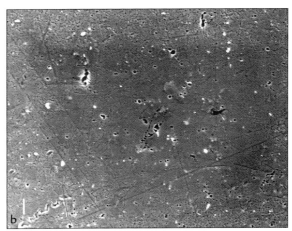

Fig 7-1 Secondary electron image of a retrieved stainless-steel orthodontic bracket showing (a) a longitudinal view of the slot wall illustrating the rough surface, and (b) the base (face view) demonstrating the formation of craters and grooves (original magnification × 40).

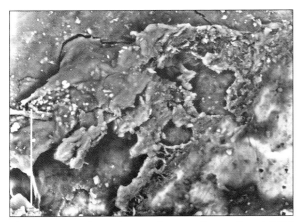
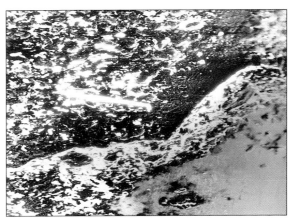

Fig 7-2 Secondary electron image of a retrieved NiTi wire demonstrating the presence of a dense film precipitated on the surface. X-ray microanalysis showed that this film consists mainly of Ca and P with traces of Na and K (original magnification × 400).

Fig 7-3 Secondary electron image of a retrieved inner/outer headgear bow junction depicting the dense precipitation of intraorally adsorbed integuments (original magnification × 50).

combination of intraoral conditions and loading attributed to the engagement of the wire into the bracket slot. Such alterations observed for retrieved wires may profoundly modify the reactivity of the archwire surface in vivo, with undetermined effects on the corrosion resistance, nickel dissolution, and frictional resistance.

Engagement of archwires to brackets bonded to crowded teeth results in increased alloy reactivity due to the local generation of tensile and compressive stresses because of the multiaxial, three-dimensional loading. Another highly important process for

the aging of orthodontic alloys is the tendency of a metal to undergo fatigue fracture under repeated cyclic stressing.[16] The process is accelerated by the reduction in the fatigue resistance induced by exposure to a corrosive medium such as saliva (corrosion fatigue) and appears to occur frequently in wires under load in the oral environment for extended periods of time. In general, this type of failure is characterized by substantial areas of smoothness on the fracture surfaces, which also have a region of increased roughness with a somewhat "crystalline" appearance. Because the same phenomena may be

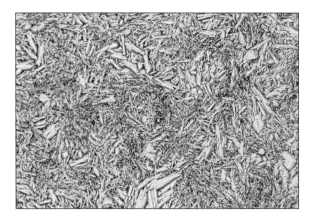

Fig 7-4 Optical microscope image of the microstructure of a retrieved, metallographically etched NiTi wire illustrating irregular spindle-like formations corresponding to the martensitic structure. (Etching solution: hydrofluoric, nitric, and acetic acids at 1:1:1 volume ratios; polarized light × 40.)

seen in other metallic orthodontic materials such as facebows[16] (Fig 7-4), fracture incidents of headgear facebow wires, especially in the inner arch where the wire segment enters the buccal tube, may be due to corrosion fatigue. While there are presently minimal reports of fatigue testing in the orthodontic materials literature, perhaps future standards for orthodontic wires used in headgear face bows should include a test for corrosion fatigue. Comparison of detailed scanning electron micrographs of clinically failed specimens with micrographs of engineering alloys that have failed by corrosion fatigue may provide unambiguous evidence of this mechanism.

In concluding this section, it seems that there is a lack of evidence of the contributory role of intraoral aging on the kinetics of nickel release and corrosion potential of stainless-steel and NiTi archwire alloys. Further research should focus on this issue to clarify a possible role of the aging process on the biocompatibility of these alloys. Adoption of in vivo experimental approaches may be instrumental in establishing clinical relevance of the reported evidence. See Eliades et al[18] for a recent comprehensive review of the intraoral aging of orthodontic materials.

Trace Metals in Environmental and Biologic Fluids: Background and General Considerations

Environmental sources of nickel

Sources of nickel intake include a wide variety of everyday life and occupational activities, ranging from airborne particulates and dust, drinking water, food, and soil, to cooking utensils and cosmetic products such as eye shadows.[19–22] The relevance of the results reported in the foregoing studies to orthodontics is questionable, however, because the binding state and formulation of nickel derivatives play a pivotal role in modulating the biologic reactions induced by nickel-containing materials.

Nickel is an important nutrient factor, as evidenced by its incorporation in dietary supplements in ionic form, typically 5 µg per tablet and at a customary dose of one tablet per day. Given the recommended daily intake of vitamins and minerals, it may be postulated that it is the reaction of nickel ions with certain chemical species that determines the hazardous nature of the nickel moieties.[23]

Of all the forms of nickel, the airborne particulate form of Ni compounds and especially the nickel carbonyls present the greatest biohazards. According to regulations for air emissions in many countries, virtually all nickel and compounds containing significant proportions of nickel are classified as "known or suspected carcinogens" because of their effects on the upper respiratory system.[24] For example, airborne nickel particulates, which are present in electroplating factories, cause nasal septum and lung lesions, including cancer. Hence most of the safety regulations address aspects of nickel mining and nickel metallurgy rather than pharmaceuticals containing nickel or Ni compounds.[25,26]

The proposal of threshold levels associated with hazardous action for a metal may often be influenced by contemporary political views. Thus, in 1993 the United States Environmental Protection Agency (USEPA) proposed a maximum contaminant level goal (MCLG) for nickel of 100 µg/L in drinking water. However, in subsequent revised directives, nickel was characterized as "another contaminant of concern" without reference to concentration levels (www. epa.gov/OGWDW/swp/vcontam3). Nonetheless, the New York State regulations for ground water continue to indicate a limit of 100 µg/L and an upper limit for nickel in soils of 15 mg Ni/kg of dry weight soil as the "clean-up standard" for contaminated soils.[27] Nickel limits for the protection and propagation of aquatic life in fresh water systems vary between 10 µg/L and 100 µg/L in different nations, with the lowest and most protective limit required by the Netherlands.[28]

Generally, the average person receives a daily amount of nickel of approximately 170 µg through ingestion and 0.4 µg through inhalation. The USEPA, focusing on the association of 20 potential carcinogens, has proposed threshold limit values since the ambient threshold limit values for nickel in air exceeded 1,400 cancer cases per million persons exposed to this element, and the aforementioned guidelines for decreased nickel concentrations were issued. Since 1996, the European Union has enforced a law requiring that materials such as earrings, watchstraps, or zippers not release nickel in amounts greater than 0.5

µg per cm^2 of material surface per week and for at least 2 years.[19]

Metals in biologic fluids

The area of metal atom or ion release from biomaterials into various sites of the human body has attracted the interest of many investigators because of the possibility that debris or degradation products would elicit a foreign body reaction or have a role in the induction of pathologic processes. Research in the general biomedical literature has focused on the release of metal ions from orthopedic and dental materials. The latter category principally consists of orthodontic materials,[2] restorative materials, and prosthetic appliances that are in contact with biologic tissues or fluids, such as saliva or blood.

To reliably assess the excretion rates of metals from an organism, Greene (as cited by Black[29]) proposed a method involving the intravenous administration of nickel, in the form of $^{63}NiCl_2$, into rabbits housed in cages and the meticulous collection of urine and feces throughout the day for specific periods of time. The relationship between the amount of nickel injected and that excreted (S) between 3 and 7 days postinjection was described by the following equation, which represents a two-stage process:

$$S \; (\mu g/L) = A_1 e^{-a_1 t} + A_2 e^{-a_2 t}$$

The first term represents the initial disappearance, while the second includes the reduced excretion rates at a later stage. The four constants (A_1, a_1, A_2, and a_2) are determined from experimental data and are species-specific. However, in this model the period of monitoring in Greene's original research was of relatively short duration, which may preclude its use for long-term predictions. For such situations, one or more additional exponential decay terms, corresponding to other processes, might be needed. This model assumes an exogenous source of metal ions, and therefore the excretion rates from individuals with an implant may be considerably different compared to those from individuals with a different type of intrinsic source of the same metal. Differences among species (eg, humans compared to laboratory primates or mice) depend upon the physiologic mechanisms of urine excretion and associated clearance rates for a metal and also upon the mass of soft tissues, which may decrease the amount of metal circulated.

The volume of plasma in contact with the trace metals, as well as the actual functional mechanisms, may also cause a variation in excretion rates among species. For example, an implanted metallic device is in contact with an interstitial pool averaging 7 L, an intracellular pool of 23 L, and a plasma water pool of 3.2 L. The entire amount of these fluids passes through the kidneys at a rate of 180 L per day.[29] The contact of metal ions accumulated in internal organs with such an enormous amount of body fluids may greatly affect its excretion kinetics. At present, most of the knowledge acquired in this field has been derived from studies of patients with total hip arthroplasties, and it is uncertain that similar elemental release patterns can be found for other biomedical applications that involve different means of implantation in which there is less invasive contact with tissues and fluids.[29,30] Although information derived from implantation of biomaterials may be irrelevant to the orthodontic analogue, where the biomaterial is placed noninvasively in the oral cavity,[2] at present such studies are the only sources of information available on this issue.

Generally, when materials are implanted or placed in contact with biologic tissues or fluids, organometallic compounds are formed. The corrosion rate of metallic materials may be enhanced by local microenvironmental factors, including pH fluctuations and temperature variants.[29] Potential alterations of the passive layer formed on the surface may also influence the corrosion rates of metallic implant materials, which rely on the formation of chromium or titanium oxide layers to resist corrosion. This factor is of paramount importance for the biologic properties of these materials. Various physiologic compounds have been tested and, while some have been found to have a neutral effect on corrosion rate, others, such as serum proteins, have been found to increase the corrosion rate by up to two orders of magnitude.[29]

An important factor that has not been studied adequately is the wear of biomaterials arising from contact with other biomaterials or tissue fluids. Such wear may affect the reactivity of adjacent biomaterials and

surrounding host tissues by two mechanisms. The first relates to the production of wear particles, which increases the effective contact surface with the tissue, thereby eliciting a reaction. Such wear is very common in orthopedic biomaterials between the stainless-steel femoral head and the ultrahigh-molecular-weight polyethylene acetabular socket. The resulting wear debris has been implicated in the shortened survival rates of these prostheses.[31]

Adhesive wear is encountered for orthodontic materials during sliding of a large cross-section rectangular archwire segment within the bracket slot walls. Kusy and Whitley[32] explained the variation of the resultant archwire-bracket friction on wear and formation of particles during sliding, which greatly affects the velocity of this movement. Evidence from more recent studies suggests that retrieved wires have been found to present delamination patterns, which are unknown to metallic biomaterials arising probably from wear between wire surfaces engaged in the slot and the slot walls.[15]

Because the size of wear debris may have a pronounced role in modifying the interfacial and biologic properties of the implanted biomaterials, efforts have focused on estimating the average particle size. Generally, wear particles may have a diameter of[29]

$$d = 6 \times 10^4 \ (W/p)$$

where (d) is the diameter, (W) is the surface energy of biomaterial, and (p) is the hardness of the wearing surfaces.

The relationship between wear debris particle size and the phagocytic capacity of leucocytes is highly important. Transfer of degradation products may be achieved via three modes: macroscopic movement, cell-mediated particulate movement, and movement through dissolution mediated by passive diffusion or active circulatory transport. The first mode of transport is movement of the entire prosthesis by macroscopic relocation in the surrounding tissues and has no relevance to most biomaterial applications.

For the other two potential modes of transporting degradation products, it is assumed that the leukocytes are the cell population that uptakes these products. Through complex modeling, it has been found that uptake and transport represent two distinctly different mechanisms.[29] While uptake can be measured ex vivo with some reliability, transport of metallic species greatly depends on physiologic mechanisms of the organism, which have yet to be revealed. The complexity of the lymphatic system and the interactions of various systems and tissues precludes a reliable approach to studying this effect.

Theoretical and experimental studies on uptake have led to the clarification of many variables involved in these phenomena. An initial phase, described by first-order kinetics, involves the engulfing of the trace biomaterial by phagocytes and is followed by a latent phase.[29] The former is described by the equation

$$1/V = 1/(K_0E) + [K_c/(K_0E)]^{1/c}$$

where (V) is the clearance uptake, (c) the concentration of particles, (E) the total available uptake sites, (K_c) the overall rate constant, and (K_0) another kinetic constant.

The second or latent phase is exponential and is dictated by the availability of particulates and the capacity of cells to uptake the trace biomaterials. An equation describing the uptake would be[29]

$$c/c_0 = e^{-kt}$$

where (c) is the uptake, (c_0) the initial colloid concentration, (t) time, and (k) the phagocytic index. Complex, higher-order kinetic relationships for the uptake process are likely because multiple pathways are expected. Further complexity is introduced by the size of the debris particles and the cell phagocytic capacity, which has not been well-defined and integrated into mathematical models. It has been shown[29] that spherical debris particles having a diameter of 0.080 μm may be phagocytosed by leukocytes to an extent of 8 μg of such particles per mg of cell mass, thus averaging about 24,000 particles per leukocyte. When the particle diameter increases to 3 μm, the uptake by cells is increased to almost 35 μg of particles per mg of leukocyte, but the number of particles per cell is now decreased to only 3. This 8,000-fold decrease in the capacity of cells to uptake multiple particles greatly modifies the kinetics of the process and also implies that large particles may be accumu-

lated directly, whereas small debris particles are collected outside the cell membrane. When a critical number or mass of debris is reached, absorption is initiated by an unknown mechanism.

Lastly, in assessing the concentrations of metallic ions present in blood serum and urine, the permeability and excretory ratios for the given ions should be considered. The former represents the ratio of the concentrations of an element in urine and plasma and is characteristic for both species and element. Ratios exceeding 1 imply a greater tendency for excretion, whereas a value less than 1 suggests binding of ions to serum proteins. An excretory ratio is defined as the relative efficiency for excretion based on a 24-hour urine volume of 1.5 L and renal infiltration of 180 L/24 h; this parameter increases with increasing excretion of dissolved species. An excellent review in greater detail for the concepts summarized in these foregoing paragraphs is provided by Black.[29]

Biologic Effects of Nickel

The major corrosion products of stainless steel are iron, chromium, and nickel. Although all three elements have potentially adverse effects, nickel and chromium have received the most attention because of their reported potential for producing allergic, toxic, or carcinogenic effects.[33–46] Caution should be used in interpreting these findings, since documented toxicities generally apply only to the soluble forms of these elements.[4] Currently, any association between release of a metal and any metabolic, bacteriologic, immunologic, or carcinogenic toxicity is considered as conjectural, since cause and effect have not been demonstrated in humans. Moreover, it is unlikely that the same pattern characterizes the orthodontic and orthopedic application of alloys.

Generally, solutions of nickel (0.05 μmol/L) and cobalt (0.01 μmol/L) have been found to impair the phagocytosis of bacteria by human polymorphonuclear leukocytes in vitro. Nickel ions may affect chemotaxis of leukocytes, mediated by a change in shape, while they stimulate neutrophils to become aspherical and move more slowly, and inhibit calcium ion–dependent contractile activity by depolarizing the neutrophil cell membrane.[40] Also, nickel has been shown to inhibit chemotaxis at a concentration of 2.5 to 50 ppm.[41] Nickel concentrations within the range of these values are released from dental alloys and have been shown to activate monocytes and endothelial cells and suppress or promote the expression of intercellular adhesion molecule 1 by endothelial cells.[40] The latter depends on the concentration of nickel. Most of the relevant literature indicates that the presence of nickel imposes a risk of promoting an inflammatory response in soft tissues.

Nickel complexes in the form of arsenides and sulfides are known carcinogens, allergens, and mutagens.[44–46] Nickel may mimic hypoxia with the upregulation of Cap43, a hypoxia-regulated gene. A different route leading to the same conclusion has been presented in which oxidative stress caused by exposure to metals and specifically nickel is mediated by induction of lactate dehydrogenase, lipid peroxidation, and induction of the Fenton reaction.[42] The latter process involves the reaction of O_2^- with an oxidative trace metal and generation of O_2, which in turn reacts with hydroxy peroxide to form the hydroxy radical and OH^-. An additional hypothesis for the oxidative stress involves the induction of acetaldehyde formation by nickel, while evidence of oxidizing action is illustrated by the increase of lactoferin receptors following exposure of cell populations to nickel. The latter constitutes an effort to diminish the active metal ions.

A plethora of studies have also established that nickel at nontoxic concentrations induces site-specific DNA base damage and single-strand scission.[45,46] The involvement of NF-kB and AP-1 transcription factors has been established through studies showing that Ni-resistant cells present reduced binding level of these two factors to their DNA sequences. Ni-mediated DNA damage may also arise indirectly by inhibition of enzymes, such as 8-oxo-2´-deoxyguanosine and 5´-triphosphate pyrophosphatase, that restore DNA breaks. At nontoxic concentrations, nickel promotes microsatellite mutations, inhibits nucleotide excision repair, and increases total genomic methylation. These contributions to genetic instability have been proposed as the basis of the carcinogenic action from nickel.[46]

Release of Wear and Degradation Products from Orthodontic Alloys

The orthodontic application of nickel alloys is unique in that the material is not implanted into tissue but is placed in an open cavity. Therefore, tests involving implantation of nickel-containing alloys and frequently used in other medical fields may bear no relevance to the clinical use of such alloys in orthodontics. Although the implantation procedure may be considered more invasive relative to intraoral placement, the reactivity of the implanted material with the environment is decreased because of the formation of a connective tissue capsule surrounding the foreign body. In contrast, intraorally placed orthodontic alloys in the form of archwires and brackets undergo continuous interaction with the local environment. In addition, there is a continuous flow of fluids (saliva or ingested liquids) that is renewed before saturation, thus increasing reactivity with the alloys.

In orthodontics, the principal sources of nickel are NiTi archwires and stainless-steel brackets, bands, and archwires. However, the entire mass of the archwires is substantially lower than that of the bonded stainless-steel brackets for a full-mouth patient case, and the duration of their use is only a relatively brief period of time.

Many investigators in the past decade have focused on the performance of alloys in the oral cavity rather than relying on in vitro laboratory tests. This is because the relatively simple storage media used in these latter tests, generally electrolyte or acidic solutions, cannot reliably simulate the complex intraoral conditions. Fluctuations in temperature, pH, and stress in vivo can accelerate the corrosion and reactivity of dental alloys under fatigue or corrosion fatigue conditions. For example, it is known that the corrosion of stainless steel is increased in acidic environments.[4] For evaluation of the corrosion of orthodontic alloys, standard protocols fail to simulate important clinical factors such as bracket-archwire ligation. Both of these components are moving elements, which may induce fretting corrosion.[2] Most importantly, there is a lack of simulation of the complex intraoral flora, plaque accumulation and its byproducts, which have proven corrosive action as previously discussed. Under clinical conditions, orthodontic alloys are in contact with these intraoral substances and with acids from degradation and decomposition of food, which can have significant effects on their reactive status and surface integrity.

Research protocols to investigate metallic ion release from orthodontic alloys can be classified in three major categories based on the experimental environment: in vitro using standard electrolyte solutions, retrieval studies, and detection of ions in biologic fluids.[2] Alternatively, these studies could be classified by experimental methodology into four categories: physical measurements, such as weight before and after immersion in media; spectroscopic analyses to identify ions in media; analytical techniques, including microscopy and spectroscopy for study of retrieved specimens; and spectroscopic analyses for investigation of ions in biologic fluids.

In vitro studies

In vitro studies are generally flawed by lack of clinical relevance due to simplifications in the models used. The majority of published in vitro studies have used various immersion solutions of different acidity to examine the variation in rate and total amount of ion release. Unfortunately, the results of such studies generally cannot be accurately applied to the clinical situation because of irrelevant methodology. For example, estimation of ion release through the use of nonagitated, nonreplenished storage media may be inconclusive with respect to release kinetics.[47] The release rate is forced to rapidly reach a plateau because of the equilibrium established between the metal ions present in the solution and the metal ions at the metal-solution interface. This leads to the conclusion that the release rate is accelerated initially and remains constant later, an observation that lacks substantiation.[18,48] Recent evidence has shown that, in multiple-phase alloys, long-term release may be higher than that occurring within the first week, while single-phase alloys have varying release patterns with increasing or decreasing rates, depending on the ele-

ment.[48] It is noteworthy that biomaterials investigators generally continue to study the short-term elemental (ion) release from alloys, when research conducted almost 3 decades ago showed that elevation of serum chromium levels continued to occur for 6 months following implantation.[29] This suggests that corrosion of such base metal implant alloys may be increasing after prolonged implantation times. A further example of the multiplicity of variables affecting metal release is illustrated by recent evidence that routine tooth brushing increases the rate of metal release from dental alloys.[49]

Retrieval studies

A method to study the alteration of biomaterial properties occurring in vivo is the analysis of used or retrieved materials. The wide range of orthodontic auxiliaries, utilities, and appliances[18] used as an integral part of daily practice present an ideal model for such study. The majority of materials (with the exception of brackets) may be removed and studied during the regular treatment visits of patients with no adverse effects on treatment outcome. Moreover, most of the orthodontic wires, elastomers, and other utilities are only periodically used during therapy. For brackets and bands, collection of used materials can take place only after the end of treatment owing to ethical concerns and technical problems arising from the intentional debonding and rebonding of these appliances.

Examination of retrieved orthodontic materials has established that biofilm adsorption and calcification may provide a protective inert surface layer, thereby reducing the incidence of host immune response as a result of decreased exposure of the alloy surface to the oral environment. Alternatively, the intraoral aging process can involve the adsorption of ions, which may accelerate corrosion and disintegration phenomena. The morphology of retrieved wire and bracket surfaces has demonstrated distinct differences compared to reference groups. Surface smoothening and deterioration, as well as increased pitting, were generally observed.[15,16,47,50] Excessive wear was observed on nickel-titanium archwires where there had been engagement to bracket slots, and characteristic patterns of delamination were observed for elastomers.

Metal content in biologic fluids

The most clinically relevant methods to study elemental release from orthodontic alloys have involved the estimation of nickel in biologic fluids (saliva, serum, and urine). Saliva is the first diluting pool for nickel, and the results have direct association with the amount of the metal leached. Urine and serum metal concentrations, however, are dependent on the excretory rate of nickel, discussed in the previous section, which is a highly individualized parameter and is species-specific.[29] Although mathematical modeling of the infusion and excretion rates of a metal by an organism can be performed, equations that predict the total body metal content do not take into account the presence of multiple compartments in the organism for these processes and the selective binding of metals to organs. For example, in rabbits nickel shows a high affinity to kidneys, while molybdenum is selectively accumulated in the spleen. Therefore, the observation that nickel levels in the blood of orthodontic patients are not different from those obtained from untreated individuals cannot rule out the possibility that nickel has been accumulated in some other organ.[2]

Most studies have confirmed that salivary metal levels of patients undergoing orthodontic treatment do not exceed daily intake levels through food and air. The concentrations of trace metals that have been found were in the range of those metals in tap water or dietary supplements.[51–54] However, large individual variations, deriving from high variability in the number of bands and brackets of each participant, precluded the detection of statistically significant differences in nickel concentration. All of the foregoing studies adopted a period of 1 month after insertion of fixed appliances to study the potential for ion release.

Because a recent investigation[51] focused on estimating the release occurring under far from routine clinical conditions, concerns have been raised pertinent to its methodology and that of the majority of articles published on this issue. Specifically, the time periods employed for saliva sampling during in vivo aging of metallic orthodontic appliances did not exceed 1 month, a time interval almost 20 times shorter than the typical duration of treatment. As a result, the effect of corrosion process and mechanical

phenomena such as wear and fatigue on the release of nickel could not be elucidated.[55] Moreover, saliva sampling in previous studies was performed at specific time periods, resulting in a lack of continuous and cumulative data extending over a wide time period. Lastly, the protocol for saliva collection, which involved stimulation though chewing of a piece of paraffin wax or gum, restricted the collection of saliva to that secreted almost directly from the gland. As a consequence, the absence of normal salivary wetting of the oral cavity, including the teeth, limited the exposure of orthodontic appliances to salivary flow, possibly inducing a false negative result in the reported[51] data.

In an attempt to address these concerns, a recent study took a different approach in selecting the patient population and obtaining salivary samples, and employed an alternative analytical method to investigate their metal content.[55] The longer-term aging of metal appliances and wires was addressed by including individuals who had been in treatment for more than 12 months. Salivary samples were obtained from patients under two different conditions: immediately upon entering the office, and following rinsing with double-distilled water to assess the effect of rinsing in altering the amount of released metals. Atomic emission spectroscopy, rather than atomic absorption spectroscopy, was chosen as the analytical procedure based on its low detection limit, which was set to 1 nm/mL or 1 ppb, along with its capacity to provide concentrations of multiple metals simultaneously. This study once again failed to detect differences in the salivary nickel and chromium content between patients and controls who were not undergoing orthodontic treatment.

The previous sampling method that was generally employed assumes that ion release follows a steady-state pattern and that the concentration found at a specific time is representative of the release for the full term of treatment, a hypothesis that requires verification. In addition, the results in previous studies were expressed as metal mass per saliva volume, thus providing no information about the time dependence of the metal release process. Since saliva secretion rates for specific patients are unknown and elemental release is additive with time, the values reported pertain only to the release for a specific time frame of

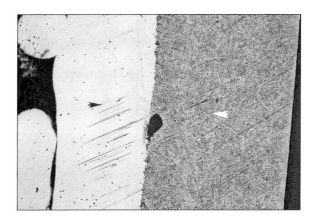

Fig 7-5 Optical microscope image of a retrieved, metallographically etched bracket section suggesting the presence of two distinct phases corresponding to different stainless-steel alloys (*black arrow*: base; *white arrow*: wing). The nominal bracket alloy is type 316L stainless steel. (Etching solution: 15 mL HNO_3, 50 mL methanol, and 5 g picric acid; polarized light $\times$ 50.)

undetermined duration. Therefore, these studies should be treated with skepticism, and no direct extrapolation to clinical conditions should be made.

Current concepts for ion release from orthodontic alloys

The foregoing data strongly suggest that this issue has not been resolved in the literature despite occasional agreement among different studies. This may be partially because of the uniformity in protocol formulation and study parameters among various investigations, leading to a repetition of the fundamental flaws existing in these protocols.

Because of the previously discussed methodologic difficulties for determining salivary levels of trace metals, a recent study[56] employed an alternative approach. Nickel leaching was measured indirectly by estimating the nickel content in new, used, and recycled brackets. Metallographic analysis and Vickers hardness measurements were used to complement the elemental analysis data. The results showed that, while the bulk elemental composition of the brackets remained stable, surface analysis of the wings revealed that the nickel content was decreased in retrieved specimens, implying ion release. Differences were noted in nickel content between bracket base and wing in all groups, implying that the base and wings may be manufactured from different stainless-steel alloys. Results from metallographic examination of etched brackets appeared to confirm the x-ray microanalysis, where the appearance of the metallurgic phases suggested that the base and wings were fabricated from two different types of stainless-steel types. Differences in Vickers hardness between the base and wing for all of the bracket groups further supported this hypothesis (Fig 7-5).[57] The results of the aforementioned studies verify the concerns expressed previously about the reliability of in vitro experiments to study the nickel release from orthodontic alloys. This review has emphasized the importance of retrieval analysis to obtain clinically relevant information. The authors hope that further research will be stimulated to obtain accurate quantitative nickel release data from orthodontic alloys and model this complex phenomenon.

Acknowledgments

The authors thank Dr Spiros Zinelis for the metallographic analyses reported in this chapter and Michael T. Kontaxis, PE, for information on USEPA guidelines.

References

1. Turpin DL. California proposition may help patients in search of better oral health [Editorial]. Am J Orthod Dentofacial Orthop 2001;120:1.

2. Eliades T, Athanasiou AE. In vivo aging of orthodontic alloys: Implications for corrosion potential, nickel release and biocompatibility. Angle Orthod 2002;74:222–237.

3. Hayes RB. The carcinogenicity of metals in humans. Cancer Causes Control 1997;8:371–385.

4. Sutow E. The corrosion behavior of stainless steel oral and maxillofacial implants. In: Eliades G, Eliades T, Brantley WA, Watts DC (eds). Dental Materials In Vivo: Aging and Related Phenomena. Chicago: Quintessence, 2003.

5. Brick RM, Pense AW, Gordon RB. Structure and Properties of Engineering Materials, ed 4. New York: McGraw-Hill, 1977:337–355.

6. Brantley WA. Orthodontic wires. In: Brantley WA, Eliades T (eds). Orthodontic Materials: Scientific and Clinical Aspects. Stuttgart: Thieme, 2001:77–105.

7. Eliades T, Eliades G, Brantley WA. Orthodontic brackets. In: Brantley WA, Eliades T (eds). Orthodontic Materials: Scientific and Clinical Aspects. Stuttgart: Thieme, 2001: 143–173.

8. Platt JA, Guzman A, Zuccari A, Thornburg DW, Rhodes BF, Oshida Y, et al. Corrosion behavior of 2,205 duplex stainless steel. Am J Orthod Dentofacial Orthop 1997; 112:69–79.

9. Torres FJ, Panyayong W, Rogers W, Velasquez-Plata D, Oshida Y, Moore BK. Corrosion behavior of sensitized duplex stainless steel. Biomed Mater Eng 1998;8:25–36.

10. Matasa CG. Biomaterials in orthodontics. In: Graber TM, Vanarsdall R (eds). Orthodontics: Current Principles and Techniques. St Louis: Mosby, 2000:305–338.

11. Matasa CG. Characterization of used orthodontic brackets. In: Eliades G, Eliades T, Brantley WA, Watts DC (eds). Dental Materials In Vivo: Aging and Related Phenomena. Chicago: Quintessence, 2003.

12. Eliades T. Passive film growth on titanium alloy: Physicochemical and biologic considerations. Int J Oral Maxillofac Implants 1997;12:621–627.

13. Ducheyne P, Healy TW. Titanium: Immersion-induced surface chemistry charges and the relationship to passive dissolution and bioactivity. In: Davies JE (ed). The Bone-Biomaterial Interface. Toronto: Univ Toronto Press, 1991:61–75.

14. Fontana MG. Corrosion Engineering, ed 3. New York: McGraw-Hill, 1986:39–152.

15. Eliades T, Eliades G, Athanasiou AE, Bradley TG. Surface characterization of retrieved orthodontic NiTi archwires. Eur J Orthod 2000;22:317–326.

16. Eliades T, Eliades G, Watts DC. Intraoral aging of the inner facebow component: A potential biocompatibility concern? Am J Orthod Dentofacial Orthop 2001;119:300–306.

17. Palaghias G. Oral corrosion and corrosion inhibition processes—an in vitro study. Swed Dent J Suppl 1985; 30:1–72.

18. Eliades T, Eliades G, Brantley WA, Watts DC. Aging of orthodontic utilities and auxiliaries. In: Eliades G, Eliades T, Brantley WA, Watts DC (eds). Dental Materials In Vivo: Aging and Related Phenomena. Chicago: Quintessence, 2003.

19. Delescluse J, Dinet Y. Nickel allergy in Europe: The new European legislation. Dermatol 1994;189(Suppl 2):56–57.

20. Basketter DA, Briatico-Vangosa G, Kaestner W, Lally C, Bontinck WJ. Nickel, cobalt and chromium in consumer products: A role in allergic contact dermatitis? Contact Dermatitis 1993;28:15–25.

21. Bennett BG. Environmental nickel pathways to man. IARC Sci Publ 1984;53:487–495.

22. Sainio EL, Jolanki R, Hakala E, Kanvera L. Metals and arsenic in eye shadows. Contact Dermatitis 2000;42:5–10.

23. Gawkrodger DJ. Nickel dermatitis: How much nickel is safe? Contact Dermatitis 1996;35:267–271.

24. New York State Department of Environmental Conservation. NY State Draft Air Guide 1. Guidelines for the control of toxic ambient air contaminants, April 5, 1994. http://www.dec.state.ny.us/website/dar/boss/toxics.html. Accessed 21 Jan 2004.

25. Barceloux DG. Nickel. J Toxicol Clin Toxicol 1999;37: 239–258.

26. Robinson JC, Paxman DG. The role of threshold limit values in U.S. air pollution policy. Am J Ind Med 1992; 21:383–396.

27. New York State Department of Environmental Conservation. Determination of soil cleanup objectives and cleanup levels. Technical and administrative guidance memorandum 4046, January 24, 1994. http://www.dec. state.ny.us/website/der/tagms/prtg4046.html. Accessed 21 Jan 2004.

28. New York Code Rules and Regulations. 6NYCRR, Part 703.5, Volume 6. http://www.dec.state.ny.us/website/regs/703.htm#703.5. Accessed 21 Jan 2004.

29. Black J. Biological Performance of Materials: Fundamentals of Biocompatibility. New York: Marcel Decker, 1999:28–44.

30. Clark GCF, Williams DF. The effect of proteins on metallic corrosion. J Biomed Mater Res 1982;16:125–134.

31. Howie DW, Vernon-Roberts B, Oakeshott R, Manthey B. A rat model of resorption of bone at the cement-bone interface in the presence of polyethylene wear particles. J Bone Joint Surg Am 1988;70:257–263.

32. Kusy RP, Whitley JQ. Effect of surface roughness on the coefficients of friction in model orthodontic systems. J Biomech 1990;23:913–925.

33. Dunlap CL, Vincent SK, Barker BF. Allergic reaction to orthodontic wire: Report of a case. J Am Dent Assoc 1989;118:449–450.

34. Staerkjaer L, Menné T. Nickel allergy and orthodontic treatment. Eur J Orthod 1990;12:284–289.

35. Greig DGM. Contact dermatitis reaction to a metal buckle on a cervical headgear. Br Dent J 1983;155:61–62.

36. Veien NK, Borchorst E, Hattel T, Laurberg G. Stomatitis or systemically induced contact dermatitis from metal wire in orthodontic materials. Contact Dermatitis 1994;30:210–213.

37. Marcusson JA, Lindh G, Evengård B. Chronic fatigue syndrome and nickel allergy. Contact Dermatitis 1999;40:269–272.

38. Costa M. Molecular mechanisms of nickel carcinogenesis. Biol Chem 2002;383:961–967.

39. Vreeburg KJJ, de Groot K, von Blomberg M, Scheper RJ. Induction of immunological tolerance by oral administration of nickel and chromium. J Dent Res 1984;63:124–128.

40. Wataha JC, Lockwood P, Marek M, Ghazi M. Ability of Ni-containing biomedical alloys to activate monocytes and endothelial cells in vitro. J Biomed Mater Res 1999;45:251–257.

41. Wataha JC, Sun ZL, Hanks CT, Fang DN. Effect of Ni ions on expression of intercellular adhesion. J Biomed Mater Res 1997;36:145–151.

42. Zhou D, Salnikow K, Costa M. Cap43, a novel gene specifically induced by Ni2+ compounds. Cancer Res 1998;58:2182–2189.

43. Chen CY, Sheu JY, Lin TH. Oxidative effects of nickel on bone marrow and blood of rats. J Toxicol Environ Health A 1999;58:475–483.

44. Salnikow K, Gao M, Voitkun V, Huang X, Costa M. Altered oxidative stress responses in nickel-resistant mammalian cells. Cancer Res 1994;54:6407–6412.

45. Lloyd DR, Phillips DH. Oxidative DNA damage mediated by copper (II), iron (II) and nickel (II) fenton reactions: Evidence for site-specific mechanisms in the formation of double-strand breaks, 8-hydroxydeoxyguanosine and putative intrastrand cross-links. Mutat Res 1999;424:23–36.

46. Lee YW, Broday L, Costa M. Effects of nickel on DNA methyltransferase activity and genomic DNA methylation levels. Mutat Res 1998;415:213–218.

47. Barrett RD, Bishara SE, Quinn JK. Biodegradation of orthodontic appliances. Part I. Biodegradation of nickel and chromium in vitro. Am J Orthod Dentofacial Orthop 1993;103:8–14.

48. Wataha JC, Lockwood PE, Nelson SK. Initial versus subsequent release of elements from dental casting alloys. J Oral Rehabil 1999;10:798–803.

49. Wataha JC, Lockwood PE, Noda M, Nelson SK, Mettenburg DJ. Effect of tooth brushing on the toxicity of casting alloys. J Prosthet Dent 2002;87:94-98.

50. Papadopoulos MA, Eliades T, Morfaki O, Athanasiou AE. Recycling of orthodontic brackets: Effects on physical properties and characteristics—Ethical and legal aspects. Rev Orthop Dento Faciale 2000;34:257-276.

51. Kerosuo H, Moe G, Hensten-Pettersen A. Salivary nickel and chromium in subjects with different types of fixed orthodontic appliances. Am J Orthod Dentofacial Orthop 1997;111:595-598.

52. Kocadereli I, Atilla A, Selin K, Durisehvan O. Salivary nickel and chromium levels in patients with fixed orthodontic appliances. Angle Orthod 2000;6:431-434.

53. Gjerdet NR, Erichsen ES, Remlo HE, Evjen G. Nickel and iron in saliva of patients with fixed orthodontic appliances. Acta Odontol Scand 1991;49:73-78.

54. Bishara SE, Barrett RD, Selim MI. Biodegradation of orthodontic appliances. Part II. Changes in the blood level of nickel. Am J Orthod Dentofacial Orthop 1993;103:115–119.

55. Eliades T, Trapalis C, Eliades G, Katsavrias E. Salivary metal levels of orthodontic patients: A novel methodological and analytical approach. Eur J Orthod 2003;25:103–106.

56. Eliades T, Zinelis S, Eliades G, Athanasiou AE. Nickel content of as-received, retrieved, and recycled stainless steel brackets. Am J Orthod Dentofacial Orthop 2002;122:217–220.

57. Eliades T, Zinelis S, Eliades G, Athanasiou AE. Characterization of as-received, retrieved and recycled stainless steel brackets. J Orofacial Orthop 2003;64:111–127.

Suggested Further Readings

Deguchi T, Ito M, Obata A, Koh Y, Yamagishi T, Oshida Y. Trial production of titanium orthodontic brackets fabricated by metal injection molding (MIM) with sintering. J Dent Res 1996;75:1491–1496.

Grímsdóttir MR, Gjerdet NR, Hensten-Pettersen A. Composition and in vitro corrosion of orthodontic appliances. Am J Orthod Dentofacial Orthop 1992;101:525–532.

Haynes DR, Crotti TN, Haywood MR. Corrosion of and changes in biological effects of cobalt chrome alloy and 316L stainless steel prosthetic particles with age. J Biomed Mater Res 2000;49:167–175.

Hensten-Pettersen A. Nickel allergy and dental treatment procedures. In: Maibach HI, Menne T (eds). Nickel and the Skin: Immunology and Toxicology. Boca Raton, FL: CRC Press, 1989:195–205.

Hensten-Pettersen A, Jacobsen N, Grímsdóttir MR. Allergic reactions and safety concerns. In: Brantley WA, Eliades T (eds). Orthodontic Materials: Scientific and Clinical Aspects. Stuttgart: Thieme, 2000:287–299.

Hunt NP, Cunningham SJ, Golden CG, Sheriff M. An investigation into the effect of polishing on surface hardness and corrosion of orthodontic archwires. Angle Orthod 1999;69:433–440.

Kim H, Johnson JW. Corrosion of stainless steel, nickel-titanium, coated nickel-titanium, and titanium orthodontic wires. Angle Orthod 1999;69:39–44.

Kotecki DJ. Welding of stainless steels. In: Olson DL, Siewert TA, Liu S, Edwards GR (eds). Welding, Brazing, and Soldering. ASM Handbook, Vol 6. Materials Park, OH: ASM International, 1993.

Kusy RP. Types of corrosion in removable appliances: Annotated cases and preventative measures. Clin Orthod Res 2000;3:230–239.

Lindsten R, Kurol J. Orthodontic appliances in relation to nickel hypersensitivity. A review. J Orofacial Orthop 1997;58: 100–108.

Maijer R, Smith DC. Biodegradation of the orthodontic bracket system. Am J Orthod Dentofacial Orthop 1986;90:195–198.

Merritt K, Brown SA. Release of hexavalent chromium from corrosion of stainless steel and cobalt-chromium alloys. J Biomed Mater Res 1995;29:627–633.

Oshida Y, Sachdeva RCL, Miyazaki S. Microanalytical characterization and surface modification of TiNi orthodontic archwires. Biomed Mater Eng 1992;2:51–69.

Pereira MC, Pereira ML, Sousa JP. Histological effects of iron accumulation on mice liver and spleen after administration of a metallic solution. Biomaterials 1999;20:2193–2198.

Sarkar NK, Redmond W, Schwaninger B, Goldberg AJ. The chloride corrosion behaviour of four orthodontic wires. J Oral Rehabil 1983;10:121–128.

Staerkjaer L, Menné T. Nickel allergy and orthodontic treatment. Eur J Orthod 1990;12:284–289.

Staffolani N, Damiani F, Lilli C, Guerra M, Staffolani NJ, Belcastro S, et al. Ion release from orthodontic appliances. J Dent 1999;27:449–454.

Steigerwald R. Metallurgically influenced corrosion. In: Davis JR (ed). Corrosion. ASM Handbook, Vol 13. Materials Park, OH: ASM International, 1987:131–134.

Polymers in Orthodontics: A Present Danger?

Claude Matasa

Polymers are the base or matrix for many plastics and devices used in orthodontics, many of which are placed in direct contact with soft human tissues, often for years. In contrast to metabolized medicines, the controls imposed on polymers by various governmental agencies are low. As a result, manufacturers are not required to disclose the ingredients or the procedures used in their production, and the specialty journals accept articles that cite commercial names instead of providing pertinent scientific information. Today, chemical compositions are disclosed only if they offer an incentive to the potential buyer. This situation needs to be remedied since some polymers, and especially their additives, are harmful to humans.

Polymer Development

Although plastics are generally regarded as a modern invention, there have always been "natural polymers," such as amber, tortoise shells, and animal horns, that behaved in a manner similar to today's manufactured plastics. Although it has been reported that the first man-made plastic, Parkesine, was introduced by Alexander Parkes at the 1862 Great International Exhibition in London, a similar material, vulcanite, was already in use in dentistry. Invented by Charles Goodyear in 1839 and made by adding sulfur to rubber, vulcanite could be used to make dentures by heating the mixture in a mold. The first attempts to commercialize the new material were not practical because it softened when heated and was partially soluble in water. It was not until 1839, when Goodyear accidentally discovered "sulfur cross-linking," that rubber became a substitute for the omnipresent plastics.

Traditionally, polymers tailored to fit the needs of industry have also been used in medicine. While many polymers have been tested over the years for their ability to enhance healing, their number has gradually decreased, as many were found to be unacceptable. With the present trend in medicine to substitute hard materials for ones that are less brittle, more biocompatible, and tissue-like, polymers have found important applications owing to their capacity to undergo large reversible deformations without the danger of catastrophic failure. Soft lenses, artificial limbs and corneas, cochlear and ophthalmic implants, vascular grafts, prostheses, and the like are used in large numbers.[1] The most common products—catheters and intravenous (IV) lines—are used nearly 100 million times a year in the US alone.[2] About two million people suffer burns each year, and almost four million diabetics who develop skin wounds are in need of elastomeric implants.[3] Facial implants include Alar (Uniroyal, Bethany, CT) cartilage in nostrils, cheeks, chin, lips, in creases above the eye and cheek-lip area, at the dorsum of the nose, in the earlobe, forehead, and glabella frown line, and in the infraorbital and infralabial grooves; most of these implant materials are elastomers.[4] While medical plastics represent less than 1% of total plastic consumption, their impact is great; in addition to auxiliary instruments and equipment, polymers can replace skin, tendons, and cartilage and can connect body tissues. For more than 40 years, plastic medical products, from disposable syringes to IV blood bags to heart valves, have helped doctors and nurses save lives. Many of the medical practices that are common today and were not even dreamed of 20 years ago are made possible by plastics.

Polymers in Orthodontics

Ever since Goodyear added sulfur to rubber to create the first synthetic materials used in the mouth, the trend has continued unabated. The polymers used in orthodontics can be divided into three classes according to their various applications: *(1)* ready-to-use devices made in their final form by manufacturers, such as brackets, retainers, and impression trays; *(2)* reformable polymers used as connecting framework for a variety of removable or functional appliances; and *(3)* polymeric materials, such as impression materials, cured adhesives, and sealant films, synthesized in situ by the orthodontist or the orthodontist's assistant. Each of these types has its unique qualities that must be treated distinctly. The latter two categories of polymers are made using kits provided by manufacturers.

Premanufactured polymers

Made in series in a controlled environment, premanufactured polymers are properly inspected and offer few surprises. Most of these polymers can be used in combination (blends) or comprise several monomers (copolymers). For hard devices (instruments, brackets) or retainers, high-molecular-weight polycarbonates, polymethacrylates, and polyurethanes are the materials of choice. For maxillofacial applications, impression trays, and mouth protectors, the materials of choice are soft and made of low-molecular-weight polyurethanes, vulcanized silicones, or copolymers of polyvinyl acetate with polyethylene, all destined to replace the controversial phthalate-plasticized polyvinyl chloride. For even softer materials like elastomers, aliphatic polyurethanes and (more recently) polyphosphazenes are replacing natural rubber. There is a growing demand for the polycarbonates, used for brackets and Invisalign retainers (Align Technologies, Santa Clara, CA). Since polycarbonates have high strength and modulus, they show little elastic deformation under load and are resistant to creep and cold flow. However, they are not as chemically resistant as nylons or polyolefins and are attacked by solvents. Accepted by the US Food and Drug Administration (FDA), polycarbonates are characteristically ductile, which accounts for their impact strength.

A general source of concern is the trend toward replacing thermoset plastics with thermoplastic materials. The former are more economical because their scraps can be easily remelted and reused, but the latter are more soluble and prone to decay due to their lack of cross links.

In office–processed polymers

Preformed sheets created for specific purposes by manufacturers are available for the orthodontist's convenience. Accompanied by step-by-step instructions, these plastic sheets help clinicians who want to spend minimal time engaged in nonclinical endeavors. The most common are made of linear (noncross-linked) polystyrene, polyurethane, or polyacrylate/polymethacrylate, with or without inorganic fillers. These fully polymerized auxiliary devices are subjected to physical transformations in the office, as is the case with the plastic sheets that are formed by heating and molding.

In situ–generated polymers

Because of the broad range of their potential applications, in situ–generated polymers require the most attention. Alginate and the less commonly used silicone and polysulfide impression materials suffer both a chain lengthening and some cross-linking in the presence of various inorganic compounds (calcium and titanium salts and lead oxide, respectively). Mixed in various proportions, the acrylic monomers are polymerized to generate adhesives, restoratives, veneers, and sealants. To initiate the process, heat, chemical reactions, or active light are used, and various organic compounds are then added according to the method of initiation. While peroxides are sufficient for the thermally cured acrylates, for those that are cold-cured, tertiary aromatic amines must be added. These enhance the decomposition of the peroxide, releasing a large number of free radicals.

To reduce shrinkage—a perpetual battle—while at the same time maintaining viscosity, the standard procedure uses mixtures of polyfunctional (and thus cross-linkable) acrylic esters of medium (such as triethylene glycol dimethacrylate [TEGDMA]) and higher (bisphenol glycidyl methacrylate [Bis-GMA]) molecular weight. To enhance bonding, acrylate esters containing hydrophilic groups (hydroxyethyl methacrylate [HEMA]) have only recently been used. Low-molecular-weight polymers of the acrylic or methacrylic acids are used in glass ionomers; due to their hydrophilic groups, these bond the enamel's calcium. The addition of copolymerizable chelating agents (N-phenylglycine [NPG], polymethyl methacrylate [PMMA]) to various composites, while quite traditional in dentistry, has found limited use in orthodontics despite the stable and insoluble complexes (better bonds) achieved when the calcium ions exist on the teeth's enamel.

Taking Polymers Seriously

While the materials currently used by orthodontists are neither invasive nor metabolized, some may remain in direct contact with the tissues for a period of many years, a potential concern. Whereas regulations in some countries require detailed information about such materials, polymers included, those used in orthodontics are neglected. Most catalogs, advertising pamphlets, and scientific journals refer to the materials used very casually, ie, only by their commercial name. Even in Germany, a country that hosts the ISO Technical Committee on dental products and publishes *Medizinproduktegesetz*, the laws governing medical products, manufacturers still present only superficial data and regard disclosure of information as a mere formality.

Thus, in a recent catalog, one of Germany's largest orthodontics manufacturers presented a table identical to the one it had published 5 years before to describe the polymers used in its products. In both, 17 polymeric materials are purported to be components of the devices advertised. Each is accompanied by an identification number that has no reference to any other data in the publication. The most widely used polymers in orthodontics—Bis-GMA and the aliphatic or polyurethane acrylates—do not even appear on the list. Nonetheless, this catalog compares well with that of other manufacturers. Table 8-1 presents the characteristics of the polymers listed in the original table.

The superficiality with which the topic is treated corresponds with the faulty terminology and other mistakes that can be found in specialty journals, advertising pamphlets, and even material safety data sheets (MSDSs) accompanying products that contain polymers. Thus, for the liquid part of a recently launched glass ionomer, Fuji Ortho LC, no information is given about the exposure limits of 2-hydroxyethyl methacrylate, 2, 2, 4 trimethyl hexamethylene dicarbonate, and triethylene glycol dimethacrylate, and no toxicity data are provided for the last two monomers. All ingredients are listed as having no mutagenic, teratogenic, or carcinogenic activity. In addition, no reproductive toxins or sensitization effects are given, in sharp contrast with what will be shown below.

One reason for the superficial treatment of polymers in advertising and even in the orthodontic literature is the fact that many of them have a long history of use, and the minor differences between the products to which they are added are hidden under various brand names. Indeed, the basic recipe for most

Table 8-1 Characteristics of plastics used in orthodontics

Material	Symbol (DIN)	Structures*	Uses
Epoxide	EP	$[CHR\text{-}CH_2\text{-}O]_n$	Water nonresistant adhesives
Polyamide	PA	$[NH\text{-}R\text{-}NH\text{-}\overset{O}{C}\text{-}R'\text{-}\overset{O}{C}]_n$	Nylon-coated wires, appliances
Polycarbonate	PC	$[O\text{-}\bigcirc\text{-}\overset{CH_3}{\underset{CH_3}{C}}\text{-}\bigcirc\text{-}\overset{O}{C}]_n$	Brackets, tools, retractors
High-density polyethylene	PE-HD	$[CH_2\text{-}CH_2]_n$	Bondable retainers, splints
Low-density polyethylene	PE-LD	$[CH_2\text{-}CH_2]_{n+}$	Matrices for models
Polymethyl methacrylate	PMMA	$[\overset{CH_3}{\underset{OC\text{-}O\text{-}CH_3}{C\text{-}CH_2}}]_n$	Appliances, plates, liners
Polypropylene	PP	$[\underset{CH_3}{CH\text{-}CH_2}]_n$	Lip bumpers, pads, shields
Polystyrene	PS	$[\underset{\bigcirc}{CH\text{-}CH_2}]_n$	Impression trays, tongue-away shields, toothbrushes
Polytetrafluoroethylene	PTFE	$[CF_2\text{-}CF_2]_n$	Nonadherent coatings
Polyurethane	PUR	$[O\text{-}R\text{-}O\text{-}\overset{O}{C}\text{-}NH\text{-}R'\text{-}NH\text{-}\overset{O}{C}]_n$	Lip expanders, mouth pieces, oral screens, brace guards, elastics
Polyvinylchloride	PVC	$[\underset{Cl}{CH\text{-}CH_2}]_n$	Morgan bumpers, tubing, soft coatings, maxillofacial appliances
Acrylonitrile butadiene styrene	ABS	Copolymer	Containers
Ethylene vinylacetate	EVA	Copolymer	Maxillofacial appliances
Synthetic isoprene rubber	IR	$[\underset{H}{}=\overset{CH_3}{}]_n$	Elastics
Natural rubber	NR	$[\underset{H}{}=\underset{CH_3}{}]_n$	Elastics
Silicone rubber	Q	$[\overset{R}{\underset{R'}{Si}}\text{-}O]_n$	Impression materials
Silicone	SI	$[\overset{R}{\underset{R'}{Si}}\text{-}O]_n$	E-chains

*Red arrows show the bonds in the polymer that are prone to break, leading to unwanted and potentially harmful byproducts.

adhesives, sealants, restoratives, and veneers used today is quite old; zinc cements, for example, have been known and used for more than 100 years, Bowen's resin has been based on Bis-GMA for almost half a century, and Wilson and Kent's glass ionomers have been around for 30 years. Because all relevant patent rights have long since expired (the life span of a patent is 20 years), anyone can manufacture and sell these products.

Manufacturers may be reluctant to give details about the composition or processing of a polymer out of concern that it would increase chances that they might be sued for health impairment. Indeed, as will be shown below, many can be harmful. According to Greenpeace International, a nongovernmental organization that monitors the environment for potential damage to human health,[5] most are lacking in data. The Greenpeace organization asserts that as of 1981 there were some 100,000 chemicals registered in the European Inventory of Existing Commercial Chemical Substances (EINECS), and little is known about the toxicity of about 75% of these. Every year variations of these products that may contain inadequately checked chemicals are launched through the support of manufacturers' lobbies against the environmentalists, between whom governments often serve as referees.

In the US in the mid-1990s, dentistry was added to the enforcement of Proposition 65, the Safe Drinking Water and Toxic Act of 1986. In California, 80 dental offices were served with 60-day notices for failing to post Proposition 65 warnings, and the California Dental Association was inundated with inquiries about what the dental offices should do to abide by the requirements.[6] In formulating materials for medical applications, the compounder should start with ingredients that are considered safe for such uses. In the US, this may mean selecting only those ingredients listed as safe for food contact in Title 21 of the Code of Federal Regulations (21 CFR) promulgated by the FDA. Compounds for medical devices involving bodily contact must also be biocompatible to prevent adverse bodily reactions. Typically, this means exhibiting no cytotoxicity in cell culture tests of conformance to the protocols of US Pharmacopoeia (USP) Class VI. In addition, the following tests are required: Ames for mutagenicity, carcinogenicity, mucus membrane irritation (hamster's pouch), and sensitization on guinea pigs. All of these tests require large funds, and the risk-takers are few: It is far easier to modify the formula a little, change the packaging, and improve or extend the advertising than to conduct research tailored to the specific needs of orthodontics.

Plastics Can Be Harmful

Are the polymers and related plastics used in orthodontics so harmless as to deserve such light and superficial treatment? Are they maintaining their initial mechanical strength and physical properties throughout treatment? The answer is a resounding no. According to the FDA's Products Classification, the dental polymers, including resin-based adhesives and restoratives (resin or glass-ionomer type), are Class II: Class I products require less control, Class III maximum control. Dental sealants, polyacrylamide and carboxy- and polyvinyl-ether maleic anhydride adhesives, however, are considered Class III, the same category as artificial hearts. ISO Standards, which also comprise three categories, consider most adhesives Class IIa and the polymers destined for implants Class IIb, in the same category as cardiac monitors.

In light of the FDA's guidelines for industry related to dental composites,[7] which requires that dental composites (in addition to being nonmutagenic, noncytotoxic, and noncarcinogenic) "should not produce adverse reproductive and developmental effects," one may be amazed to learn the products currently used. Indeed, the FDA's classification (Dental Cements and Dental Composites, ADA/ANSI #66, ISO 7489) indicates that while these devices deserve moderate control, they should not, either directly or through the release of their material constituents, (1) produce significant adverse local or systemic effects; (2) be carcinogenic; or (3) produce adverse reproductive and developmental effects. Therefore, evaluation of any new device intended for human use requires data from systematic testing to ensure that the benefits provided by the final product will exceed any potential risks produced by dental cement materials. The ISO standard (ISO-109993, Part 1) uses an approach to test selection that is very similar to Tripartite Guidance used by the FDA in the past. It also uses a tabular format (matrix) for laying out the test requirements based

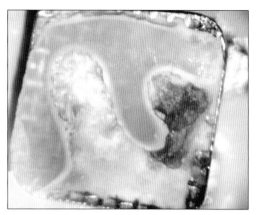

Fig 8-1 Orthodontic adhesive consumed by aerobic microbes.

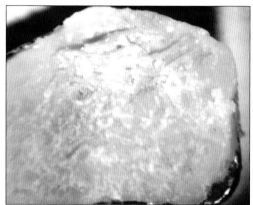

Fig 8-2 Orthodontic adhesive attacked by anaerobic microbes.

on the various factors discussed above. The matrix consists of two tables: Initial Evaluation Tests for Consideration and Supplementary Evaluation Tests for Consideration. To harmonize biologic response testing with the requirements of other countries, the FDA has recognized the ISO standard.[8,9]

The reasons for polymer control are many. First, freshly made polymers release ingredients that are harmful. Thus, monomers almost never fully polymerize, and consequently the unreacted component and some of their various ingredients (which should be entrapped and kept in the macromolecule) are allowed to leach out. The degree of conversion into the final, presumably insoluble, polymer is currently measured with the help of the residual unsaturation (unreacted double bonds) and amounts to up to 45%, with an equivalent degree of conversion of up to 15%.[10] While it is true that the monomers used today are polyunsaturated, that only one of the double bonds participating in the final macromolecule is sufficient, it is also true that some monomers remain either un-polymerized or have too high a content of oligomers (polymers of low molecular weight and bearing a short chain) that are readily soluble. While the maximum accepted weight loss of a restorative material (which, astonishingly, may contain up to 80% insoluble filler) has been recommended to be under 5 µg/mm^3 (ISO Standard 4048), amounts of 9 µg/mm^3 have been reported.[11] The elution occurs quite fast: 50% of the leachable species from a dental polymer is found after 3 hours in water, and 75% after mixture with ethanol. The leaching from various dental composites and its effects, which have been exposed over the years, confirm at least a cytotoxic effect.[11–23] In addition to the studies directed at the dental polymers, there are journals and books dedicated entirely to the general problem of polymer degradation.[23,24]

Another reason for concern is the effects of polymer biodegradation. Through exposure to light, air, warm temperatures, and moisture, polymers suffer mechanical and chemical transformations. Enzymes attack polymers to a degree that varies by product[25]; as a result, plaque accumulates,[26] and both aerobic and anaerobic microbes consume them (Figs 8-1 and 8-2). These microbes attack not only the polymer but also the teeth's enamel. Fortunately, this type of attack can be avoided by adding bactericides such as quaternary to the polymer ammonium salts.[27]

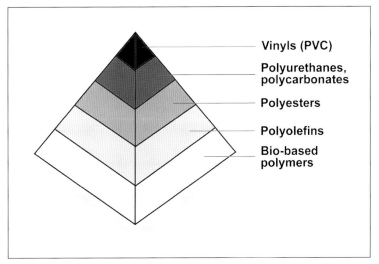

Fig 8-3 Hazardous properties of plastics according to Greenpeace International.

Polymer Toxicity

According to Greenpeace, plastics can be ranked according to their hazardous characteristics (Fig 8-3).

Polyvinyl chloride

Polyvinyl chloride (PVC), considered the most harmful type of plastic, is at the top, and the bio-based plastics, the least harmful, are at the bottom of the pyramid. This classification is based on the impact of the plastic on the environment, on general perception, and on human exposure, and can serve as a crude ranking criterion.

Polyurethanes

Polyurethanes (PUR) can be dangerous due to oligomers (low-molecular-weight polymers, unreacted monomers, and additives).[28] When subjected to hydrolysis, PUR elastomers depolymerize. The least stable type is the polyether polyurethanes.[28] Another mechanism that leads to polyurethane decay and cracking is proximity to metals, the corrosion of which could generate a metal ion–induced oxidation (MIO). Attempts to prevent this complex interaction between metal-polyurethane-body have focused on using noncorrosive metals and coating them with polymers that are less soluble and incorporating antioxidants in them.[29] When proper caution is taken, polyurethanes can be successfully used in critical FDA Class III devices, such as the self-contained AbioCor heart (Abiomed, Danvers, MA). Polyurethane elastomers have been proven to be cytotoxic in at least one study.[30]

The toxic acrylic and methacrylic derivative of polyurethanes, sometimes used as alternatives to Bis-GMA polymers (see below), have undergone less scrutiny and exhibit poorer performances with regard to leaching concerns.[31] Their aliphatic structure should, however, place them in the less-controlled polyesters category, as shown by their comparative testing in suppressing macrophage activity.[32]

Polycarbonates

Although polycarbonates are polyesters and theoretically derive from the inoffensive carbonic acid, they are considered much more potentially harmful than

119

their composition would suggest. The reason is that they are also derivatives of bisphenol A (BPA), into which they are converted during hydrolysis. Also in the same category are other polyesters that release BPA, such as bisphenol A dimethacrylate (BAD) and bisphenol A diglycidyl dimethacrylate (Bis-GMA), etc. However, in deference to Greenpeace's classification, the latter will be discussed under the polyesters category.

Known chemically as 4,4'-isopropylidenediphenol, BPA is currently used in the manufacture of resins and fungicides. Recognized for over 70 years as an estrogenic,[33–35] its derivative use in health-related fields is controversial. Allegations have been made that it triggers premature puberty in young girls (and possibly cancer) and influences male fertility as a result of its structural analogy to estrogen. True or not, Japan's environmental agency has not allowed the manufacture of polycarbonate bottles, citing fears of BPA contamination. In defense of BPA, a special web site has been launched (www.bisphenol-a.org) by the Bisphenol A Global Industry Group of the American Plastics Council; the Association of Plastics Manufacturers in Europe; and the Japan Chemical Industry Association. Many baby bottle processors, however, have switched from polycarbonates to polyether-sulfones (PS). In the US, a study performed at the request of the American Dental Association (ADA) examined some 30 blood samples from dentists who had sealants put on their teeth; no BPA was found.[36] In another study,[37] only 1 of 12 brands of dental sealants accepted by the ADA leached a trace amount of BPA (5 parts per billion); since then, its manufacturer has changed the formula. Devices made of polystyrene or acrylonitrile-butadiene-styrene (ABS) copolymers have little exposure to human tissues and therefore do not raise much concern.

Aliphatic polyesters

Aliphatic polyacrylates and methacrylates, particularly PMMA, have a relatively low toxicity when compared to the aromatic polyesters and especially to those releasing BPA. While the amount of methyl methacrylate released by a PMMA composite denture plate has been determined to be as high as 0.18% from the polymer, its presumable effect is to act only as an allergen.[38] Added often to Bis-GMA to render it more

fluid, triethyleneglycol dimethacrylate (TEDGMA) has been found to leak the most.[39]

The polymers of TEGDMA and 2-hydroxyethyl methacrylate (HEMA) have been shown to be more toxic than some mercury compounds to lung cells.[40] Extracts from some composites containing high amounts of TEGDMA and HEMA were found to be extremely cytotoxic,[41] generating adverse systemic effects in patients. Both monomers are known to produce allergies in dental assistants and dentists.[17]

Because it is water soluble, HEMA may cause more problems than the other monomers. It disturbs the human dental pulp cycle,[42] suppresses the mitochondrial activity of macrophages,[33] and can generate inflammatory reactions within the connective tissues.[43]

Aromatic polyesters

As noted above, the derivatives of BPA are discussed in this less-controlled category in deference to Greenpeace's classification system and because the amount of basic monomer (eg, Bis-GMA) is relatively small (high cross-linking, low solubility).[32] According to the Dental Investigation Service of the US Air Forces,[44] each of the following products contains Bis-GMA: AEliteflo (Bisco Dental), Fl Restore (Den-Mat), Flow-It (Jeneric-Pentron), Revolution (E&D Dental), UltraSeal XT Plus (Ultradent), Star Flow (Danville Engineering), VersaFlo (Centrix), and Tetric Flow (Ivoclar). Since few other flowable resins are used to make dental products, there is a high probability that most of these materials contain Bis-GMA.

The aromatic components in the early resins were found to be mutagenic.[45,46] Up to 14% of the total mass of the direct-bonding adhesive can leach out, and the discharge may continue for up to 2 years.[47,48] In addition, the monomers and oligomers released by the resins were found to be cytotoxic.[49,50] It is reasonable to deduce that the leaching decreases in the following order, in proportion to the content in the inert filler: sealants>liquid-solid>liquid-paste>paste-paste systems. The cured adhesive is significantly less toxic since it may have up to 80% inert filler. Completely polymerized resins are also described to be insoluble.[51]

Shrinking less and exhibiting a lower solubility in water, polyesters containing benzenic cycles should, however, be controlled as much as the polycarbonates. Indeed, the category comprises most of the polyacrylates and the polymethacrylates used in adhesives. Tests comparing several heat-, cold-, and light-cured acrylic materials under the ISO Standard 10993-5 have shown all of them to be cytotoxic; only the prosthetic acrylic (heat-cured) could be graded nontoxic.[52] While the cytotoxicity response of acrylic-based restorative materials cured chemically and with light may not be the same at all time periods, it equalizes after a 24-hour exposure.[53] The higher cytotoxicity exhibited by the oxygen-inhibiting layer that forms above the polymer clearly demonstrates a major contribution by the unpolymerized monomers and related oligomers. Interestingly, the Bis-GMA–based composites were found to release less basic, aromatic monomer than other ingredients.[32]

In animals, a study performed on a classic estrogen target tissue, rat vaginae, showed a response in some of the animals tested.[54] Further studies confirmed that Bis-GMA is indeed weakly estrogenic in mice[37] and that BPA influences the growth of the rats' mammary glands.[55] Answering such criticisms, a Spanish team supported with in vitro research the results obtained in vivo,[56] while trying to determine the relationship of the structure of BPA to estrogenicity.[57] The controversy is far from over. Although some studies have concluded that dental resins in general do not represent a significant source of BPA or BAD exposure[58] and that even if a weak estrogenic effect is not impossible, the effects are small and the risk assumable,[59] the clinician should not become complacent since newer studies are likely to dispute these findings.

Indeed, the potential harm produced by the resins commonly used in orthodontics seems to have far-reaching effects. While the layer of low-molecular-weight polymers (oligomers), known as the oxygen-inhibiting layer (OIL), is considered the most cytotoxic and the most active,[60] this effect was found to be significant even 2 years after the initial polymerization.[49] No-mix materials as well as sealants exhibit greater toxicity both immediately after mixing and 30 days after mixing.[50]

Glass-ionomer and phosphate cements have been found to exhibit effects similar to those of the composites, except that they are less cytotoxic than the carboxylate cements that contain polyacrylic acid.[11]

The cytotoxic effect of resin-modified glass-ionomer cements, which contain two types of acrylates (Bis-GMA and TEGDMA) in the resin (hydrophobic part) and an oligomer of acrylic acid (in the aqueous part), has been attributed not only to the unpolymerized monomers but also to the heavy metals contained in the glass.[61] As newer formulations are used, findings about the toxicity of their ingredients are expected. Thus, recently 4-methacryloxyethyl trimellitate anhydride (4-META), an aromatic monomer, has started to be used in the composite formulation, although until recently it was only an additive.[62] It was claimed not only to suppress the mitochondrial activity of macrophages, but also to have a residual effect.[33]

An important health-related issue is the polymers' extraction in view of removing harmful components. While some researchers claim that the restorative materials' elution with water for 3 days[52] or merely by boiling[63] shows a significant reduction in toxicity, another study has shown that sufficient components are released to kill or alter cellular functions even after 2 weeks of exposure in artificial saliva.[19] While lengthy rinsing with an alcohol solution also alleviates the problem,[32] the clinician should always provide the maximum degree of polymerization attainable regardless of the cost of longer chair time. To paraphrase J. Perkins,[64] "speed is a militant force against not only sterilization, but also proper cure."

Polyethylene, polypropylene

Polyolefins such as polyethylene (PE) and polypropylene (PP) and in particular ultra-high-molecular-weight polyethylene (UHMWPE) are used as fibers in splints: silane-treated reinforcements did not show health problems after 18 months.[65]

Bio-based polymers

This last, less-controlled category may cause more problems than some of the preceding ones since it comprises, along with the polymers made by fermenting sugars from corn or starch, those made of natural rubber. The first is used for onplants and implants, and the second is found in the ubiquitous gloves. While the dearth of information about corn- and starch-based polymers leads to the assumption that their use is safe, complaints regarding latex products abound. Named for its source, the milk of *Hevea brasiliensis* (latex, from Latin for milk), this polymer causes problems ranging from urticaria to asthma, and from allergic eczemas to anaphylaxis due not only to its constitution but also to its additives (discussed below). More than 19% of the dental personnel examined in a study showed some positive history of hand dermatitis.[66] If the latex gloves become contaminated with orthodontic adhesives, the combined toxic effect on cultured cells exceeds that of the washed gloves alone.[67] Between 1988 and 1992, more than 1,000 reports of allergic reactions to latex-containing products were received by the FDA, including 15 deaths; as a result, the National Institute for Occupational Safety and Health published an alert in June 1997 recommending the use of nonlatex gloves.[68] Interestingly, latex gloves have been found to have better barrier properties than the vinyl (PVC) used as a substitute.[69]

Cytotoxicity studies of plain and colored elastics and rubber bands have shown that all are cytotoxic.[70] The allergen responsible for such reactions has been identified as a protein, profilin, that exists in both fruits and pollen. People allergic to these have a higher risk of developing latex allergy.[71]

Toxicity of Additives

Greenpeace did not limit its campaign to the actual plastics, but included the solvents used in their manufacture (eg, methylene chloride for polycarbonates) and their raw materials (eg, isocyanates for polyurethanes). In some instances, plastics were condemned not for the polymers but for the additives they contain. Indeed, when referring to the various plastics, usually only the polymers are mentioned, and little information is given concerning the chemistries and additives that enable these products to be as useful as they are. Additives comprise plasticizers, impact modifiers, heat stabilizers, lubricants, biocides, antioxidants, antiblocking agents, slip agents, light stabilizers, clarifying agents, flame retardants, organic initiators, and blowing and coupling agents.

Many of these additives can leach into the human body, and even the fillers can leach from cross-linked composites.[72] Immersed in water or synthetic saliva, composites leach, in addition to monomers, additives such as ultraviolet stabilizers (TInuvin P), plasticizers (dicyclohexyl phthalate and bis [2-ethylhexyl] phthalate), initiators (triphenyl stibine), coupling agents (gamma-methacryloxypropyl trimethoxysilane), and phenyl benzoate. Interestingly, the chief polymerizing monomer, Bis-GMA, was not found.[32] While most composite additives are cytotoxic, including the inhibitor butylated hydroxytoluene (BHT) and the photo-stabilizer 2-hydroxy-4-methoxy benzophenone (HMBP), little effort is spent in seeking a replacement with less harmful additives.[18] Benzoyl peroxide (BPO) and hydroquinone have also been found to be allergenic.[73]

Additives and their decomposition products are usually more toxic than the polymers to which they are added. In orthodontics, however, with few exceptions, their amount is significantly smaller and therefore often overlooked. In one notable exception, that of plastisols (softened PVCs), plasticizers can often reach over half of the total weight and deserve special attention. Table 8-2 shows some additives used in various plastics and their LD_{50} values (lethal dose for a 50% kill, given in mg/kg for the oral dose in the rat). In several instances, no data were found for special additives; products having a similar structure were used instead.[74]

Plasticizers

Without plasticizers or softeners, PVC is hard and brittle, and so are PMMA plates, dentures, and linings. The best and most commonly used plasticizers are the phthalates, aromatic esters suspected to mimic hormones.[16,32,75–79]

In high dosages, dibutyl phthalate (DBP) acts as a testicular toxicant in three species of young adult laboratory animals, while adult females' functional reproductive toxicity (ie, decreased fertility) has been evidenced in rats.[80] Such substances can affect the hormonal system of an organism in a wide variety of ways, blocking a hormone's action and accelerating

Table 8-2 Additives used in various plastics and their LD$_{50}$ values

Additive	Use	Toxicity*
Benzoyl peroxide	Initiator (Polyesters, PUR)	7,710 mg/kg, poison, questionable carcinogen
Butylated hydroxyanisole	Inhibitor (Polyesters)	29 mg/kg, poison
Dibutyl-bis(lauroyloxy) stannate	Initiator, PUR	175 mg/kg, poison, strong irritant
Mercaptobenzoic acid	Accelerator, rubber latex	50 mg/kg, poison
Na-Diethyl dithiocarbamate	Accelerator, rubber latex	1,500 mg/kg, toxic, questionable carcinogen
1-Naphthol	Colorant base	134 mg/kg, poison
NN-Diethylaniline	Curing agent, kicker (Polyesters)	782 mg/kg, toxic
NN-Dimethylaniline	Curing agent, kicker (Polyesters)	1,410 mg/kg, poison, nervous depressant
Octyl-isothiazoline	Antimicrobial (PUR, PVC)	550 mg/kg, toxic, irritant
Phenols, base	Curing agents, inhibitors	300 mg/kg, poisons, teratogens
Phenyl hydroxylamine	Antioxidant (Polyesters, PVC, PC, PE)	100 mg/kg, poison
Phenyl-naphthylamine	Antioxidant (Polyesters, PVC, PC, PE)	1,625 mg/kg, toxic, questionable carcinogen
Stannous 2-ethylhexanoate	Initiator, PUR	90.7 mg/kg, poison
Tetramethyl thiourea	Accelerator, rubber latex	920 mg/kg, toxic, questionable carcinogen
Tetramethyl-ethylene diamine	Curing agent (Polyesters, epoxy, PUR)	1,580 mg/kg, toxic
Thio-bis (butyl, cresol)	Antioxidant (Polyesters, PVC, PC, PE)	6,540 mg/kg, toxic
Triphenyl tin	Initiator, PUR	491 mg/kg, poison
Triphenyl phosphite	Antioxidant (Polyesters, PVC, PC, PE)	1,600 mg/kg, toxic, skin irritant
Zinc pyridine-thiol-oxide	Antimicrobial (PUR, PVC)	177 mg/kg, poison

*LD$_{50}$ values: lethal dose for a 50% kill in the rat.

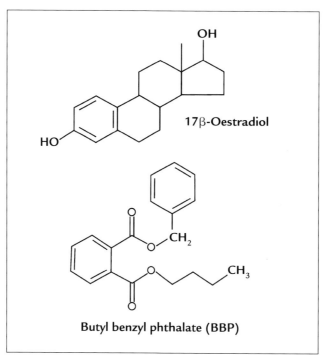

Fig 8-4 Similarity in structure between estrogens and phthalates.

its breakdown, eventually causing cancer and death. The relative similarity in structure between estrogens and phthalates is shown in Fig 8-4.

Publication of the book *Our Stolen Future* in 1996,[81] with a foreword written by then-Vice President Al Gore, stirred emotions as well as controversies. The book fueled a campaign against plastics that had long been sustained by organizations such as Greenpeace, Chemical Impact Project, the World Wildlife Fund, World Resources Institute, and Friends of the Earth. Among its successes is the fact that in all of the construction related to the 2000 Olympic games in Sydney, no PVC was used.

The controversy continues despite assurances from the American Plastics Council that intermediate products, such as BPA, and plastic additives, such as the phthalates (and especially di [2-ethylhexyl] phthalate [DEHP]) have been used without problems for over 40 years. The use of the latter has received an endorsement from former US Surgeon General Dr C. Everett

Koop[82] and the American Council on Science and Health panel, which concluded that "DEHP and DINP (phthalate esters) are not genotoxic" and that the current human exposure levels in products containing them are "not harmful." It was pointed out that "there is a critical difference between the toxicology and mechanisms for these chemicals between rodents and humans." According to the FDA, DEHP can be used only as a flow promoter at a level not to exceed 2 w/w based on the monomers.[83]

Curing agents

For polymerization of the monomers to occur as desired, a variety of ingredients must be added. In some cases (eg, condensations), no curing agents are needed because the macromolecule results from an interaction of the ingredients (eg, between an isocyanate and a compound-bearing hydroxyl group for polyurethanes, or the opening of an oxyrane group–containing compound when reacting to an amine for epoxies). In some industrial uses, amines and their derivatives also work as curing agents (ie, additives), despite the large amount used.

To polymerize in the absence of light acrylic monomers, peroxides (initiators) are commonly used with or without tertiary aromatic amines (kickers). In cases where the process is light-activated, the additive is a benzoin alkyl ether or a quinone. Also used are some metallo-organic compounds, recently forbidden for use in coatings on boats for being too toxic.[84]

Aromatic amines (peroxide decomposition accelerators) have been shown to be carcinogenic as well as toxic.[85] The lethal doses for some representative aromatic amines are shown in Table 8-2.

Cross-linking agents

Because natural rubber is too weak to be used in the manufacture of many products, including gloves, a series of cross-linking agents delivering sulfur must be added, as per Goodyear's vulcanization. Among these are compounds such as 2-mercaptobenzthiazole, dithiocarbamates, tetramethyl thiuram disulfide, and sulfenamide. The lethal doses for some representative cross-linking agents are shown in Table 8-2.

Inhibitors

To prevent monomers from setting prematurely, compounds that neutralize the free radicals that are accidentally generated must be added. Among these are various phenols or their derivatives, such as hydroquinone and butylated hydroxy toluene (BHT). The lethal doses for phenols are shown in Table 8-2.

Antioxidants

If exposed to air in moist and warm conditions, polymers such as acrylics, PVC, PC, and PE are subjected to an oxygen attack that lowers their physical properties. Such generated hydroperoxides are compounds that decompose under the influence of metals, lead-

ing to a premature setting. To protect the polymer against this type of decay, an array of phenols as well as organic phosphites and sulfur-containing compounds must be added. The lethal doses for some representative antioxidants are shown in Table 8-2.

Ultraviolet light stabilizers

To prevent decay due to light, amines, or organometallic or sulfur-containing compounds, benzophenones, or benzotriazole derivatives (Tinuvin P) must be added.

Coloring agents

Subsequent to the banning of toxic cadmium derivatives, organic pigments such as various azo-compounds and the derivatives of naphthol, quinacridone and anthraquinone are now the main additives used to provide the various shades desired by patients. Since some are also used in food, modern coloring agents are of less concern than other types of additives.

Biocides

In addition to the additives needed to provide adequate mechanical properties, medical biocides with antimicrobial agents are added to protect plastics when exposed to dark, moist, and warmer conditions. After consuming the plasticizers, various microbes, fungi, and algae produce enzymes and byproducts that cause the plastic to become brittle, lose tensile strength, smell, and even become toxic. While industrial antimicrobials may contain arsenic or sulfur compounds, medical grades contain ammonium quaternary salts and microcapsules capable of freeing silver ions. Whereas in nonmedical applications additives must be noncarcinogenic, nonallergenic, and have very low or no toxicity in recommended concentrations, in medical applications additives also must be nonmutagenic, ie, they must hinder bacteria from easily developing resistance to them and thus becoming a greater health threat.[86]

125

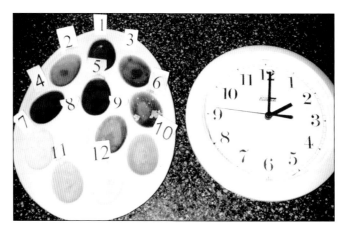

Fig 8-5 Change in color after 30 minutes of a potassium permanganate solution in contact with various plastics.

Testing Plastic's Leachability

Testing of the undesirable materials released in water from various sources has been the object of both the ISO[87] and the FDA,[83] and testing of the materials released by solvents has been conducted by the American Society for Testing and Materials (ASTM).[88] The chemical oxygen demand (COD) indicates the quantity of oxygen required for the chemical oxidation of organic matters present in water. The value measured provides a quantitative estimate of everything that can be oxidized, ie, most of the organic compounds and some oxidizable mineral salts. A related test, the Permanganate Index (value) is an international method used to monitor the water pollution caused by oxidizing organic and inorganic matters.

While all of these methods use either spectrophotometer measurements or advanced analytical chemical skills, the obvious change in color of the potassium permanganate occurring in the process allows the evaluation of the amount of leachate. Based on this commonly used disinfectant, a do-it-yourself method has been developed by Ortho-Cycle Co (Hollywood, FL).[89] Although only an approximation and not specific to toxic substances, this method allows a quick visual evaluation of the organic materials leaching from various plastics used in the mouth. As shown in Fig 8-5, a marked color variation of a solution of permanganate from purple (control) to clear (increased leaching) takes place in direct rapport with the amount and nature of the leachate. In the process, the permanganate has been reduced from Mn^{VII} to the practically colorless Mn^{II} salts resulting from the reduction of the permanganate in contact with the leached materials.

Conclusions

The potential health risks of many plastics and polymers used in orthodontics have been under scrutiny for over 40 years, and its workhorse, Bowen's resins or Bis-GMA, for almost half a century. A comparison of the adult exposure to some of the Bis-GMA degradation products, such as formaldehyde and methacrylic acid, and the average level of exposure to these chemicals yields the results that the formaldehyde is 1/10,000 times and the methacrylic acid is 1/1,600,000 times, respectively, lower than the admissible level.[90]

Summing up the situation, Dr Gordon J. Christensen, founder and director of Clinical Research Associates and a respected clinician who has a strong interest in dental biomaterials, takes the same position as the FDA: "We must weigh the known benefits against the alleged risk" (1998 Chicago Dental Society meeting).

This is no excuse for paying less attention to the possible nociceptive effects of the polymers: *un homme averti en vaut deux* (a warned man is worth two). New products should be launched only after undergoing thorough investigation, and manufacturers should provide as much information about their products as is feasible. When one considers the large number and variety of products that are launched, the limitations of the various governmental agencies treating those used in orthodontics is obvious. While polymers in general present a relatively low risk, the clinician should feel responsible for the iatrogenic effects they may induce and should be willing to go an extra mile by using do-it-yourself methods to test them, if necessary.

Continual awareness of the risk incurred should lead manufacturers to strive to replace the older, more harmful products with new ones that are less harmful, even if this requires them to incur additional expenses. The public should appreciate such efforts while not succumbing to hysterias such as those caused by the use of amalgam.

References

1. Defosse M. Growth is steady. Modern Plastics 2001;78:34–35.
2. National Research Council. Polymer Science and Engineering. Washington DC: National Academy, 1994.
3. Silver FH. Biomaterials, medical devices and tissue engineering: An integrated approach. London: Chapman & Hall, 1993.
4. Glasgold AI, Silver FH. Applications of Biomaterials in Facial Plastic Surgery. Boca Raton, FL: CRC, 1991.
5. Http://www.greenpeace.org.
6. Pichay TJ, Seifert LI. Proposition 65 in the dental office. Calif Dent Assoc 2001;29:501–506.
7. Center for Devices and Radiological Health. Guidance for Industry and FDA Staff: Dental composites—Premarket notification. November 27, 1998. http://www.fda.gov/cdrh/ode/642.pdf.
8. American National Standards Institute/American Dental Association. Document No. 41 for Recommended Standard Practices for Biological Evaluation of Dental Materials. Washington DC, 1982.
9. ISO/TR, 1984(E), Biological Evaluation of Dental Materials, Geneva, Switzerland, 1984.
10. Brantley WA, Eliades T, eds. Orthodontic Materials: Scientific and Clinical Aspects. Stuttgart, NY: Thieme, 2001.
11. Schedle A, Franz A. Cytotoxic effect of dental composites. Dent Mater 1998;14:429–440.
12. Oyesaed H, Ruyter IE, Sjovic KI. Release of formaldehyde from dental composites. J Dent Res 1998;67:1289–1294.
13. Koch MJ, Alves M, Stein G. Formaldehyde release from sealant materials [abstract no. 1533]. J Dent Res 1994;73 (Spec issue):293.
14. Ruyter IE, Sjovik, KI. Formaldehyde release from light-cured glass ionomer restorative materials [abstract no. 1534]. J Dent Res 1994;73(Spec issue):293.
15. Larsson KS. Potential teratogenic and carcinogenic effects of dental materials. Int Dent J 1991;41:206–211.
16. Lygre H, Hol PH, Solheim E. Organic leachables from polymer-based dental filling materials. Eur J Oral Sci 1999;107:378–383.
17. Geurtsen W. Biocompatibility of resin-modified filling materials. Rev Oral Biol Med 2000;11:333–355.
18. Geurtsen W, Lehmann F, Spahl W. Cytotoxicity of 35 dental resin composite monomers/additives in permanent 3T3 and three human fibroblast cultures. J Biomed Mater Res 1998;41:474–480.
19. Wataha JC, Rueggeberg FA, Lapp CA. In vitro toxicity of resin-containing restorative materials after aging in artificial saliva. Clin Oral Invest 1999;3:144–149.
20. Leyhausen G, Lehmann F, Geurtsen W. Cytocompatibility of 38 composite monomers/additives in human oral primary cell cultures [abstract no.3985]. J Dent Res 1997; 76(Spec issue):382.
21. Sletten GBG, Dahl JE. Cytotoxic effects of extracts of compomers. Acta Odontol Scand 1999;57:316–322.
22. Costa CAS, Teixera HM, Nascimento ABL. Biocompatibility of two current adhesive resins. J Endo 2000;23:512–516.
23. Polymer Degradation and Stability [journal]. The Hague, Netherlands: Elsevier Science.
24. Hamid HS. Handbook of Polymer Degradation. New York: Dekker, 2000.
25. Santerre JP, Shajii L, Tsang H. Biodegradation of commercial dental composites by cholesterol esterase. J Dent Res 1999;78:1459–1468.
26. Sukontapatipark W, El-Agroudi M, Selliseth NJ, Thunold K, Selvig KA. Bacterial colonization associated with fixed orthodontic appliances. A scanning electron microscopy study. Eur J Orthod 2001;23:475–484.
27. Matasa CG. Microbial attack of orthodontic adhesives. Am J Orthod Dentofacial Orthop 1995;108:132–134.
28. Toxicity and Safe Handling of Diisocyanates and Ancillary Chemicals. A Code of Practice for Polyurethane Flexible Foam and Elastomer Manufacture. 2nd ed. Shrewsbury: Rapra Technology Ltd, 2000.
29. Lelah MD, Cooper SL. Polyurethanes in Medicine. Boca Raton, FL: CRC, 1986.
30. Matasa CG. Are all cytotoxic materials a real danger for the patient? J Orthop Orthod Pediatr 196;3:25–34.
31. Lee SY, Huang HM, Lin CY, Shih YH. Leached components from dental composites in oral simulating fluids and the resultant composite strengths. J Oral Rehabil 1998; 25:575–588.
32. Rakich DR, Wataha JC, Lefebvre CA, Weller RN. Effects of dentin-bonding agents on macrophage mitochondrial activity. J Endod 1998;24:528–533.

33. Allan H, Dickens F, Dodds EC. Observations on the standardization of the water-soluble, oestrus-producing hormone. J Physiol 1930;68:348–363.

34. Dodds EC, Lawson W. Synthetic estrogenic agents without the phenantrene nucleus. Nature 1936;137:996.

35. Solmssen UV. Synthetic estrogens and the relation between their structure and their activity. Chem Rev 1945;137:481–589.

36. Nathanson D, Lertpitayakun P, Lamkin MS, Mahnaz EB, Lee-Chou L. In vitro elution of leachable components from dental sealants. J Am Dent Assoc 1997;128:1517–1523.

37. Soderholm KJ, Mariotti A. Bis-GMA–based resins in dentistry: Are they safe? J Am Dent Assoc 1999;130:201–208.

38. Lassila LV, Vallittu PK. Denturebase polymer Alldent Sinomer: Mechanical properties, water sorption and release of residual components. J Oral Rehabil 2001;28:607–613.

39. Geurtsen W. Substances released from dental resin composites and glass ionomer cements. Eur J Oral Sci 1998;106:687–689.

40. Kehe K, Reichl FX, Durner J. Cytotoxicity of dental composite components and mercury compounds in pulmonary cells. Biomaterials 2001;22:317–320.

41. Geurtsen W, Spahl W, Muller K, Leyhausen G. Aqueous extracts from dentin adhesives contain cytotoxic chemicals. J Biomed Mater Res 1999;48:772–777.

42. Lin N, Miao X, Takugavwa M, Sato K, Sato A. Effect of dental materials HEMA monomer on human dental pulp cells. Biotechnol 1999;27:85–90.

43. Costa CA, Teixeira HM, Do Nascimento AD, Hebling J. Biocompatibility of an adhesive system and 2-HEMA. J Dent Child 1999;66:337–342.

44. Dental Investigation Service of the US Air Forces: www.brooks.af.mil/dis/DIS51/attach1.htm. Accessed 21 July 2003.

45. Fredericks HE. Mutagenic potential of orthodontic bonding materials. Am J Orthod Dentofacial Orthop 1981;80:316–324.

46. Cross NG, Taylor RF, Nunex LJ. "Single-step" orthodontic bonding systems: Possible mutagenic potential. Am J Orthod Dentofacial Orthop 1983;84:344–350.

47. Thompson LR, Miller EG, Bowels WH. Leaching of unpolymerized materials from orthodontic bonding resins. J Dent Res 1982;61:989–992.

48. Ferracane JL, Gordon JR. Rate of elution of leachable components from composites. Dent Mater 1990;6:282–287.

49. Tell RT, Sydiskis RJ, Isaacs RD, Davidson WM. Long-term cytotoxicity of direct-bonding adhesives. Am J Orthod Dentofacial Orthop 1988;93:419–422.

50. Terhune WF, Sydiskis RJ, Davidson WM. In vitro cytotoxicity of orthodontic bonding materials. Am J Orthod Dentofacial Orthop 1983;83:501–506.

51. Williams DF. Introduction to the toxicology of polymer-based materials. In: Williams DF (ed). Systemic Aspects of Biocompatibility. Boca Raton, FL:CRC, 1981.

52. Rose EC, Bumann J, Jonas IE, Kappett HF. Contribution to the biological assessment of orthodontic materials. J Orofacial Orthop 2000;61:246–257.

53. Ergun G, Mutlu-Sagesen L, Karaoglu T, Dogan A. Cytotoxicity of provisional crown and bridge restoration materials: An in vitro study. J Oral Sci 2001;42:123–128.

54. Long X, Steinmetz R, Ben-Jonathan N, et al. Stain differences in vaginal responses to the xenoestrogen Bisphenol A. Environ Health Perspect 2000;108:243–247.

55. Colerangle JB, Deodutta R. Profound effects of the weak environment estrogen-like chemical bisphenol A on the growth of the mammary gland of Noble rats. J Steroid Biochem Mol Biol 1997;60:153–160.

56. Olea N, Pulgar R, Olea-Serrano F, et al. Estrogenicity of resin-based composites and sealant used in dentistry. Environ Health Perspect 1996;104:298–305.

57. Pulgar R, Olea-Serrano MF, Novillo-Fertrel A, Rivas A, Pazos P, Pedraza V, et al. Determination of bisphenol A and related aromatic compounds released from Bis-GMA-based composites and sealants by high performance liquid chromatography. Environ Health Perspect 2000;108:21–27.

58. Lewis JB, Rueggeberg FA, Lapp CA, Ergle JW, Shuster GS, Identification and characterization of estrogen-like components in commercial resin-based dental restorative materials. Clin Oral Investig 1999;3:107–113.

59. Schuurs AH, Moorer WR. Hormone dysregulators. Pseudo-estrogens in dental composite resins and sealants. Ned Tijdschr Tandhelkd 2000;107:290–495.

60. Tang ATH, Liu Y, Björkman L, Ekstrand J. In vitro cytotoxicity of orthodontic bonding resins on human oral fibroblasts. Am J Orthod Dentofacial Orthop 1999;116:132–138.

61. Stanislawski L, Daniau X, Lauti A, Goldberg M. Factors responsible for pulp cell cytotoxicity induced by resin-modified glass-ionomer cements. J Biomed Mater Res 1999;48:277–288.

62. Miwa H, Miyazawa K, Goto S, Kondo T, Hasegawa A. A resin veneer for enamel protection during orthodontic treatment. Eur J Orthod 2001;23:759–767.

63. Koutis D, Freeman S. Allergic contact stomatitis caused by acrylic monomer in a denture. Australas J Dermatol 2001;42:203–211.

64. Perkins J. Principles and Methods of Sterilization in Health Sciences. Springfield, IL: Charles Thomas, 1982.

65. Karacaer O, Dogan OM, Tincer T, Dogan A. Reinforcement of maxillary dentures with silane-treated ultra high modulus polyethylene fibers. J Oral Sci 2001;43:103–107.

66. Hill JG, Grimwood RE, Hermesh CB, Marks JG Jr. Prevalence of occupationally related hand dermatitis in dental workers. J Am Dent Assoc 1998;129:212–217.

67. Afsahi SP, Sydiskis RJ, Davidson WM. Protection by latex or vinyl gloves against cytotoxicity of direct bonding adhesives. Am J Orthod Dentofacial Orthop 1988;93:47–50.

68. Muto CA, Sistrom M, Strain B. Glove leakage rates as a function of latex content and brand: Caveat emptor. Arch Surg 2000;135:982–985.

69. Rego A, Roley L. In-use barrier integrity of gloves. Am J Infect Control 1999;27:542–560.

70. Holmes J, Barker MK, Walley EK, Tuncay OC. Cytotoxicity of orthodontic elastics. Am J Orthod Dentofacial Orthop 1993;104:188–191.

71. Gangleberger E, Radauer C, Wagner S, et al. Hev b 8, the *Hevea brasiliensis* latex profiling. Intern Arch Allergy Immunol 2001;125:216–227.

72. Soderholm KJ, Yang MC, Garcea I. Filler particle leachability of experimental dental composites. Eur J Oral Sci 2000;108:555–560.

73. Kanerva L, Jokanki R, Alanko K, Estlander T. Patch-test reactions to plastics and glue allergens. Acta Derm Venereol 1999;79:296–300.

74. Lewis RJ Sr. Sax's Dangerous Properties of Industrial Materials, 8th ed. New York: Van Nostrand, 1992.

75. Jobling S, Reynolds T, White R, Parker MG, Sumpter JP. A variety of environmentally persistent chemicals, including some phthalate plasticizers, are weakly estrogenic. Environ Health Perspec 1995;103:582–587.

76. Toppari J, Larsen JC, Christiansen P, et al. Male reproductive health and environmental xenoestrogens. Environ Health Perspec 1996;104(suppl 4):741–803.

77. Kavlock RJ, Daston GP, DeRosa C, et al. Research needs for the risk assessment of health and environmental effects of endocrine disruptors: A report of the US EPA-sponsored workshop. Environ Health Perspec 1996;104(suppl 4): 714–740.

78. Albro PW, Thomas RO. Enzymatic hydrolysis of di(2-ethylhexyl) phthalate by lipases. Biochem Biophys Acta 1973;360:380–390.

79. Carpenter CP, Weil CS, Smith HFJ. Chronic oral toxicity of di(2-ethylhexyl) phthalate for rats, guinea pig, and dogs. Am Med Assoc Arch Ind Hyg Occup Med 1953;8: 219–226.

80. DBP Center for the Evaluation of Risks to Human Reproduction. Expert Panel Report on di-n butyl Phthalate. National Toxicology Program. US Dept Health and Human Services, Government Printing Office, 2000.

81. Colborn T, Dumanoski D, Myers JP. Our Stolen Future. New York: Penguin, 1996.

82. Koop E. The latest phony chemical scare. Wall Street J 22 June 1999.

83. FDA, 21CFR 177.2600, Chapter I, Sec. 177.1010:333–338.

84. Matasa CG. Biomaterials in Orthodontics. In: Graber TM, Vanarsdall RL (eds). Orthodontics: Current Principles and Techniques. St Louis: Mosby, 2000.

85. Weisenburger EK, Russfield AB, Homburger F, et al. Testing of twenty-one environmental aromatic amines or derivatives for long-term toxicity or carcinogenicity. J Environ Pathol Toxicol 1978;2:325–356.

86. Smith J. Stunting microbial growth. Mod Plas 2000; October:22.

87. Water quality: Determination of permanganate index. ISO 8467:1993.

88. American Society for Testing and Materials (ASTM). Test Method D1363–94(1997). Standard Test Method for Permanganate Time of Acetone and Methol.

89. Matasa CG. A do-it-yourself detection of leaching polymers. The Orthodontic Materials Insider 14;(2):5–7.

90. Richardson GM. An assessment of adult exposure and risks from components and degradation products of composite resin dental material. Human Ecolog Risk Assessment 1997;3/4:683–697.

Pain and Discomfort in Orthodontics

Stavros Kiliaridis and Marianne Bergius

According to the clinical literature and a number of systematic research studies, discomfort and pain during orthodontic treatment are common. It has been reported that nearly 10% of patients interrupt their orthodontic therapy due to early pain experiences.[1] In addition to the actual experience of pain, fear of pain is also a significant problem since it contributes to patients' reluctance to seek orthodontic treatment.[2] However, despite claims that it is a significant area of concern, few investigators study, report, analyze, or discuss causes, manifestations, or consequences of pain reactions in orthodontic treatment. Perhaps this is because most patients are highly motivated to undergo treatment and therefore do not report pain or ask for pain alleviation. Clinical experience shows that most patients report pain and discomfort during the first day(s) of treatment. Therefore, it may not be clearly identified by the orthodontist since recall visits and check-ups are usually carried out during a period

when the symptoms are weak or have disappeared. Even if the orthodontist does not recognize the pain, however, it still exists for the patient.

Several general dental procedures incident to orthodontic treatment may also elicit pain and/or discomfort (eg, extraction and other surgical procedures, grinding for reshaping of the form and size of the tooth, dental impressions). Furthermore, discomfort or pain may accompany some symptoms induced by allergic-immunologic reactions. However, these subjects will not be addressed in this chapter. To understand patients' pain reactions in orthodontics, this chapter will discuss general principles of pain physiology, methods to measure and evaluate pain, and the factors that influence the perception of pain. Moreover, the prevalence, manifestations, cause-related factors, and alleviation of the pain during orthodontic treatment will be addressed.

Prevalence of Pain in Orthodontics

Pain is frequently associated with dental care. Though many dentists may be unaware of their patients' pain experiences during treatment,[3] up to 77% of dental patients report some degree of pain during their visits to the dentist.[4] In a Norwegian study of 2,384 adults, 60% reported having had at least one unpleasant painful dental experience during their life, and 6% reported that dental treatment was always very painful.[5]

Orthodontic treatment does not seem to be any less painful. In a retrospective study of dental discomfort and pain among 203 adult Chinese patients in Singapore, 91% reported discomfort caused by their fixed orthodontic appliances. In 39% of these patients, discomfort was experienced during each step of the treatment, when a new archwire or elastic force was applied.[6] Prospective investigations of children and adults by Scheurer et al[7] in Switzerland and Kvam et al[8] in Norway revealed that 95% of the patients in both studies reported pain experiences during orthodontic treatment.

The main cause of the pain appears to be the application of orthodontic forces inducing tooth movement.[2,7,9,12] However, rapid palatal expansion (RPE) resulted in at least some pain in almost all of the 97 children examined (ages 5 to 13 years). The highest levels of pain were reported during the first 2 mm of expansion, especially in those expanded at a rate of 0.5 mm per day.[13] Posterior displacement of the condyle, which can be induced by chin cup therapy, may cause anterior disc displacement as well as pain. In a retrospective study, 16% of the patients responding to a questionnaire reported pain during chin cup use.[14] It was found that during correction of anterior crossbite, the posterior occlusion remained open because of an unstable mandibular position, which in turn may have caused muscular dysfunction with concomitant temporomandibular joint (TMJ) pain. Similarly, treatment with Herbst appliances has been reported as a possible factor in the occurrence of pain in the masticatory system.[15]

Soft tissue lesions and wounds caused by orthodontic appliances may be one of the factors contributing to pain. In a study of 161 patients aged 12 to 17 years, Kvam et al[8] reported that lesions caused by fixed appliances were present in 76% of the patients while severe ulcers were present among 2.5% of the patients.[8] Complaints of tongue soreness were found in 72% of the 46 adults wearing bonded lingual orthodontic appliances in both arches.[16] Another cause of pain during orthodontic treatment was an increase in the frequency of recurrent aphthous ulceration (RAU) among adolescents.[8] However, the underlying mechanisms for increased frequency of RAU and orthodontic treatment are not clear.

Definition of Pain

According to the International Association for the Study of Pain (IASP), pain is "an unpleasant sensory and emotional experience associated with actual or potential damage or described in terms of such damage."[17] The IASP stresses the importance of the psychologic aspects of the experience of pain. Thus, pain is recognized and accepted as subjective and unpleasant, not necessarily connected with a stimulus, reported even in the absence of direct tissue damage, and possibly an effect of emotional or cognitive factors. In a subjective report, it is impossible to distinguish experiences that do not have a pathophysiologic cause from those caused by actual tissue damage. This may also be the case in orthodontics when a patient suddenly complains of pain in spite of a lack of physical reason for this complaint. However, although pain is an unreliable indicator of pathology, self-reports of pain should be an important diagnostic tool in orthodontics, TMD therapy, and dentistry in general.[18]

In principle, pain serves as a "warning signal," enabling the organism to sense impending tissue damage and thus avoid harm.[19] The pain threshold is the smallest pain experience that is recognized by an individual. Similarly, the pain tolerance level is the greatest level of pain that one is prepared to tolerate. However, as with the pain threshold, the pain tolerance level is a subjective experience. Thus, neither pain threshold nor pain tolerance level is defined in terms of the external stimulation, but rather in terms of the individual's subjective report.

Gate Control Theory of Pain

An understanding of general pain physiology can help us to better understand the reactions to pain observed among dental patients and relate them to the orthodontic treatment situation. In 1965, the Gate Control Theory was proposed by Melzack and Wall[20] and provided explanations for many of the phenomena associated with the experience of pain. The neurophysiology behind this theory explains how impulses from peripheral nerves are modulated (inhibited) by a gating mechanism located in the dorsal horn of the spinal cord. Information from the periphery is received through either large- or small-diameter fibers, each of which has a different action on the spinal cells—ie, the gate mechanism. Activity in the large fibers tends to inhibit transmission (close the gate), whereas activity in the small fibers tends to facilitate transmission (open the gate). In the regions of the face and mouth, the anatomic organization is somewhat different. Impulses carried by the trigeminal nerve enter directly into the brain stem pons to synapse in the trigeminal spinal nucleus. This region of the brain stem may be considered an extension of the spinal cord dorsal horn.[21]

All impulses that enter the central nervous system (CNS) are subject to modulation as they ascend to the higher centers. This modulation enhances or diminishes nociceptive input, resulting in either an increase or a decrease in the pain experience. There are several different sites within the CNS where modulation can occur. As the impulse ascends, it passes through several interneurons, which "filter" the impulses that enter the brain stem. It has been shown that nociceptive input, in particular, increases the activity of these "filters" and can strongly excite the brain to attention.

It is important for the clinician to appreciate that pain is not a simple conduction of noxious impulses via several synapses to the cerebral cortex, where it is sensed and acted upon. What is sensed as pain may not even arise from a noxious stimulation. Normal ongoing somatosensory input that ordinarily would not be perceived at all, or at least not as a painful sensation, may be sensed as pain if the inhibitory influences are not effective. Also, the general intensity of suffering relates to the preconditioning experience, attention, attitude, and temperament of the subject.

Thus, the phenomenon of central pain modulation is an important factor in orofacial pain. It helps explain the enormous variation in the experience of pain from individual to individual.

The trigeminal corresponding mechanism parallel to the gate control may be the underlying mechanism when, on the recommendation of their orthodontists, patients chew on something hard to decrease or inhibit pain after forces have been applied to the dentition.[22] However, an alternative explanation may be that chewing possibly alleviates the constant orthodontic pressure that has been applied and temporarily restores the normal vascular and lymphatic circulation. This may prevent or relieve the acute inflammation and edema caused by orthodontic forces, as discussed below.[23]

Subjective Experience of Pain

As noted earlier, there is little or no relation between the objective strength of a pain stimulus and the response to or personal experience of pain. This is due to the complexity of the sensory reaction when it becomes an experience modulated by higher structures of the CNS. Thus, the pain experience is influenced not only by emotional and cognitive factors, but also by environmental factors including culture, gender, and age.

Among emotional factors the most obvious in dentistry concern patients' worries, fears, and anxieties. Between 3% and 21% of the child and adolescent population, depending on different populations and survey methods, have reported being fearful or anxious when visiting the dentist.[24] It is frequently stated that elevated anxiety levels are paralleled by increased pain reports.[25–27] This is mainly explained by the notion that anxiety creates an expectation of future pain created by previous pain memories.[28] Williams et al[29] studied the differences between children who had a history of refusing dental treatment in the community and control children, as rated by their parents. A history of treatment refusal was found to be associated with a general fear of "medical people," intolerance of any pain or discomfort, and greater difficulty in approaching novelty or adapting to change. These children were also rated by their parents as being generally more negative in their mood and having greater difficulty in playing with unfamiliar children. Recently, Litt,[30] in a literature review of pain and anxiety in the dental setting, argued that anxiety and pain may be indistinguishable. Anxiety, according to Litt, lowers the pain threshold and may lead to the perception of normally non-painful stimuli as painful; for example, the mere vibration of drilling on an anesthetized tooth may still be perceived as a painful stimulus.[30]

While emotional factors such as fear and anxiety are probably not as important in orthodontic treatment as in other areas of dentistry, cognitive factors probably are. It is reasonable to believe that factors such as motivation and expectations may play a particularly important role in orthodontic treatment. Such factors constitute a powerful filter that acts upon the perception, appraisal, and experience of pain. Other important cognitive aspects of pain relate to the dimension of beliefs, attention/distraction, and feeling of control, which in turn relates to factors such as receiving information, prediction, and memory.

The possibility of an individual being able to control or influence a situation has frequently been proposed to reduce the experience of both stress and pain.[30] A sense of control can be achieved not only by direct control over the dentist's actions, but also by means of information about the anticipated or ongoing treatment. Patients usually search for information to give meaning to an experience, and fear of uncontrolled pain is a primary concern for most dental patients.[31] However, the concept of providing information is not entirely clear-cut with regard to young children, where lack of abstract thinking may hamper or counteract the intended message.

In a study by Wardle,[32] it was shown that a sense of increased control by means of hand signals during dental treatment as well as pretreatment information and distraction were all effective ways to reduce both anxiety and pain experiences in an average dental patient. It was shown that, with regard to pain reduction, increased control and treatment information were equally effective as and more effective than distraction, respectively. Talking to the patient during treatment or providing background music is probably the most common distraction method used in dentistry. However, it is important to understand that distraction is most effective in reducing stress in mild but not in intense pain situations.[33]

Cultural differences in reaction to pain also reflect the role of learning in pain behavior. Evidence exists that some dimensions of pain are universal while others are culture-specific.[34] Thus, several studies have reported differences among ethnic and cultural groups in their responses to pain. People of Mediterranean origin, such as Italians and Jews, for example, are apt to report pain before people of northern European descent and to tolerate less intense levels of laboratory-induced pain before refusing to continue.[35,36] Some ethnic groups encourage stoic attitudes and behavior, whereas in other groups a person in pain is expected to express pain responses openly and receives sympathy and attention for this behavior. These patterns are socially learned and transmitted largely by the family. Thus, we might expect the family to be the most important source of early learning about pain perception and appropriate behavior in response to pain.

Yet another important predictor of pain is gender. While there is strong general consensus of a gender difference in response to pain, Riley et al[37] underlined the ambiguity of these findings in a meta-analysis of the results. Tradition says that women are fragile and sensitive to pain, while men are more stoic than women and can "take more pain." As a result, research has shown that among postoperative patients, women are likely to be given pain killers earlier than men.[38] In addition, men must complain more than women about pain before being given pain medication.[39] Most studies of pain tolerance have found that men are willing to tolerate more pain than women. However, other studies have shown that when pain threshold measures are used, men and women do not differ in reporting the feeling of pain.[40] Thus, it is plausible to believe that sex differences in pain behavior may reflect the influence of culture rather than differences in physiology. The orthodontic literature seldom points to any correlation between gender and perception of pain during orthodontic treatment.[10,41,42] However, some studies have found that girls report more discomfort/pain than boys[7,8] and that girls more often than boys report ulcerations caused by fixed appliances.[8]

There are several indications that pain in general is related to age, and it seems that pain thresholds increase with age. To assess pain thresholds in the general population, a study was performed by Tucker et al[43] among 520 healthy individuals aged 5 to 105 years. A constant current electrical stimulator that did not produce tissue damage but a clearly defined "pricking pain" was used to measure the cutaneous pain threshold. It was found that pain thresholds increased rapidly to the age of 25 years, followed by a plateau with a very gradual rise to the age of 75 years. Above this age there was another rapid mean rise, but with a wide scatter of values.[43]

In orthodontics, it is difficult to compare different studies concerning the relation between age and how the patient perceives pain during orthodontic treatment. This is because the treatment plan may differ depending on age. Patients at the mixed dentition stage do not always get the same appliances as the older patients. However, some studies concluded that there is a difference in the perception of pain due to age. It appears that younger patients perceive less pain than older patients.[7,9–11,41] The most vulnerable ages seem to be 13 to 16 years of age. Not all situations fit into this pattern. Thus, when RME is used to expand the midpalatal suture, it initiates more pain in adolescents older than 15 years of age.[44] When the discomfort was estimated based on visual analogue scale indices related to different situations as they have been perceived by individuals during treatment with fixed appliances, no differences were reported among the individuals of different ages.[42]

Pain Assessments

It is impossible to evaluate precisely what someone else's pain feels like. Since pain is a complex perceptual phenomenon and a subjective experience, it can be assessed only indirectly. Thus, a number of different methods have been used to assess pain. The most common method for assessing pain in orthodontics is the visual analogue scale (VAS)[7,10,41,42] and the verbal rating scale (VRS).[11,45,46] The VAS is one of the most common tools for measuring pain intensity. The scale consists of a 100-mm horizontal or vertical line with two endpoints labeled, for example, "no pain" and "worst ever pain." The patient places a mark on the line at a point that corresponds to the level of pain intensity she or he currently feels.

The VRS scale consists of a list of adjectives describing different levels of pain intensity. An adequate VRS of pain intensity should include adjectives that reflect the extremes of this dimension (eg, from no pain to extremely intense pain) and sufficient additional adjectives to capture the gradations of pain intensity that may be experienced. Patients are asked to read over the list of adjectives and select the word or phrase that best describes their level of pain. In the 4-point VRS used by Seymour,[47] for example, no pain would be given a score of 0, mild pain a score of 1, moderate pain a score of 2, and severe pain a score of 3.[47] A criticism frequently raised with respect to the rank scoring method is that it assumes equal intervals between the adjectives, even though it is extremely unlikely that equal intervals exist.[48] Another method for assessing pain is the numerical rating scale (NRS). This scale is not common for evaluating pain perception in orthodontics. When using the NRS, the patients rate their pain from 0 to 10 or from 0 to 100; 0 represents no pain and 10 or 100 represents pain as bad as it could be.

For adolescents and adults, the three most commonly used methods for assessing pain intensity are the VRS, the VAS, and the NRS. Generally, children over 5 years of age are able to use the VAS in a reliable and valid manner to rate their pain intensity, regardless of their gender or health status.

Discomfort and Pain During Orthodontic Tooth Movement

The words "discomfort" and "pain" are often used in the literature to describe the unpleasant experience of the patient during an orthodontic procedure. Although these two words are often used synonymously, they do not express the same magnitude or intensity of the perceived unpleasant feeling. For example, the discomfort caused by an unstable or modified occlusion during the progress of an orthodontic treatment may be annoying, but it can hardly be considered painful. Similarly, the unpleasant taste of adhesives may lead to discomfort after the bonding procedure, but this too is definitely not a painful experience. This lack of distinction between the use of these two words may create some confusion among different studies in the evaluation of how the patient perceives the different stages of an orthodontic treatment.

When a force is applied to a tooth, the patient usually experiences 1 or 2 days of discomfort/pain. Few studies have assessed the patient's experience of pain earlier than 4 hours after insertion of an appliance. Fernandes et al[10] assessed pain/discomfort in 128 patients 9 to 16 years of age (mean 12 years, 6 months) for routine placement of an initial archwire. Assessments were made daily by means of a 100-mm VAS over the first 7 days after bonding. On the first day, recordings were made every hour for the first 11 hours. They found that the level of discomfort/pain increased continuously every hour after insertion of nickel-titanium wires.

The pain intensity in general increases with time at 4 hours and at 24 hours but falls to rather normal levels at 7 days.[7,10,41,42] However, when treated with different fixed appliances, some patients reporting severe pain had the highest scores within the first 3 days, often peaking at night. In patients reporting moderate pain, the worst was over by the second day, peaking in the evening and night. In those reporting mild discomfort, this continued for about a week, evenly distributed through mornings, afternoons, and evenings, but little at night.[11] There is a great variety of findings concerning the duration of pain. A number of patients describe much longer periods of pain than the initial 1 or 2 days of discomfort/pain.

However, studies using different evaluating procedures and definitions have created confusion regarding the duration of discomfort and pain. In a study by Ngan et al,[42] 70 patients ranging from 10.5 to 38 years of age were selected for comprehensive orthodontic treatment. Each patient completed questionnaires before insertion of separators and initial archwires and after placement at 4 hours, 24 hours, and 7 days. An index card based on VASs was created to evaluate the discomfort of treatment during different functions such as chewing, biting, and fitting the teeth together. The VAS assessments ranged from "very comfortable" to "very uncomfortable." This study included a control group, which also completed the initial questionnaires and the discomfort index card but received no treatment. There was a significant increase in the level of discomfort associated with the two kinds of treat-

ment at 4 hours and 24 hours. The discomfort then decreased to pretreatment levels at 7 days, which is the same as what the control group reported. This study also indicated that patients who initially reported a high level of discomfort continued to report a high level of discomfort throughout the study.

Scheurer et al[7] investigated the intensity, location, and duration of discomfort/pain in 170 patients (ages 8 to 53 years) following insertion of different orthodontic appliances. The patients received eight questionnaires; the first one they completed and returned 4 hours after insertion and the others once daily for 7 days. Sixty-five percent reported pain after 4 hours, and 95% after 24 hours. Typically, pain intensity decreased at day 3, but at day 7, 25% of the patients still reported discomfort. Patients' pain-intensity scores were significantly higher for the anterior than for the posterior teeth.[7]

Since emotional and cognitive factors probably play an important role in how patients perceive the orthodontic treatment, the motivation level of the patients and their expectations for treatment should be considered when evaluating the pain characteristics during an orthodontic procedure. As noted earlier, other important cognitive aspects of pain relate to the dimensions of beliefs, attention/distraction, and the feeling of control, which relates to factors such as receiving information, prediction, and memory.

In a recent study, the present authors[49] undertook to investigate in a standardized fashion the pain characteristics of patients entering orthodontic treatment. A total of 55 teenagers, each of whom had all permanent teeth present excluding the third molars, were selected from patients starting comprehensive orthodontic treatment due to crowding in one or both jaws. Gender, dental anxiety, previous experience of other types of pain, and motivational factors were studied in relation to the patient's perceived pain after insertion of separators mesial and distal to the first molars. After the placement of the elastic separators, the pain intensity was assessed on a VAS scale. In contrast to most studies, where unselected orthodontic treatments were used, the perception of pain was measured among the patients after separators were placed in order to create a simple and homogeneous research model procedure. Telephone interviews were conducted every second evening to collect information regarding experience

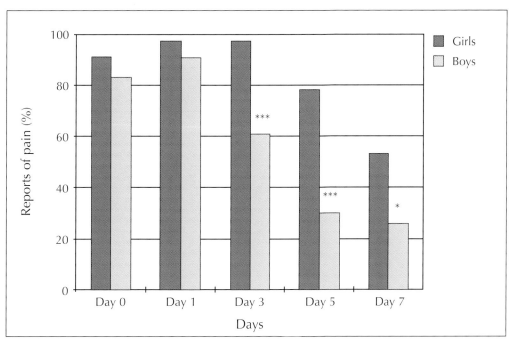

Fig 9-1 Distribution of patients, boys and girls, reporting pain during the evenings of the follow-up week after placement of separators (Day 0).

of pain, pain medication, and character of pain. The patients were also asked to put the VAS assessments into separate envelopes marked for each day and to bring them to the clinic at the next appointment. The character of pain was indicated using four descriptors according to the McGill Questionnaire.[50]

In concurrence with previous studies, the great majority of the patients reported pain during the first 2 days. The pain started almost immediately after placement of the separators. More than 80% of the patients reported pain on the evening of the treatment day (day 0). The peak degree of pain occurred 1 day after placement of the separators, when 91% of the boys and 97% of the girls reported pain. At day 3, these frequencies dropped to 60% of the boys, while 97% of the girls continued to report pain. Still, at day 7, more than half of the girls and every fourth boy reported pain. Significantly, more girls than boys experienced pain during days 3, 5, and 7 (Fig 9-1).

The intensity of the pain showed a similar pattern (Fig 9-2). The pain assessments on the first evening after the placement of the separators averaged 30 (range 0 to 78; median 26) for boys and 26 (range 0 to 82; median 14.5) for girls on the 100-mm VAS scale. One day after the start of treatment, the average pain intensity reached 41 (range 0 to 93; median 38) for the boys and 46 (range 0 to 100; median 40.5) for the girls. The patients' experience of pain varied considerably, but girls scored consistently higher with the exception of day 0. There was a significant drop in mean scores after day 1. It should be mentioned that when pain intensity peaked one day after the procedure, 27% of the patients relieved the pain by taking painkillers. Thus, there is a possibility that pain medication curtailed the most intense pain reaction among patients who medicated and thus confounded the "true" pain assessments, which in fact may have been more pronounced.

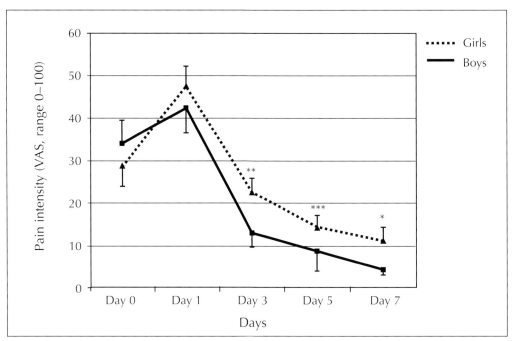

Fig 9-2 Reported intensity of pain (mean and standard deviation) among boys and girls during the evenings of the follow-up week after placement of separators (Day 0).

Pain intensity gradually decreased, but even at day 7 a considerable proportion still reported pain (>50% of the girls and 25% of the boys). However, average pain levels were low, and only one girl at day 7 still reported pain comparable to that of the average peak score level. This was in agreement with Scheurer et al,[7] who reported 25% "discomfort" (rather than pain) after 1 week. However, it should be noted that, whereas Scheurer used a variety of treatment methods, the present study used only patients who were subjected to one uniform treatment with separators.

The patients described the character of pain (without differences according to gender) only as either constant pain or as pain when chewing/biting; "shooting" and "dull" were never used to describe pain. Less than every fifth patient experienced constant pain during the first 2 days except at day 1, when 41% of the girls reported constant pain. The frequency decreased during the rest of the week, and at day 7 nobody reported constant pain. The picture was completely different regarding pain during chewing/biting. A majority of patients already reported this type of pain on the first night after treatment. It peaked at day 1

when more than 82% of the patients reported this type of pain. At day 7, about 30% still reported pain when chewing/biting. During the first 2 days, boys experienced more chewing/biting pain than did girls, while girls reported higher levels during the last 5 days of the follow-up week.

It has been shown that patients who perceive their malocclusion as severe report less pain during treatment.[51] This was not validated in our study. The peak level of pain experience in this study was comparable to the highest-ranked general pains (spraining one's ankle, vaccination, and wasp sting). Thus, both the frequency and intensity showed that pain reactions during orthodontic treatment could not be ignored. In this study, the present authors found a group of patients who reported a significant reaction to placement of the separators. This group consisted mainly of girls experiencing prolonged pain during the end of the week (days 3, 5, and 7). These girls also assessed the experience of general pain, especially from vaccination, higher than did the boys, and they reported elevated dental anxiety. Thus, it seems that there are some patients who are prone to experience stronger pain during a longer period of time after placement of separators. It has been shown that patients who initially reported a high level of discomfort continued to report a high level of discomfort throughout the week.[11,42] However, this was not substantiated by our results, where no such significant correlations were found.

Physiology of Pain During Orthodontic Tooth Movement

It is still not entirely clear why pain arises during orthodontic tooth movement and what subjective and objective factors influence the perception of pain. It is a common observation that there is no pain for at least 2 hours after the placement or activation of orthodontic appliances. After the pain is initiated, it generally lasts for about 3 days. Furstman and Bernick[23] concluded that pain in the surrounding tissues during orthodontic tooth movement may depend on a combination of pressure, ischemia, inflammation, and edema. The periodontal ligament has a rich nerve supply, where pressure receptors are mainly located in the apical two thirds of the root. The increased tenderness to pressure suggests an inflammation at the apex and a mild pulpitis. These generally appear soon after orthodontic forces have been applied and probably also contribute to the pain.[52]

In one study, Burstone[53] noted both an immediate and a delayed pain response. He speculated that the former was related to the initial compression of the periodontal ligament immediately after the placement of the wire. The latter response, which started a few hours later, was attributed to hyperalgesia of the periodontal ligament, an increased sensitivity of nerve fibers to noxious stimuli such as prostaglandins, histamines, and substance P.[53] Substance P is a neuropeptide released from receptors in the region of tissue damage. This peptide increases the firing rate of neurons that relay nociceptive information. In an experimental study by Nicolay et al,[54] substance P appeared to increase markedly after application of an orthodontic force in the cat. This phenomenon occurred rapidly within 3 hours in the dental pulp but later (24 hours to 14 days) in the periodontal ligament, mainly at compression sites.[54]

Influence of Type of Orthodontic Force Used

The level of the force magnitude has been considered to be essential in the perception of pain in orthodontics. According to Reitan,[55] pain is the result of compression of the periodontal ligament. It may indicate that hyalinized zones are about to be formed in the periodontal ligament. To reduce pain, Reitan suggested that it is favorable to use lighter forces for tooth movement. However, patients seem to respond to different orthodontic forces to varying extents. Andreasen and Zwanziger[56] found no relationship between reported pain and increased forces. In their study, different forces were applied between the canine and the molars on each side using light force (100 to 150 g) on one side and heavier force (400 to 500 g) on the other.[56]

Clinical experience suggests that there is a relationship between the severity of crowding and the forces applied by a fully engaged initial archwire, which means the more severe the crowding, the heavier the forces applied, the more intense the pain. However, in a study by Jones and Richmond,[45] no relationship was found between pain, applied forces, and degree of crowding. Thus, further studies are required to better understand pain during treatment of crowding. Pain in relation to different levels of applied forces has also been investigated in studies using different archwire materials. Nickel titanium (NiTi) alloys deliver lighter forces compared to the stiffer steel wires. However, in concurrence with the study by Jones and Richmond, recent studies have shown no differences in pain perception when comparing NiTi wires with multistranded steel wires[41] and superelastic NiTi wires with conventional NiTi wires.[10] Thus, it seems that the "clinical feeling" that the perception of pain during orthodontic tooth movement is directly related to the level of the applied force is not fully supported by evidence in the literature, at least when the normal range of clinical orthodontic forces has been considered.

The type of force in terms of the way it is applied has been considered to elicit different levels of pain. Fixed appliances mostly create continuous forces on the teeth, while removable appliances create intermittent forces. Both appliances cause pain. However, in a study by Stewart et al,[46] the patients reported that fixed appliances created more severe problems than removable appliances (ie, active plate in the maxilla). The initial problems associated with fixed appliances included sensitivity, tightness, and pain in the teeth. However, other types of problems were associated with removable appliances, including salivary flow, swallowing problems, and speech, and these could continue for more than 3 months.[46]

Nevertheless, orthodontic treatment with fixed appliances includes an additional painful procedure, the debonding of brackets. When the finishing phase is reached and it is time for debonding, patients seem to experience some discomfort/pain. It has been reported that the discomfort threshold is influenced by the mobility of the tooth and the direction of force application. Patients withstand significantly more intrusive forces than forces applied in a mesial, distal, labial, lingual, or extrusive direction.[57] However, it should be noted that taking place at the end of the orthodontic treatment, this procedure may be perceived as less severe due to the very positive attitude of the patient than it might be in the middle of the treatment, when correction of the position of some brackets requires a similar debonding procedure.

Pain Alleviation

Ideally, pain would be avoided completely in orthodontics. While this is not a realistic goal, nonetheless it is the orthodontist's responsibility to minimize any risk or unnecessary cause of pain. Still, some patients will experience pain and report it according to their personal previous pain experiences and motivational attitude. These responses are influenced by a number of factors previously discussed. Thus, the orthodontist first must be aware of which treatments can cause pain and second be able to identify the patients most susceptible to negative pain reactions and to have strategies for helping those patients.

In a practical sense, some pain can be avoided by taking care in the application and adjustment of the appliances and by performing any treatment sequence with the risk of pain in mind. To carefully and thoroughly inform the patient about the treatment and to be sure that he/she is prepared for each step in the treatment also is important, and the orthodontist must be sensitive to the reactions of the patients. If the patient perceives or reacts with pain, additional information should be offered, and he/she should be calmly reassured. These simple rules are all commonly and intuitively used by most dentists, and they are effective since they let the patient feel that he/she has control over the situation (an informed, prepared, and motivated patient). Most patients need only this basic information. However, patients who are more anxious or afraid may need more extensive information, possibly in combination with some simple relaxation exercises. The patient should also be informed that the pain is not dangerous and that it will decrease with time.

Recent years have seen major developments in our understanding of pain mechanisms and new approaches to the management of pain. Consequently, substantial progress has been made in our ability to control pain in the clinical situation. The effect of soft laser irridiation of the periodontal tissues has been studied as a way to reduce pain in patients undergoing orthodontic treatment with a fixed appliance.[58] The irridiation was applied from the labial and lingual sites for a total of 1 minute after the appliance was inserted. Reduction in pain was found in some patients, and delay in the pain occurrence was noted as compared to control groups. However, none of these observations reached a statistically significant difference level.

Transcutaneous electrical nerve stimulation (TENS) is another method of reducing pain in orthodontics. It has been found that pain is decreased significantly for those patients treated with TENS during 24-, 36-, and 48-hour assessment periods.[59]

Also, some have reported that chewing something hard after appliance adjustments may be used as a means of reducing pain.[25,52] One suggestion was to chew on a plastic wafer for 10 to 12 minutes within 1 hour following an orthodontic adjustment. This method successfully reduced pain in several patients, but a large number reported increased discomfort after chewing the wafers.[22] Chewing sugarless gum has also been recommended.

In orthodontics, the most common way to reduce pain is to use different analgesic agents. The nonsteroidal anti-inflammatory drugs, aspirin and ibupro-

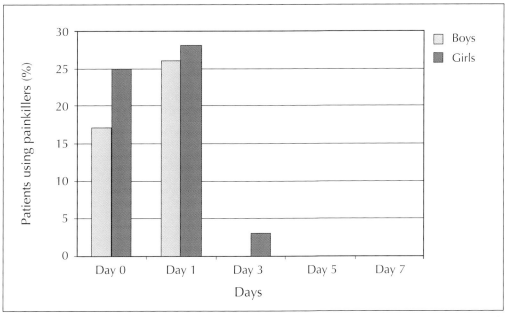

Fig 9-3 Distribution of patients medicating for pain according to gender during the follow-up week after placement of separators (Day 0).

fen, have been studied for their ability to reduce pain in orthodontics. It was found that ibuprofen relieved discomfort/pain better than aspirin in patients treated with separators and archwire placement.[60] Though common, effective, and simple to handle, painkillers are not used by the majority of orthodontic patients in spite of their frequent pain experiences. In a study by Scheurer et al,[7] it was shown that 16% of the patients used analgesics the first day and 13% the second day after insertion of a fixed appliance.[7]

Similarly, in a recent study[49] on teenagers who underwent a uniform orthodontic treatment procedure, ie, placement of elastic separators mesial and distal to the first molar, pain medication was most frequently used during the first 2 days, and the type and dosage of medication indicated a moderate need for pain alleviation (Fig 9-3). Less than 20% of the boys and 25% of the girls used painkillers the day of placement of the elastic separators, which increased somewhat the next day when 26% of the boys and 28% of the girls used analgesics. However, 3 days after the placement of the separators, all patients but one girl had already stopped using pain medication. In light of these results, it should be stressed that the use of pain medication may reflect not only the perception of pain but also a "habit" of using such relief.

In view of the high level of reported pain in orthodontics, the relatively low use of pain medication indicates that these patients are highly motivated and expect or are prepared to endure necessary treatment pain. This, however, does not excuse any orthodontist from carefully analyzing pain attitudes and from providing proper care that is as pain-free as possible. The importance of these aspects was shown in follow-up studies of adult individuals who had been subjected to dental trauma during childhood.[61] What remained as common patient memories after several years were painful emergency and follow-up treatments, not enough information, and the behavior (especially if unpleasant) of the dental staff. It is reasonable to believe that the common long-term perspective of orthodontic treatments and the frequent orthodontist-patient interaction make these aspects even more important in orthodontic dental care.

References

1. Patel V. Non-completion of Orthodontic Treatment: A Study of Patient and Parental Factors Contributing to Discontinuation in the Hospital Service and Specialist Practice. Heath Park: Univ of Wales, 1989.
2. Oliver RG, Knapman YM. Attitudes to orthodontic treatment. Br J Orthod 1985;12:179–188.
3. Dangott L, Thornton BC, Page P. Communication and pain. J Commun 1978;28:30–35.
4. Klepac RK, Dowling J, Hauge G, McDonald M. Reports of pain after dental treatment, electrical tooth pulp stimulation, and cutaneous shock. JADA 1980;100:692–695.
5. Vassend O. Anxiety, pain and discomfort associated with dental treatment. Behav Res Ther 1993;31:659–666.
6. Lew KK. Attitudes and perceptions of adults towards orthodontic treatment in an Asian community. Commun Dent Oral Epidemiol 1993;21:31–35.
7. Scheurer PA, Firestone AR, Burgin WB. Perception of pain as a result of orthodontic treatment with fixed appliances. Eur J Orthod 1996;18:349–357.
8. Kvam E, Gjerdet NR, Bondevik O. Traumatic ulcers and pain during orthodontic treatment. Commun Dent Oral Epidemiol 1987;15:104–107.
9. Brown DF, Moerenhout RG. The pain experience and psychological adjustment to orthodontic treatment of preadolescents, adolescents, and adults. Am J Orthod Dentofacial Orthop 1991;100:349–356.
10. Fernandes LM, Ogaard B, Skoglund L. Pain and discomfort experienced after placement of a conventional or a superelastic NiTi aligning archwire. A randomized clinical trial. J Orofacial Orthop 1998;59:331–339.
11. Jones ML. An investigation into the initial discomfort caused by placement of an archwire. Eur J Orthod 1984;6:48–54.
12. Kvam E, Bondevik O, Gjerdet NR. Traumatic ulcers and pain in adults during orthodontic treatment. Commun Dent Oral Epidemiol 1989;17:154–157.
13. Needleman HL, Hoang CD, Allred E, Hertzberg J, Berde C. Reports of pain by children undergoing rapid palatal expansion. Pediatr Dent 2000;22:221–226.
14. Deguchi T, Uematsu S, Kawahara Y, Mimura H. Clinical evaluation of temporomandibular joint disorders (TMD) in patients treated with chin cup. Angle Orthod 1998;68:91–94.
15. Pancherz H, Anehus-Pancherz M. The effect of continuous bite jumping with the Herbst appliance on the masticatory system: A functional analysis of treated Class II malocclusions. Eur J Orthod 1982;4:37–44.
16. Miyawaki S, Yasuhara M, Koh Y. Discomfort caused by bonded lingual orthodontic appliances in adult patients as examined by retrospective questionnaire. Am J Orthod Dentofacial Orthop 1999;115:83–88.
17. International Association for the Study of Pain. Pain terms: A list with definitions and notes on usage. Pain 1979;6:249–252.
18. Horowitz LG, Kehoe L, Jacobe E. Multidisciplinary patient care in preventive dentistry: Idiopathic dental pain reconsidered. Clin Prev Dent 1991;13:23–29.
19. Sternbach RA. Acute versus chronic pain. In: Wall PD, Melzack R (eds). Textbook of Pain. London: Livingstone, 1989.
20. Melzack R, Wall PD. Pain mechanisms: A new theory. Science 1965;150:971–979.
21. Okeson JP, ed. Orofacial Pain. Chicago: Quintessence, 1996.
22. Hwang JY, Tee CH, Huang AT, Taft L. Effectiveness of Thera-bite wafers in reducing pain. J Clin Orthod 1994;28:291–292.
23. Furstman L, Bernick S. Clinical considerations of the periodontium. Am J Orthod 1972;61:138–155.
24. Klingberg G. Dental fear and behavior management problems in children. A study of measurement, prevalence, concomitant factors, and clinical effects. Swed Dent J Suppl 1995;103:1–78.
25. Chapman CR, Turner JA. Psychological control of acute pain in medical settings. J Pain Symptom Manage 1986;1:9–20.
26. Melzack R. The Puzzle of Pain. New York: Basic Books, 1973.
27. Weisenberg MI. Pain and pain control. Psychol Bull 1977;84:1008–1044.
28. Leventhal H, Everhart D. Emotion, pain and physical illness. In: Izard CE (ed). Emotions in Personality and Psychopathology. New York: Plenum Press, 1979:263–298.
29. Williams JM, Murray JJ, Lund CA, Harkiss B, de Franco A. Anxiety in the child dental clinic. J Child Psychol Psychiatry 1985;26:305–310.
30. Litt MD. A model of pain and anxiety associated with acute stressors: Distress in dental procedures. Behav Res Ther 1996;34:459–476.
31. Lindsay SJ, Humphris G, Barnby GJ. Expectations and preferences for routine dentistry in anxious adult patients. Br Dent J 1987;163:120–124.
32. Wardle J. Psychological management of anxiety and pain during dental treatment. J Psychosom Res 1983;27:399–402.
33. McCaul KD, Malott JM. Distraction and coping with pain. Psychol Bull 1984;95:516–533.
34. Moore RA, Dworkin SF. Ethnographic methodologic assessment of pain perceptions by verbal description. Pain 1988;34:195–204.
35. Hardy JD, Wolff GH, Goodell H. Pain Sensation and Reactions. New York: Hafner, 1952.
36. Sternbach RA, Tursky B. Ethnic differences among housewives in psychophysical and skin potential responses to electric shock. Psychophysiology 1965;1:241–246.
37. Riley JL III, Robinson ME, Wise EA, Myers CD, Fillingim RB. Sex differences in the perception of noxious experimental stimuli: A meta-analysis. Pain 1998;74:181–187.
38. Loan WB, Morrison JD. The incidence and severity of postoperative pain. Br J Anaesth 1967;39:695–698.
39. Pilowsky I, Bond MR. Pain and its management in malignant disease. Elucidation of staff-patient transactions. Psychosom Med 1969;31:400–404.

40. Ingersoll BD. Behavioral Aspects in Dentistry. East Norwalk, CT: Appleton-Century-Crofts, 1982.

41. Jones M, Chan C. The pain and discomfort experienced during orthodontic treatment: A randomized controlled clinical trial of two initial aligning arch wires. Am J Orthod Dentofacial Orthop 1992;102:373–381.

42. Ngan P, Kess B, Wilson S. Perception of discomfort by patients undergoing orthodontic treatment. Am J Orthod Dentofacial Orthop 1989;96:47–53.

43. Tucker MA, Andrew MF, Ogle SJ, Davison JG. Age-associated change in pain threshold measured by transcutaneous neuronal electrical stimulation. Age Ageing 1989; 18:241–246.

44. Timms DJ. Rapid Maxillary Expansion. Chicago: Quintessence, 1981.

45. Jones ML, Richmond S. Initial tooth movement: Force application and pain—A relationship? Am J Orthod 1985; 88:111–116.

46. Stewart FN, Kerr WJ, Taylor PJ. Appliance wear: The patient's point of view. Eur J Orthod 1997;19:377–382.

47. Seymour RA. The use of pain scales in assessing the efficacy of analgesics in post-operative dental pain. Eur J Clin Pharmacol 1982;23:441–444.

48. Tammaro S, Berggren U, Bergenholtz G. Representation of verbal pain descriptors on a visual analogue scale by dental patients and dental students. Eur J Oral Sci 1997; 105:207–212.

49. Bergius M, Berggren U, Kiliaridis S. Experience of pain during an orthodontic procedure. Eur J Oral Sci 2002; 110:92–98.

50. Melzack R. The McGill Pain Questionnaire: Major properties and scoring methods. Pain 1975;1:277–299.

51. Sergl HG, Klages U, Zentner A. Pain and discomfort during orthodontic treatment: Causative factors and effects on compliance. Am J Orthod Dentofacial Orthop 1998; 114:684–691.

52. Proffit WR. Contemporary Orthodontics. St Louis: Mosby, 1992:280–281.

53. Burstone CJ. The biomechanics of tooth movement. In: Kraus BS, Riedel RA (eds). Vistas in Orthodontics. Philadelphia: Lea & Febiger, 1964:197–213.

54. Nicolay OF, Davidovitch Z, Shanfeld JL, Alley K. Substance P immunoreactivity in periodontal tissues during orthodontic tooth movement. Bone Miner 1990;11:19–29.

55. Reitan K. Biomechanical principles and reactions. In: Graber TM, Swain BF (eds). Current Orthodontic Concepts and Techniques. Philadelphia: Saunders, 1975.

56. Andreasen GF, Zwanziger D. A clinical evaluation of the differential force concept as applied to the edgewise bracket. Am J Orthod 1980;78:25–40.

57. Williams OL, Bishara SE. Patient discomfort levels at the time of debonding: A pilot study. Am J Orthod Dentofacial Orthop 1992;101:313–317.

58. Harazaki M, Isshiki Y. Soft laser irradiation effects on pain reduction in orthodontic treatment. Bull Tokyo Dent Coll 1997;38:291–295.

59. Roth PM, Thrash WJ. Effect of transcutaneous electrical nerve stimulation for controlling pain associated with orthodontic tooth movement. Am J Orthod Dentofacial Orthop 1986;90:132–138.

60. Ngan P, Wilson S, Shanfeld J, Amini H. The effect of ibuprofen on the level of discomfort in patients undergoing orthodontic treatment. Am J Orthod Dentofacial Orthop 1994;106:88–95.

61. Robertson A, Noren JG. Subjective aspects of patients with traumatized teeth. A 15-year follow-up study. Acta Odontol Scand 1997;55:142–147.

Temporomandibular Disorders and Orthodontics

Athanasios E. Athanasiou and
Thomas M. Graber

Definition and Classification of TMD

Temporomandibular disorders (TMD) is a collective term for a number of clinical problems involving the masticatory musculature, the temporomandibular joint (TMJ), or both. The term is synonymous with craniomandibular disorders.[1] Extensive research during the last 20 years and relevant scientific consensus support the view that TMD is a cluster of related disorders in the masticatory system that share many common features.[2–5] Therefore, old concepts that viewed them as one syndrome have been discarded.

TMD can be associated with headaches, nonpainful muscle hypertrophy, abnormal occlusal wear, and osseous alterations of the TMJ; they can also be related to stressful habits, parafunctional activities, emotional disorders, structural malrelationships, trau-

ma to the face or head, occlusal disharmonies, and other medical problems. The most common clinical markers of TMD in the general population are abnormal mandibular motion, muscle and TMJ tenderness, and TMJ sounds.[1,6]

Despite the voluminous amount of literature written and continuing education activities devoted to TMD, a vast chasm separates many dental professionals and groups on subjects ranging from etiology to treatment procedures.[3,7] A clear and complete understanding of all facets of TMD is currently lacking.

Classification systems have been based on signs and symptoms, tissues of origin, etiology, structural and functional disorders, frequency, and medical classification. Currently, a consensus regarding the classification of TMD is notably lacking, and it seems unlikely that such a system would ever be uniformly accepted.[8] According to a minimally accepted classification,[2] TMD represents a broad range of conditions that involve medical, dental, and psychologic factors and can be divided into five main categories:

1. Masticatory muscle disorders
2. Disc-interference disorders
3. Inflammatory disorders of the joint
4. Chronic mandibular hypomobilities
5. Growth disorders of the joint

The complex nature of TMD, the great variety of symptoms and signs that it encompasses, and its countless pathologic and functional manifestations on the stomatognathic system require that orthodontists possess adequate relevant knowledge and experience to perform accurate diagnoses and to identify potentially at-risk patients. The risk-management implications are obvious and form a fertile field for contingency-fee lawyers.

TMD Epidemiology

The prevalence of TMD is considerable if nonspecific symptoms and moderate clinical signs are included. The frequency of severe disorders accompanied by headache and facial pain and characterized by an urgent need for treatment is 1% to 2% in children, about 5% in adolescents, and 5% to 12% in adults.

TMJ sounds are the most common clinical criterion. However, due to its very poor reliability and reproducibility, this clinical sign does not by itself indicate either a serious health problem or a treatment need.[3,9–12]

Studies of the prevalence of signs and symptoms of TMD have found that mild problems are equally distributed among men and women in the general population. Severe problems, however, are much more common among women in clinical populations, and more women than men seek care for TMD by a ratio of about 8:1.[13]

Independent studies examining patients who requested care for TMD at Scandinavian institutions concluded that there was a common peak in the age distribution of the patients, specifically during the period between 20 and 40 years.[14] One of the possible explanations for this finding may relate to the emotional aspects and stressful lifestyles that characterize this age period.

There have been several studies on the prevalence of symptoms and signs of TMD in different countries or ethnic groups; the findings indicate a lack of significant deviation. Ethnic origin should be no reason for expecting significant differences in the prevalence of TMD between populations in the industrialized world, where lifestyles, nutrition, and health-delivery systems do not differ significantly.

TMD patients constitute a significant portion of the population in industrialized societies. Consequently, orthodontic practices receive many patients who present TMD signs and symptoms regardless of their chief complaint, their level of awareness concerning the dysfunction, the malocclusion characteristics, and the orthodontic treatment priority need.

TMD Etiology: Current Knowledge and the Role of Occlusion

TMD does not constitute one single, specific, abnormal condition, although the term embraces a number of clinical problems that involve the masticatory musculature, the TMJs, or both. Because it is considered a cluster of related disorders in the stomatognathic system that have many features in common, TMD should be considered as having a multifactorial etiology. TMD might be associated with stressful activities, emotional aberrations, parafunctional activity, structural malrelationships, trauma to the craniofacial region, malocclusion, and medical problems related to various types of arthritis or viral diseases. The role that occlusion plays in the development of TMD is controversial.[15,16] Today, its role is widely considered as contributory by initiating, perpetuating, or predisposing to TMD.[17] Initiating factors lead to the onset of the symptoms and are often related to trauma or adverse loading of the masticatory system. A survey of the voluminous literature indicates that the perpetuating factors may include the following subcategories:

1. Behavioral factors including grinding, clenching, abnormal oral behavior, and abnormal jaw and head posture

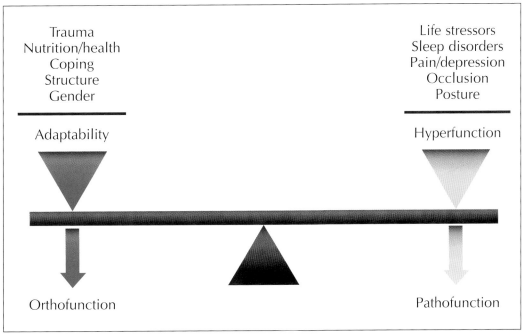

Fig 10-1 Model demonstrating a balance in the stomatognathic system between destructive overloading that leads to craniomandibular disorders and homeostatic adaptability that promotes normal function. The model includes five factors that prescribe the potential for the system to adapt homeostatically and five factors that predispose to destructive hyperfunction. The five factors on each side of the model interrelate to determine whether the balance tilts toward dysfunction or normal function of the stomatognathic system. (Redrawn with permission from Parker.[18])

2. Social factors that affect perception and influence learned response to pain
3. Emotional factors characterized by prolonged, negative feelings (ie, depression and anxiety)
4. Cognitive factors, ie, thoughts or attitudes that, when negative, can make resolution of the illness more difficult
5. Predisposing factors, namely pathophysiologic, psychologic, or structural processes that alter the masticatory system sufficiently to increase a risk of the development of TMD.

The stomatognathic system, like any other part of the body, undergoes continuous structural and functional influences and changes that are of significance to the physiology of all tissues involved. A dynamic model on the etiology of TMD presented by Parker describes how a continuous interplay exists between factors that tend to increase the adaptability of the stomatognathic system or to produce hyperfunction (Fig 10-1).

Thus, morphologic, functional, and behavioral alterations that influence factors such as general health, nutrition, stress, posture, and occlusion and induce physical trauma can produce changes in the status of the stomatognathic system in either an orthofunctional or a pathofunctional direction.

The concept of adaptation regarding the ability of occlusion to withstand stress was presented earlier by Amsterdam.[19] He defined physiologic occlusion as the one that adapts to the stress of function and can be maintained indefinitely, in contrast to pathologic occlusion, which cannot function without contributing to its own destruction.

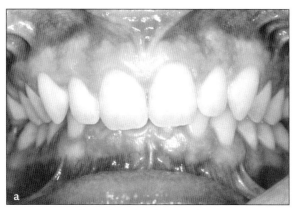 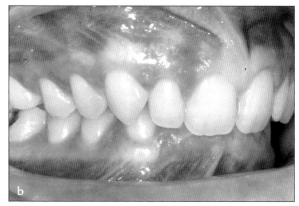

Figs 10-2a and 10-2b Malocclusion characterized by increased overbite, minimal overjet, and palatal inclination of maxillary incisors in a young adult female suffering from masticatory myalgia. This condition can be related to the excessive muscle action necessary to produce mandibular muscular guidance and avoid incisal interferences. (Reprinted with permission from Athanasiou.[33])

There are certain conditions or prerequisites that characterize a physiologic occlusion:

a. It could very well be a malocclusion, but in a state of health.
b. It has adapted well to its environment.
c. It has no pathologic manifestations or dysfunctional problems.
d. It is in a state of harmony and requires no therapy.

A significant debate concerning etiologic factors of TMD involves the contribution of various types of malocclusions or occlusal factors. In most instances, the methodologic weaknesses of the studies aiming to correlate occlusal factors with TMD (ie, lack of reliable measures or heterogeneous samples) made the results inconclusive.[5] On the other hand, there are instances where occlusal abnormalities can be considered as predisposing or initiating factors to the occurrence of TMD.

Signs of dysfunction may be the result of how the individual uses the occlusion and not a result of its structural features.[1,20] Thus, the term *nonphysiologic occlusion* does not imply a cause-and-effect relationship. For example, in subjects with increased overbite, minimal overjet, and palatal inclination of maxillary incisors, a precise mandibular muscular guidance in the closing phase of mastication is necessary to avoid incisal interferences. Such a response may be associated with strong action of the posterior temporal muscles caused by an increased overlap between the elevators and the lateral pterygoid and digastric muscles in the shift from opening to closing and vice versa (Fig 10-2).[21–23]

Although the role of occlusion in TMD is mired in disagreement, its potential effects on the biomechanics of the craniofacial complex cannot be ignored. McNeill et al[24] and McNeill[25] theorized that a broader array of biomechanical factors rather than occlusal factors alone contributes to the development of TMD. Pullinger et al[26] applied multiple factor analysis, which indicated the low correlation of occlusion to TMD. However, there were some occlusal factors that did have a slight relation:

1. Apertognathia (open bite)
2. Overjets greater than 6 to 7 mm
3. Retruded contact position/intercuspal position slides greater than 4 mm
4. Unilateral lingual crossbite
5. Five or more missing posterior teeth

With regard to the distribution of occlusal contacts, symmetry of their intensity (stress) rather than symmetry of their number in the posterior occlusion per se seemed to be important in relation to temporomandibular function.[27] Also, more frequent headaches in individuals with few occlusal contacts have been noted.[28]

Pullinger and Seligman[29] estimate that occlusal factors contribute about 10 to 20% to the total spectrum of multifactorial factors, differentiating between healthy persons and patients with TMD.

Subjects who have a malocclusion over a long period of time tend to report more symptoms of TMD and show a higher dysfunction index than those who do not. This was the conclusion of a superb 20-year follow-up study of subjects with and without orthodontic treatment in childhood.[30]

Our profession's scientific inability to exactly assess the contribution of occlusion in the etiology of various types of TMD does not justify ignorance or underestimation by orthodontists regarding the existence of certain important biomechanical relationships between functioning dentition and various components of the stomatognathic system. Again, this uncertainty fosters litigious action. The number of malpractice suits brought against orthodontists is significant.

TMD Diagnosis

The American Academy of Orofacial Pain has published consensus-based guidelines that outline principles for TMD diagnosis and evaluation.[1] Of particular importance is the classification containing diagnostic criteria consistent with the International Headache Society's Classification of Headache, Cranial Neuralgias and Facial Pain.[1,31]

The aim in evaluating TMD is to determine the chief complaint, the diagnosis, the contributing factors, and the level of complexity.[1] All major textbooks dealing with the subject of TMD describe extensively and systematically the screening evaluation, comprehensive history, comprehensive physical examination, behavioral and psychosocial assessment, and additional clinical or laboratory tests. Application of a well-organized, comprehensive, and systematic approach is absolutely mandatory for the problem list, differential diagnosis, treatment planning, management, and assessment of treatment.[1]

With regard to the history, special attention should be given to (a) familial history, (b) inflammatory bone diseases, (c) muscle disorders, (d) nocturnal parafunctional activity, (e) face and head trauma, and (f) chronic facial pain.

The clinical examination must detail the issues of pain, limitations, noises, and deviations. The clinical examination should minimally include evaluation of mandibular mobility, impaired function of the TMJs, stress-strain-tension release manifestations, detection for masticatory and neck muscle pain, and TMJ pain, as well as assessment of head and body posture.

At present, the only available and logical gold standard that can be used to identify the presence or absence of TMD is the evaluation of the patient's chief complaint, history, clinical examination, and, when indicated, radiographs and imaging. Thorough temporomandibular and medical history and head and neck clinical examinations are the first, and in most cases the only, procedures that provide sufficient diagnostic information.[32]

Methodological and clinical studies indicate that TMJ radiology and imaging should be used only when the patient presents developmental facial asymmetries, continuously changing intermaxillary relationships, no response to conservative treatment, history of trauma, crepitation of the TMJ, or history of rheumatic disease.[33,34] A thorough knowledge of the diagnostic possibilities and limitations of the various radiographic techniques must always precede a decision for referring the patient for such an examination. Current digital radiography techniques may offer significant nondamaging diagnostic information.[35]

Accumulation of unnecessary diagnostic data, overinterpretation of "abnormal findings," excessive exposure to radiation, increased cost of treatment, and an inaccurate diagnosis may otherwise be among the resulting consequences of the "routine" application of imaging techniques of TMD.[23,36] Clinicians should not refer a patient to the radiologist without first having formulated a diagnostic hypothesis and an understanding of what they are looking for. The ideal imaging technique for the diagnosis of TMJ disorders should provide information about the osseous structures, the articular disc, and the joint dynamics. Improper use fosters litigious consequences.

Conventional radiography is of limited value because only the osseous components of the TMJ can be evaluated. Moreover, in most joints with internal derangements, the findings of conventional radiography are either noncontributory or nonspecific.

Computed tomography (CT) is an excellent imaging modality that provides images with very good bony details. CT is of particular value in evaluating trauma and developmental abnormalities of the craniofacial region using three-dimensional technology. Unfortunately, CT is not the most appropriate method for imaging the soft tissues of the TMJ.

Both arthrography and magnetic resonance imaging (MRI) are of proven value in evaluating internal derangements of the TMJ. Arthrography has the advantages of providing a dynamic display of TMJ mechanisms and easy detection of disc perforation. However, its technical difficulties, invasive nature, and poor visualization of the disc in the mediolateral direction limit this method. MRI of the TMJ provides excellent soft tissue detail and demonstrates mediolateral disc displacements more readily than arthrography. MRI also enables both TMJs to be examined at the same time using dual superficial coil technology. MRI usually does not, however, reveal perforations of the disc or the ligaments, and the bony anatomy is not shown as clearly as on plain radiography or CT. In addition, real-time dynamic imaging of joint mechanics is not possible with MRI.

At present, the choice of TMJ imaging is based on the presence of a clearly understood diagnostic objective and the availability of arthrography and, especially, MRI.[37]

Caution should be exercised in using electronic devices for the interpretation of the recorded mandibular movements and TMJ sounds. Several of these instruments have not been adequately tested concerning their sensitivity, specificity, reliability, and validity. Furthermore, none of these magnetic jaw-tracking devices can produce a discrete clinical diagnosis of TMD in the absence of a thorough history and physical examination.[23,38,39] Overinterpretation of gnathologic, mechanistic, articulator-oriented diagnoses should be avoided. Applied biology and physiology are always dominant considerations.

Diagnostic procedures appropriately applied and cautiously interpreted are absolutely necessary for developing an all-inclusive problem list, a specific differential diagnosis, a reasonable treatment plan, effective management, and an accurate assessment of treatment outcome.

Principles of TMD Management

Management of TMD should have the primary goals of eliminating or significantly reducing pain or discomfort, improving mandibular motion, and addressing any other serious symptoms by establishing normal condyle-disc-fossa relationships and/or physiologic muscle function. It should be noted that a significant number of TMD symptoms are expressed as mainly muscular. A thorough understanding of TMJ metabolism and means of enhancement is imperative.[23]

Some problems of internal TMJ derangements, such as mild disc displacement with reduction or disc displacement without reduction during their acute phase; myofacial pain associated with parafunction; or muscle hypertonicity or secondary to trauma can usually be successfully managed by means of flat (Fig 10-3) or repositioning (Fig 10-4) occlusal acrylic splints.[9]

For controlling TMD pain, multiple strategies in addition to the use of splints are usually necessary. These may include biofeedback training, physical therapy and exercises for restoring function, strengthening the muscles, and stopping stressful traumatic habits and parafunctional activities. Occasionally, medication should be used. Also, 3 to 5% of TMD patients with TMJ internal derangements or osseous degeneration may require surgery to repair, remove, reconstruct, or reconfigure the joint.

The choice of one or more nonsurgical approaches to managing TMD should depend on the information collected by the clinical examination, the history of the patient, and the findings of radiographs or imaging examinations, if available.

In addition to the dental specialties, medical specialties (eg, neurology; ears, nose, and throat; physical medicine; psychiatry; rheumatology; and ophthalmol-

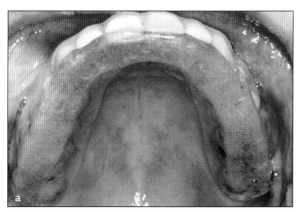
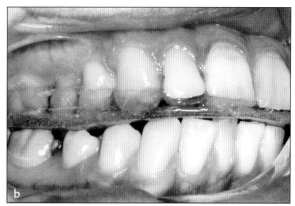

Fig 10-3 Full-coverage flat occlusal maxillary splint: *(a)* occlusal view and *(b)* lateral view.

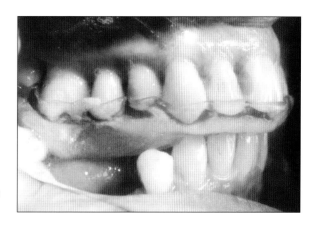

Fig 10-4 Full-coverage repositioning occlusal maxillary splint. (Reprinted with permission from Athanasiou.[33])

ogy) may often contribute significantly to the successful management of TMD patients. Also, chronic pain syndromes are known to affect patients with orofacial pain, leading to the development of interdisciplinary teams for chronic orofacial pain management.[6]

With the use of the occlusal acrylic splint, disarticulation of the occlusion takes place, thereby eliminating existing occlusal interferences; this has an effect on the maxillomandibular relations, muscle function, parafunctional activity, and TMJ internal arrangements. There are many opinions as to how a splint works, including claims for changing the position of the tongue and other soft tissues as well as the placebo effect. The major working hypotheses for the mechanism of action of splints are occlusal disengagement, intercepting parafunctional activity, alteration of vertical dimension, maxillomandibular realignment,

condylar repositioning, muscle relaxation, stress-strain-tension release, and cognitive awareness.[23,40,41]

No "cookbook" approach is available for using occlusal splints, and different concepts, guidelines, and techniques have been suggested; a detailed guide to the types of splints that are available and how to use them is available elsewhere.[33,42] Acrylic splints are usually placed flat in the maxillary arch, have full coverage, and are made in a way that permits the mandible to move in all directions without any particular guidance. Graber[9,23] stresses the need to intercept deleterious consequences of parafunction or to allow stress-strain-tension release activity. A repositioning splint is an alternative type of splint that varies both in design and manner of function, changing condylar position unilaterally or bilaterally. However, depending on the occlusal characteristics and the specific symptomatology, a maxillary or mandibular splint may be prescribed based on practicality, optimal function, stability, and esthetics. In some partially edentulous patients, the dental arch that has enough teeth will be selected to accommodate the splint.

Opinions and concepts also vary regarding the degree to which the bite should be opened by the splint. In some patients with excessive overclosure who lack adequate posterior occlusal support, an increase in the vertical dimension, even with a violation of the existing freeway space, may be indicated. In other patients, increased vertical dimension by means of a splint should aim at restoring proper internal TMJ function by re-establishing normal condyle-disc-fossa relationships. In such patients, the amount of vertical increase can sometimes transitionally induce muscle discomfort. Accurate diagnosis is the key.

Instructions concerning how much time a splint must be worn also vary considerably. Full-time use usually is not indicated when the problems are related solely to masticatory muscle hyperactivity and dysfunction. On the other hand, when signs and symptoms of TMJ internal derangements are dominant, full-time use of the splint is often recommended.

All patients undergoing TMD management involving the use of splints must be prepared for the changes in occlusion that may occur as well as for the possibility of a second phase of treatment to re-establish optimum occlusion to the new maxillomandibular relationship.

Hawley bite plates have recently been shown to be effective in decreasing ipsilateral masseter and anterior temporal muscle activities at rest and in maximum closure.[43] However, full-time use of a Hawley bite plate for an extensive period is usually not indicated except in deep bite patients with infraocclusion of posterior teeth. Indiscriminate use may produce uncontrolled eruption of the posterior teeth and lead to an unbalanced occlusion.

Physical therapy and exercises can either supplement splint therapy or be prescribed independently. Physical self-regulation primarily involves training in breathing, postural relaxation, and proprioceptive re-education.[25,44] This method of management can be used to restore function, strengthen weak muscles, instruct the patient on how to alter oral habits, and reduce stress and anxiety. The patient may be referred to a physical therapist who can be fully responsible for this management, especially when the need for strengthening the muscles is not limited to those of the stomatognathic region. There are, however, exercise devices and instruments that can be used in the office for a short period or on a regular basis at home.[45] Opening, closing, protrusion, and laterotrusive movements can be prescribed as needed. For patients with anterior disc displacement without reduction who have a low prognosis for recapturing the disc, priority may be given to increasing the amount that the patient can open the mouth. This goal can be accomplished by performing regular physical exercises. Resistance against the opening movement can be created by placing the fist beneath the chin and is often effective in strengthening the associated musculature.[46]

Medication plays a specific role in the treatment rationale for managing the symptoms of TMD and especially orofacial pain. However, such management is an important adjunct to other treatment modalities. Proper medical therapy can have a positive influence on the treatment outcome of patients with certain types of TMJ internal derangements.[47] As with all therapies, establishing a proper diagnosis is crucial to determining the appropriate medication. Several categories of medications may be prescribed for patients with TMD, including anti-inflammatory agents, muscle relaxants, anti-anxiety agents, antihistamines, opiate-narcotic analgesics, local anesthetics, and antidepressants. An example of when medication is crucial would be the use of anti-inflammatory agents for patients with polyarthritides.[48]

There is a long history of using occlusal adjustment in the management of TMD; however, there is a lack of evidence from randomized controlled trials that occlusal adjustment treats or prevents TMD. Occlusal adjustment seldom can be recommended for the management or prevention of TMD.[49,50]

Conservative management of TMD problems in a clinic or private practice environment is reported to be the most logical approach, and the same would hold true for orthodontic practices.[51]

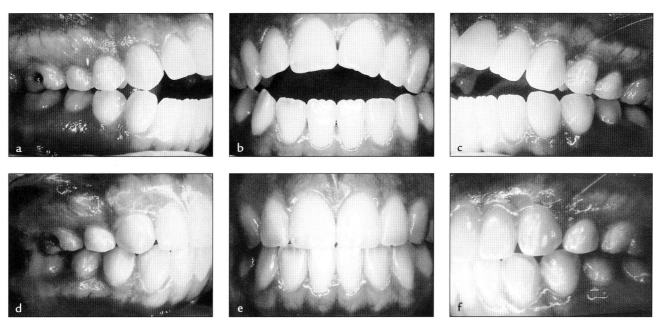

Fig 10-5 Anterior open bite, Class II malocclusion, in a young female adult. *(a–c)* Before and *(d–f)* after, right frontal and left intra-oral views. No interocclusal clearance, with overeruption of posterior segments. Tongue thrust present on swallowing. Orthodontist had maxillary first premolars removed and closed the open bite extraction space, with an end-to-end incisal relationship. Lower third molars were then removed by the oral surgeon. Patient records show that TMD complaints essentially started with third molar removal and increased subsequent to appliance removal. It is well established that surgical removal of impacted third molars, using a bite block for access, can at times cause overstretching of TMJ ligaments and even articular disc displacement. With increased TMD sequelae, the patient sought legal redress and claimed that treatment caused TMD problems, even though this is not reflected in the written record. She settled for $2,500 in her suit against the oral surgeon but was awarded close to $1 million from the orthodontist by the jury because of "expert" claims of orthodontic malpractice, trapping the mandible and forcing it posteriorly, due to removal of the maxillary first premolars only. The post-treatment views clearly indicate an end-to-end incisor relationship, which opened slightly during retention, so functional retrusion was not possible. Nonetheless, an *amicus curiae* appeal by the American Association of Orthodontists, with the support of expert testimony, failed to obtain a reversal of the litigious decision. There has been a flurry of TMD cases in court since this well-publicized decision.

TMD and Orthodontic Treatment Planning

Orthodontists have traditionally sought to improve esthetics and oral health as well as the stability and function of the treated dentition. Brodie,[52] Thompson,[53] Ricketts,[54] and Graber[22,55] each have taken a leadership role in the American orthodontic community in emphasizing the interrelationship between occlusion and TMJ.

In a malpractice trial in the United States, an orthodontist was found liable by a jury for a patient's suffering from TMD symptoms following treatment (Fig 10-5). It was the first in a series of "million-dollar cases." This case prompted the American Association of Orthodontists to support research related to orthodontic treatment and its effects on the TMJ. Numerous studies discounted orthodontic treatment as an etiologic factor and provided some noteworthy caveats for the orthodontic practitioner. A subsequent National Institute of Health conference in 1995 substantiated the results.[3,11]

The evidence overwhelmingly supports the conclusion that orthodontic treatment performed on children and adolescents generally does not place the patient

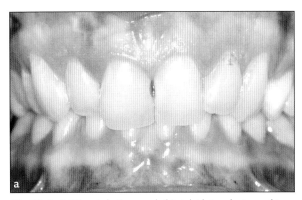 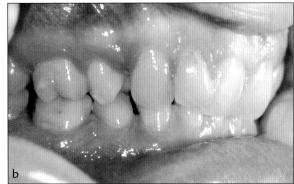

Fig 10-6 *(a)* Frontal view and *(b)* right lateral view of inappropriate post-treatment occlusal relationships in a 21-year-old female presenting occlusal trauma, severe signs of TMJ internal derangements, and muscle hyperactivity. The patient had received orthodontic treatment by means of removable appliances and extractions of the four first premolars at a younger age. In this case, litigation against the general practitioner was initiated by the patient claiming that the signs of TMD were related to the previous orthodontic treatment and led to the conviction of the dentist. (Reprinted with permission from Athanasiou.[33])

at risk for the development of TMD at a later age.[5,30,56,57] Two main explanations have been advanced: *(1)* a multiplicity of factors may be responsible for producing or exacerbating a craniomandibular disorder, and *(2)* orthodontic mechanotherapy produces gradual changes in an environment that is generally quite adaptive.

On the other hand, if orthodontic therapy or any other dental treatment compromises the ability of the stomatognathic system to adapt to it, the treatment may well predispose the patient to TMD or it may perpetuate an existing dysfunction. Examples of iatrogenic origin related to the occurrence of TMD include inappropriate post-treatment occlusal relationships, which cause trauma; severe mandibular displacement; and/or muscle hyperactivity (Fig 10-6). Also, significant orthodontic relapse that creates a functional imbalance between the TMJ, muscles, and occlusion may contribute to the occurrence of signs and symptoms of TMD in some patients. However, a clear distinction must be made between individual TMD cases caused by, on the one hand, orthodontic misdiagnosis and/or treatment failure, and on the other, unjustified attempts to systematically associate any type of orthodontic treatment with the etiology of TMD. Furthermore, there is no scientific proof that any particular method of orthodontic treatment, whether it involves extractions or not, has any causative effect on TMD.[58,59] On the contrary, studies have shown that individuals who underwent orthodontic treatment during childhood had a significantly lower clinical dysfunction index during adulthood than those who had not received orthodontic therapy.[57] Furthermore, many successfully managed TMD patients subsequently underwent orthodontic treatment to achieve the final occlusal stabilization (Fig 10-7).

An increasing number of patients with TMD are being seen in orthodontic offices. There may be several explanations for this phenomenon. Orthodontic treatment is now routinely available to adults, who have a higher prevalence of TMD than children. Also, adjunctive orthodontic treatment is often used to facilitate other dental procedures necessary to control disease and restore function. Furthermore, the specialty of orthodontics is better prepared to detect, diagnose, and manage TMD as a result of better undergraduate and postgraduate training as well as continuing education programs.

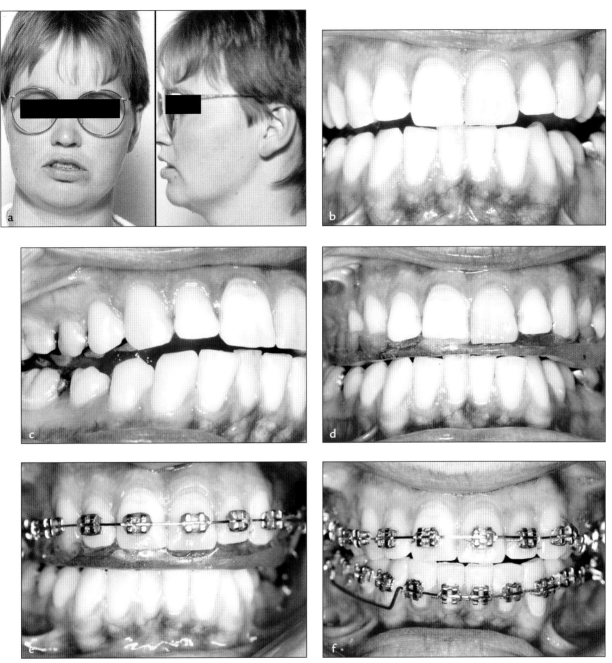

Figs 10-7a to 10-7f *(a)* Frontal and profile, *(b)* frontal, and *(c)* right lateral views of the occlusal relationships in a 25-year-old female patient. *(d)* The patient used a full-coverage flat occlusal maxillary splint 24 hours a day, became symptom-free, and was referred by a TMD clinic for orthodontic treatment to achieve final occlusal stabilization. Review of the history and the previous treatments of this patient revealed a diagnosis of anterior disc displacement with reduction on the right TMJ, unsuccessful splint therapy, unsuccessful surgical repositioning of the disc, surgical removal of the disc, and subsequent use of a splint to achieve occlusal stability and joint unloading. *(e)* The patient was treated by means of fixed orthodontic appliances with the splint in place *(f)* until stable interocclusal relationships were established. (Reprinted with permission from Athanasiou.[33])

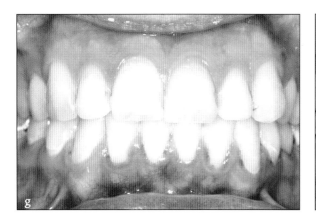

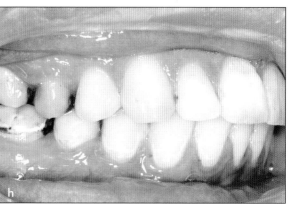

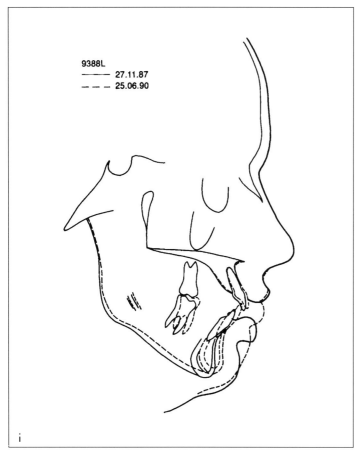

Figs 10-7g to 10-7i Optimal occlusal relationships were achieved post-treatment, as shown in the *(g)* frontal and *(h)* right lateral views. *(i)* Overall superimposition of the cephalometric tracings indicates that minor tooth movements took place in the sagittal plane. However, the significant anterior rotation of the mandible, which contributed to the closure of the bite, can be attributed mainly to the correction of the transverse occlusal malrelationships in the molar regions. (Reprinted with permission from Athanasiou.[33])

Like any other health problem, TMD can be present during the initial examination of orthodontic patients or it can occur during treatment, post-treatment, or post-retention periods. Based on extensive clinical experience in treating hundreds of TMD patients, one of the authors (TMG) is convinced that parafunctional activity is a major common denominator and may require adjunctive treatment during orthodontic appliance wear.

All patients, independent of their type of malocclusion and their reasons for seeking orthodontic treatment, must receive the same attention during the initial screening prior to the initiation of therapy. This must include a thorough temporomandibular and medical history and head and neck clinical examination. When taking the history, special attention should be given to inflammatory bone or muscle disorders (eg, rheumatoid arthritis), craniofacial trauma, and chronic facial pain (Fig 10-8). Referral to an orthopedic surgeon may at times be indicated.

If there is no evidence of TMD, the orthodontist should proceed with the orthodontic treatment as planned. If there is evidence of TMD, a differential diagnosis must be attempted, and the severity of the disorder should be assessed. The first step is to inform the patient and to document the findings in the patient's file. Special TMD forms are available to record the multiple diagnostic observations. This is imperative on a risk-management basis (see chapters 12 to 15). Then, depending on the preliminary diagnosis, a decision must be made about whether to manage the problem in the orthodontic office or refer the patient to a colleague who is more specialized or involved in this field.

In general, orthodontic therapy must not be performed on patients presenting with acute and severe signs and symptoms of TMD until these problems are under control. In cases of minor signs or symptoms (ie, TMJ clicking with no pain), orthodontic treatment can be recommended and initiated, but the TMD should be observed and monitored.[33,60]

Following the management of TMD by means of one or a combination of the various therapeutic modalities discussed earlier, orthodontic treatment should proceed only if the patient is free of pain, can function adequately, and has a stable mandibular position for at least 3 to 6 months. In addition, the patient should continue to be regularly observed by the clinician who initially treated the TMD.

Not every patient who undergoes TMD therapy requires orthodontic treatment for functional/occlusal reasons. Following TMD therapy, some patients have acceptable stomatognathic function with their existing occlusal relationships, without any orthodontic intervention. However, there are other patients who have minimal or no TMD symptoms after the initial splint therapy, but their attempts to discontinue the splint are unsuccessful because of reccurrence of discomfort (ie, persistent parafunctional activity). When a patient cannot function with the existing occlusal relationships, occlusal treatment may be necessary to provide stability during function. Minor or major occlusal changes can be achieved by means of equilibration, resin or amalgam dental restorations, prosthodontics, orthodontics, or orthognathic surgery (Fig 10-9).

Of course, there may be other reasons for seeking and performing orthodontic therapy after the initial phase of management of TMD, including dental or facial esthetics and to prepare for restorative, prosthodontic, or periodontal dental treatment.

Following successful management of TMD, the orthodontist should respect the new functional balance between the TMJ, the masticatory muscles, and the therapeutic occlusal relationships. Subsequently, proper interocclusal registrations, articulator mounting of the casts, and monitoring of all functional aspects are required. In this increasingly litigious world, it cannot be overemphasized that proper documentation of all procedures and communication with both the patient and referring dentist are essential.

Orthodontic treatment cannot be justified as an effective means of preventing TMD. However, it may be indicated to reduce existing signs and symptoms of TMD in certain carefully selected cases or to provide a morphologically and functionally optimum occlusal environment following successful management of TMD.[61]

Examination Protocol

Patient's Name _____   Dr. _____

Address _____   Address _____

_____   _____

Occupation: _____

Examination date: _____   _____

Chief complaint: _____

_____

_____

CM–history

		yes
Pain:	face	☐
	head	☐
	ear	☐
	eye	☐
	neck	☐
	regular headache	☐
TMJ sounds:	clicking	☐
	other noises	☐
Disturbances of mandibular functions:	difficulties in opening, closing, chewing, muscular tiredness, stiffness of the jaw	☐
Oral habits:	nail-lip biting, smoking etc.	☐
Previous extensive dental treatments:	prosthodontics	☐
	orthodontics	☐
	surgery	☐
	equilibration	☐

Are you comfortable with the way your teeth fit together?   yes ☐   no ☐

Medical history

Do you have or did you have a history of ?

	yes
infection (hepatitis)	☐
heart and cardiovascular diseases	☐
blood diseases	☐
respiratory tract diseases	☐
digestive tract diseases	☐
urinary and genital diseases	☐
neurological diseases	☐
metabolism	☐
allergies	☐
rheumatoid diseases	☐
psychological problems	☐
hormonal problems	☐
pregnancy	☐
trauma	☐
drugs _____	☐
general anaesthesia or surgery	☐

a

Figs 10-8a and 10-8b In an effort to develop *(a)* a standard history form and *(b)* a form for clinical findings for examination of CMD patients, in 1985 the European Academy of Craniomandibular Disorders produced the protocol reproduced here. (Reprinted with permission from Praktische Kieferorthopadie.[33])

Clinical Findings

Range of motion* opening (with overbite) ☐ mm

Deviation on movement R ☐   L ☐

Laterotrusion to the right ☐

Laterotrusion to the left ☐

Protrusion ☐

R   L

Auscultation TMJ clicking R ☐   L ☐

TMJ crepitation R ☐   L ☐

Tenderness to palpation

	R	L		R	L
TMJ laterally during movements	☐	☐	Temporalis M. insertion	☐	☐
Temporalis M.	☐	☐	Pterygoid M. complex	☐	☐
Masseter M.	☐	☐	Tongue	☐	☐

Provocation test positive ☐   negative ☐

Inspection Excessive facial asymmetries ☐

Dentition Shiny facets ☐ —————|—————   fractures ☐ —————|—————

Manipulation of the mandible in CR (RP)
easy ☐   difficult ☐   impossible ☐

Slide CR — CO (RCP — ICP)
sagittal ☐ mm   lateral ☐ mm   vertical ☐ mm

Contacts on movements

—————|—————   —————|—————   —————|—————
to the left   to the right   in protrusion

Conclusion Can you explain the chief complaint of the patient by your findings?   yes ☐   no ☐

Diagnosis (provisional) _____

Important

If you cannot explain the chief complaint do not start to treat! Refer your patient to a specialist!

X—rays are always to be taken when you suspect

- growing facial asymmetries
- continuously changing intermaxillary relationship
- no response to the treatment
- history of trauma
- crepitation of the joint

If you cannot interpret an X—ray do not take it! Refer your patient to an X—ray specialist with your specific questions.

*Please fill the appropriate box with the amount of movement in mm. In the right hand diagram draw deflections or deviations from the midline during the opening and/or closing movements as well as the position where TMJ sounds occur.

b

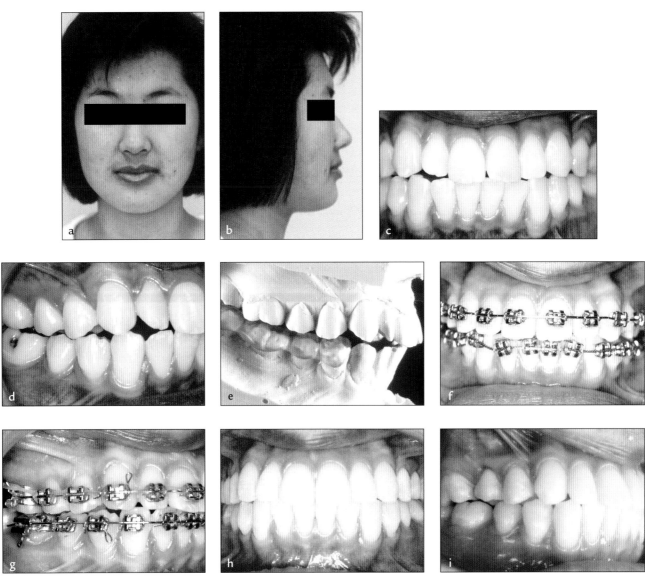

Fig 10-9 *(a)* Frontal and *(b)* profile views, *(c)* frontal and *(d)* right lateral views of the occlusal relationships in a 14-year-old female patient. The patient presented with severe signs of anterior disc displacement with reduction. A partial-coverage flat occlusal mandibular splint was utilized during the first phase of the treatment. After 4 months of splint therapy, the patient became symptom-free. Since the patient was not able to function in the maximum intercuspal position without reoccurrence of the symptoms, it was decided to proceed with orthodontic treatment in order to achieve final occlusal stabilization. Following articulator mounting, both without and *(e)* together with the splint, a three-dimensional assessment of the occlusal relationships was made. This procedure detected premature interferences in the anterior occlusion. *(f,g)* The patient was treated initially by means of fixed orthodontic appliances in the maxillary dental arch and with the splint in place in the mandible until stable interocclusal relationships were established. Optimal occlusal relationships were achieved post-treatment as they appear in the *(h)* frontal and *(i)* right lateral views. (Reprinted with permission from Athanasiou.[42])

TMD Management During and After Orthodontic Treatment

Clinical examination of the function of the stomatognathic system should take place regularly throughout the period of orthodontic treatment. If severe signs and symptoms of TMD occur during orthodontic therapy, the differential diagnosis will influence the decisions of the orthodontist either to (a) postpone treatment, (b) alter occlusion with corrective orthodontic tooth movements, (c) refer to an orthopedic surgeon or TMD specialist, or (d) discontinue treatment.

A differential diagnosis should be made before any decision concerning the continuation of orthodontic treatment. In some cases, the clinician may consider the postponement of treatment until the TMD is under control. In such cases, all TMD management modalities discussed earlier need to be applied.

Transient TMD symptoms during orthodontic treatment may be associated with traumatic occlusal interferences or with the movement of teeth. In these instances, appropriate corrective orthodontic procedures may be required. In some cases, the use of heavy intermaxillary elastics (Class II or Class III) may need to be discontinued if muscular and TMJ pain have developed following their use.[33,42] Similar adjustment may also be necessary during the initial phase of extraoral force.

Retention procedures for patients who have had orthodontic treatment and presented with TMD should aim to minimize orthodontic relapse and preserve the existing functional balance between the TMJs, the muscles, and the established occlusion. Retention appliances that incorporate a full-coverage acrylic splint for nighttime use may contribute to the reduction of detrimental influences of parafunctional activities on the occlusion, muscles, and TMJs.[23,33,42]

The occurrence of dysfunctional signs and symptoms in young or adult patients during orthodontic treatment, post-treatment, and post-retention should be addressed by applying the same comprehensive diagnostic and management procedures as are used in TMD patients who did not receive orthodontic therapy. These TMD signs and symptoms are not likely to be related to the orthodontic treatment. However, both patients and referring general dentists may not have the same opinion. Be sure the written record reflects symptoms and steps taken to control any sequelae. Risk management ramifications are discussed in chapters 12, 13, 14, and 15.

Guidelines on What to Do and What Not to Do

The complex nature of TMD, the great variety of its symptoms and signs, and its potential pathologic and functional manifestations on the stomatognathic system require orthodontists to possess adequate relevant knowledge and experience to perform an accurate diagnosis and to identify potentially at-risk patients. Continuing educational activities providing advanced and evidence-based knowledge relevant to stomatognathic function, TMD, and orofacial pain must be a high priority for orthodontists.

Regardless of the chief complaint, the level of awareness concerning the dysfunction, the malocclusion characteristics, and the orthodontic treatment recommendations, patients with TMD signs and symptoms require comprehensive diagnosis before, during, and after active therapy.

Diagnostic procedures appropriately applied and cautiously interpreted are absolutely essential for developing an all-inclusive problem list, a specific differential diagnosis, a reasonable treatment plan, effective management, and an accurate assessment of treatment outcome. This information must be communicated to both the patient and the attending dentist. TMD patients whose signs and symptoms have been ignored, underestimated, or inadequately addressed or managed impose a potential litigious risk and may cause problems for the orthodontist.

Orthodontic treatment cannot be justified as an effective means of preventing TMD. Development of TMD cannot be predicted. No method of TMD prevention has been demonstrated, though properly designed splints during and after orthodontic treatment can control unfavorable TMD sequelae and parafunctional activity. However, harmony of the interface between the teeth, muscles, nerves, supporting tissue, and TMJs must be established to provide health, functional efficiency, esthetics, and stability to the entire stomatognathic system.[22,23,55] An optimum condyle/disc position during optimum integrated muscle activity with maximal occlusal stability should constitute the functional goal of any orthodontist.[21]

Once TMD is present, cure cannot be assumed or assured. Conservative management of TMD problems is the most logical approach for orthodontic practices.[51] Given that 50% of the population may resort to uncontrolled nocturnal parafunctional activity at one time or another as a stress-strain-tension release mechanism, protection of the TMJ is essential. A simple splint, worn at night, may be all that is necessary. If there is functional impingement on the retrodiskal pad during the day, other measures must be taken by the clinician. Nature has provided an efficient mechanism for the multifunctional stomatognathic system. Understanding the physiologic aspects of this system is a prime requisite.[23]

Orthodontic treatment may be indicated to reduce existing signs and symptoms of TMD in certain carefully selected cases or to provide a morphologically and functionally optimum occlusal environment following successful management of TMD. According to existing literature, the relationship of TMDs to occlusion and orthodontic treatment is minor. The important question that still remains in dentistry is how this minor contribution can be identified within the population of TMD patients.[11] Orthodontists should always have in mind the existence of certain important biomechanical relationships between the functioning dentition and various components of the stomatognathic system. Occurrence of dysfunctional signs and symptoms in young or adult patients during or after orthodontic treatment should be addressed with extreme caution. While most TMD problems are unrelated to the orthodontic treatment itself, the orthodontist should show the same level of concern to provide optimal care.

References

1. Okeson JP, ed. Orofacial Pain: Guidelines for Assessment, Diagnosis, and Management. Chicago: Quintessence, 1996.
2. Bell WE. Temporomandibular Disorders. Classification, Diagnosis, Management. Chicago: Year Book Medical, 1990.
3. National Institute of Health. Technology Assessment Conference Statement. Management of Temporomandibular Disorders. Washington, DC: NIH, April 29– May 1, 1996.
4. Perry HT. Orthodontics and TMD: Past and present. In: Sachdeva RCL, Bantleon H-P, White L, Johnson J (eds). Orthodontics for the Next Millennium. Gendora, CA: Ormco, 1997:189–206.
5. Kim MR, Graber TM, Viana MA. Orthodontics and temporomandibular disorder: A meta-analysis. Am J Orthod Dentofac Orthop 2002;121:438–446.
6. Fricton JR. Recent advances in temporomandibular disorders and orofacial pain. J Am Dent Assoc 1991;122: 25–32.
7. National Library of Medicine. Management of Temporomandibular Disorders. Current Bibliographies in Medicine. Bethesda, MD: National Institute of Health, US Department of Health and Human Services, CEM 96–2, 1996.
8. Kaplan AS. Classification. In: Kaplan AS, Assael LA (eds). Temporomandibular Disorders. Diagnosis and Treatment. Philadelphia: WB Saunders, 1991:106–117.
9. Graber TM. Occlusal splints. J Am Dent Assoc 1980;100: 171.
10. Bakke M, Moeller E. Craniomandibular disorders and masticatory muscle function. Scand J Dent Res 1992;100: 32–38.
11. McNamara JA, Seligman DA, Okeson JP. Occlusion, orthodontic treatment and temporomandibular disorders: A review. J Orofacial Pain 1995;9:73–90.
12. Sato S, Goto S, Nasu F, Motegi K. Natural course of disc displacement with reduction of the temporomandibular joint: Changes in clinical signs and symptoms. J Oral Maxillofac Surg 2003;61:32–34.
13. Rugh JD, Solberg WK. Oral health status in the United States: Tempromandibular disorders. J Dent Educ 1985; 49:398–405.
14. Carlsson GE, Magnusson T, Wedel A. Patientmaterialet vid en bettfysiologisk avdeling. Swed Dent J 1976;69:115–121.
15. Greene CS. Occlusion and temporomandibular disorders (TMD): Still unsolved question? J Dent Res 2002;81:732.
16. Rabie AB, Tsai MJ, Hagg U, Du X, Chou BW. The correlation of replicating cells and osteogenesis in the condyle during stepwise advancement. Angle Orthod 2003;73: 457–465.
17. McNeill C, ed. Temporomandibular disorders: Guidelines for Classification, Assessment, and Management. Chicago: Quintessence, 1993.
18. Parker MW. A dynamic model of etiology in temporomandibular disorders. J Am Dent Assoc 1990;120:283–290.

19. Amsterdam M. Periodontal prosthesis: Twenty-five years in retrospect. Part II. Occlusion. Compend Contin Educ Dent 1984;5:325–334.

20. Okeson J. Fundamentals of Occlusion and Temporomandibular Disorders. St. Louis: CV Mosby, 1989.

21. Moeller E. The myogenic factor in headache and facial pain. In: Kawamura Y, Dubner R (eds). Oral-Facial Sensory and Motor Functions. Chicago: Quintessence, 1981:225–239.

22. Graber TM. The anatomical and physiological aspects in the treatment of temporomandibular joint disorders. Fortschr Kieferorthop 1991;52:126–132.

23. Graber TM. The clinical implications of the unique metabolic processes in the human temporomandibular joint. In: Sachdeva RCL, Bantleon H-P, White L, Johnson J (eds). Orthodontics for the Next Millennium. Glendora, CA: Ormco, 1997:181–187.

24. McNeill C, Mohl ND, Rugh JD, Tanaka TT. Temporomandibular disorders: Diagnosis, management, education and research. J Am Dent Assoc 1990;120:253–255, 257.

25. McNeill C. Current Concepts of TMJ Diagnosis and Treatment. Illinois Society of Orthodontists, Chicago, October 20, 2003.

26. Pullinger AG, Seligman DA, Gornbein JA. A multiple regression analysis of risk and relative odds of temporomandibular disorders as a function of common occlusal features. J Dent Res 1993;72:968–979.

27. Giannizi AI, Melsen B, Nielsen L, Athanasiou AE. Occlusal contacts in maximum intercuspidation and craniomandibular dysfunction in 16–17-year old adolescents. J Oral Rehabil 1991;18:49–59.

28. Wanman A, Agerberg G. Etiology of craniomandibular disorders: Evaluation of some occlusal and psychological factors in 19-year-olds. J Craniomandib Disord 1991;5:35–44.

29. Pullinger AG, Seligman DA. Quantification and validation of predictive values of occlusal variables in temporomandibular disorders using a multifactorial analysis. J Prosthet Dent 2000;83:66–75.

30. Egermark I, Magnusson T, Carlsson GE. A 20-year follow-up of signs and symptoms of temporomandibular disorders and malocclusions in subjects with and without orthodontic treatment in childhood. Angle Orthod 2003;73:109–115.

31. Okeson J, ed. International Headache Society classification of headache disorders, cranial neuralgias, and facial pain. Cephalalgia 1990;8 (Supplement 7).

32. Greene CS. Can technology enhance TMD diagnosis? Calif Dent Assoc J 1990;18:21–24.

33. Athanasiou AE. TM disorders, orthodontic treatment and orthognathic surgery. Prakt Kieferorthop 1993;7:269–286.

34. Capurso U, Marini I, Alessandri Bonetti G, Athanasiou AE. Stomatognathic function in patients with chronic juvenile rheumatoid arthritis. Kieferorthopaedie 1997;11:27–34.

35. Papadopoulos MA, Christou P, Athanasiou AE, Bouttchez P, Zeilhofer HF, et al. Three-dimensional craniofacial reconstruction imaging. Oral Surg Oral Med Oral Pathol Oral Radiol Endod 2002;93:382–393.

36. Athanasiou AE. Use and misuse of radiographic imaging techniques in the diagnosis and treatment of temporomandibular joint disorders. Orthod Rev 1990;4:24–25.

37. Elefteriadis JN, Athanasiou AE. Guidelines for temporomandibular joint imaging. Eur Dent 1995;4:19–21.

38. Mohl ND, Lund JP, Widmer CG, McCall WD. Devices for the diagnosis and treatment of temporomandibular disorders. Part II: Electromyography and sonography. J Prosthet Dent 1990;63:332–335.

39. Mohl ND, McCall WD, Lund JP, Plesh O. Devices for the diagnosis and treatment of temporomandibular disorders. Part I: Introduction, scientific evidence, and jaw tracking. J Prosthet Dent 1990;63:198–201.

40. Clark GT. A critical evaluation of orthopedic interocclusal appliance therapy: Design, theory and overall effectiveness. J Am Dent Assoc 1984;108:359–364.

41. Landulpho AB, de Silva WA, de Silva FA, Vitti M. The effect of the occlusal splints on the treatment of temporomandibular disorders—A computerized electromyographic study of masseter and anterior temporali muscles. Electromyogr Clin Neurophysiol 2002;42:187–191.

42. Athanasiou AE. Orthodontics and craniomandibular disorders. In: Bishara SE (ed). Textbook of Orthodontics. Philadelphia: WB Saunders, 2001:478–493.

43. Greco PM, Vanarsdall RL, Levrini M, Read R. An evaluation of anterior temporal and masseter muscle activity in appliance therapy. Angle Orthod 1999;69:141–146.

44. Carlson CR, Bertrand PM, Ehrlich AD, Maxwell AW, Burton RG. Physical self-regulation training for the management of temporomandibular disorders. J Orofacial Pain 2001;15:47–55.

45. Dunn J. Physical therapy. In: Kaplan AS, Assael LA (eds). Temporomandibular Disorders. Diagnosis and Treatment. Philadelphia: WB Saunders, 1991:455–500.

46. Capurso U, Marini I, Alessandri Bonetti G. I Disordini Cranio-Mandibolari Fisioterapia Speciale Stomatognatica. Bologna: Martina, 1996.

47. Stiesch-Scholz M, Fink M, Tschernitschek H, Rossbach A. Medical and physical therapy of temporomandibular joint disk displacement without reduction. Cranio 2002;20:85–90.

48. McMullen RD. Pharmacologic management of psychiatric disorders. In: Kaplan AS, Assael LA (eds). Temporomandibular Disorders. Diagnosis and Treatment. Philadelphia: WB Saunders, 1991:535–548.

49. Koh H, Robinson PG. Occlusal adjustment for treating and preventing temporomandibular joint disorders. Cochrane Database Syst Rev 2003;CD003812.

50. Graber TM. Nobel Prize Research and Its Impact on Growth Guidance and TMJ Metabolism. American Association of Orthodontics, Hawaii, May 6, 2003.

51. Randolph CS, Greene CS, Moretti R, Forbes DP, Perry HT. Conservative management of temporomandibular disorders: A post treatment comparison between patients from a university clinic and from private practice. Am J Orthod Dentofacial Orthop 1990;98:77–82.

52. Brodie AG. Differential diagnosis of joint conditions in orthodontia. Angle Orthod 1934;34:160.

53. Thompson JR. Function, the neglected phase of orthodontics. Angle Orthod 1956;26:129.

54. Ricketts RM. Variations of the temporomandibular joint as revealed by cephalometric laminagraphy. Am J Orthod 1950;36:877.

55. Graber TM. Normal occlusion. Dent Clin North Am 1968; 273–290.

56. Gavakos K, Witt E. The functional status of orthodontically treated prognathic patients. Eur J Orthod 1991;13:124–128.

57. Sadowsky C. The risk of orthodontic treatment for producing temporomandibular disorders: A literature overview. Am J Orthod Dentofacial Orthop 1992;101:79–83.

58. Gavakos K, Witt E. The head-chin cup—A functional risk? Fortschr Kieferorthop 1989;50:268–275.

59. Franco AA, Yamashita HK, Lederman HM, Cevidanes LH, Proffit WR, Vigorio JW. Frankel appliance therapy and the temporomandibular disc: A prospective magnetic resonance imaging study. Am J Orthod Dentofacial Orthop 2002;12:447–457.

60. Gaynor G. Orthodontic therapy. In: Kaplan AS, Assael LA (eds). Temporomandibular Disorders. Diagnosis and Treatment. Philadelphia: WB Saunders, 1991:576–625.

61. Mohlin B, Kurol J. To what extent do deviations from an ideal occlusion constitute a health risk? Swed Dent J 2003;27:1–10.

Orthodontic Treatment for the Medically Compromised Patient

Carla A. Evans

Orthodontic patients who have medical conditions often face greater risks, limitations, and complications than normal healthy people undergoing routine orthodontic treatment. These difficulties will be considered in terms of how they relate to diagnosis, prognosis, and compliance.

Diagnosis

Since a successful treatment outcome should improve the patient's physical and emotional well-being, it is important that oral health, functional relationships, and psychosocial needs all be assessed during the diagnostic phase of treatment. It is important to diagnose not only craniofacial anomalies of congenital, tumor, or traumatic origin, but also systemic conditions that may affect orthodontic tooth movement, healing, or patient compliance.

A clinician must have a sound knowledge of normal anatomy, growth, and development to recognize abnormalities. For example, bulimia may be detected by the loss of tooth structure on the lingual surfaces of maxillary teeth. Knowledge of the behavioral sciences is needed to understand attitudes and prejudices toward facial disfigurement and to motivate patients to adopt good health practices and follow instructions. Knowledge of statistics and epidemiology is necessary for the clinician to understand cause and effect. Today, so many people wear orthodontic appliances that almost anything can happen to an orthodontic patient. Just as an orthodontic patient who skis may break a leg, orthodontic patients may contract any number of disease processes, and nearly all are unlikely to be linked causally to the appliances or treatment.

During the first appointment, the orthodontist listens to the patient's chief complaints and expectations. If the patient's concerns are within the scope of the clinician's practice, arrangements are made for a thorough evaluation of the patient's problems. Medical, dental, and social histories are obtained as part of the information collected by the orthodontist, and these records are updated periodically throughout treatment. It is important to evaluate medical conditions, allergies, medications, previous hospitalizations or traumatic injuries, history of alcoholism and substance abuse, mental status, and attitude toward treatment. Allergies to nickel, latex, and antibiotics and other drugs should be prominently noted in the chart to prevent adverse sequelae that may result from orthodontic treatment. Such information can help the clinician determine at a future time whether gingival hyperplasia is the result of a drug side effect, hormones, or a third cause such as poor oral hygiene. Likewise, if a patient requires antibiotic prophylaxis, that should be documented. The physician's recommendations about conditions that potentially may affect orthodontic treatment should be obtained.

The clinical examination includes general observation of the patient's gait, speech, respiration, function of the temporomandibular joints (TMJs), hands, ears, skin, facial motion, symmetry, skull shape, oral health, and behavior. It is easy to rely on photography to document the patient for future assessment and limit the direct examination of the patient. However, many findings are not visible in photographs, particularly those that are found by palpation or probing or that relate to function. For example, periodontal pockets, dental interferences, and TMJ noises cannot be observed in photographs.

Diagnosis is a four-dimensional puzzle in which time serves as the fourth dimension. Determining the timing of treatment may be especially difficult in young patients who have complex medical conditions since dental age, skeletal age, and chronological age all may differ. Height, weight, skeletal maturity, dental maturity, and emotional development should be assessed to form the basis for clinical judgments. Some typical timing-related decisions are whether primary teeth should be extracted to promote tooth eruption and whether early surgery should be performed for psychosocial reasons with the expectation that it may need to be repeated at a later time.

The radiographs and computed tomography (CT) scans necessary for evaluation of the patient are ordered, while at the same time care is taken to minimize the patient's exposure to x-ray radiation. If abnormal growth is suspected, as in condylar hyperplasia, a bone scan may be requested from the nuclear medicine department of the hospital. Other diagnostic tests that may be needed include blood samples, microbiology cultures, magnetic resonance imaging, three-dimensional laser surface scans, and so forth. Ordinary cephalometric radiographs may be used to evaluate areas beyond the jaws, such as the spinal column.[1]

Photographs are used for documentation, patient education, and communication with other providers and insurance carriers and for reference during surgical procedures. An important application of photography is its use in evaluating the patient's esthetic expectations. Some practitioners draw on an enlarged photograph of the patient to point out problems or indicate areas of concern. Others use digital photography and computer imaging to manipulate an image of the patient's face for the purpose of demonstrating potential changes that may result from various orthodontic or surgical maneuvers. These imaging procedures must be conducted with great care because the results can be so realistic that the patient might regard them as predictions of the treatment result. The changes preferred by the patient cannot be guaranteed and indeed may not be possible at all. Patients must realize that photographs are used primarily for documentation, education, and communication. Orthodontic patients find imaging beneficial for understanding the magnitude of their skeletal disharmonies and how orthodontic masking or camouflage procedures affect facial appearance.

Computer morphing software has been developed as a means for patients to express an esthetic preference.[2] Patients watch a series of changing images, similar to a slow-motion movie (Fig 11-1), and indicate which ones they consider most pleasing and a range of acceptability by clicking a button on a computer mouse. The computer records the choices for use by the clinician. Thus, patients can communicate their preferences to the clinician, but the clinician does not risk making an "implied guarantee." If the patient's preferences are not realistic, then referral of the patient for learning coping strategies may be beneficial. Another use of photographs is for determining the patient's level of acceptable risk. Some clinicians show pre- and post-operative photos demonstrating a range of results including good, average, and those with potential complications. However, viewing a

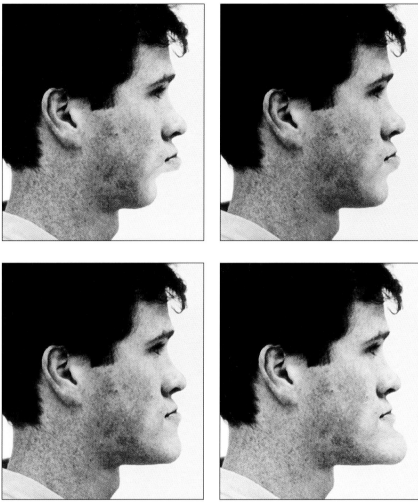

Fig 11-1 Morphing software can be used by clinicians to acquire information about patient preferences.

clinician's work has become less common now that privacy regulations limit the unauthorized use of photographs and other elements of the patient chart. Likewise, since technology permits misuse, it is difficult for a patient to know for certain if the images viewed are authentic.

The diagnostic phase of treatment planning can be both lengthy and costly. When the patient has a complex medical condition, a comprehensive, accurate diagnosis may evolve only after multiple consultations with many specialists and extensive interviewing of the patient. Ultimately, the level of orthodontic intervention is based on many physical, functional, and psychosocial considerations. For patient convenience and to facilitate communication between specialists, treatment teams have been formed for the more common craniofacial disorders, such as cleft lip/palate and craniofacial pain. Team members for cleft lip/palate typically include the orthodontist, plastic surgeon, pediatrician, speech and hearing specialists, pediatric dentist, prosthodontist, psychologist, social worker, etc, all of whom work together to provide coordinated long-term treatment. The orthodontist who works alone and tries to "save the patient money" by skipping necessary consultations may miss important diagnostic findings. Similarly, restrictions imposed on patients by insurance companies may limit the patient's access to clinical expertise.

Common deficiencies in diagnosis are missed diagnoses and errors in diagnosis. The busy practitioner who overlooks or minimizes diagnostic findings may underestimate the seriousness of medical conditions or propose flawed treatment plans. Complex conditions require considerable knowledge and education about medical conditions, more than the single practitioner is likely to have. Documentation from other specialists about diagnostic findings and their treatment recommendations, including dated notes taken during telephone conversations, should become part of the patient's permanent record. When lack of insurance or personal funds for adjunctive appointments jeopardizes the patient's access to needed information, the orthodontist is placed in a precarious position. It may be a serious mistake to place brackets and bands without first having a comprehensive overall plan.

Prognosis

The problem list generated during the diagnostic phase of treatment planning should be comprehensive and accurate. Whether a specific problem actually warrants treatment depends on the nature of the chief complaints, therapeutic modifiability of the problem, the risks of treatment, and its cost in terms of both time and finances. Therapeutic modifiability refers to the likelihood that the problem can be changed as desired with treatment. Some problems, such as restoration of caries, can be addressed predictably. Others, such as a short upper lip, most speech disorders, and chronic disease status, are not changed easily.

Some limitations affecting prognosis are related to the status of the local periodontal tissues, such as those accompanying advanced periodontal disease, previous traumatic damage to teeth, and gingival recession. In amelogenesis imperfecta (Fig 11-2), the poor quality of the enamel prevents conventional bonding of attachments to the teeth; instead, cemented bands and modified appliances are placed when orthodontic tooth movement is desired and skeletal fixation

methods are used for orthognathic surgery fixation. In congenital tooth agenesis (Fig 11-3), closing spaces to reduce the need for prosthodontic replacement of the missing teeth may flatten the profile and narrow the dental arches. Palatal scars such as those in clefts may limit expansion and make it less stable as well as limit the amount of surgical maxillary advancement possible because of safety concerns having to do with blood supply. Severely scarred palatal tissue may be an indication for maxillary osteodistraction when surgical advancement of the maxilla is required so that the tissue can be stretched gradually without jeopardizing the blood supply. Patients who have severe facial and oral burns may have similar limited adaptability of soft tissues and high risks for relapse. Electrical burns of the mouth can limit access to the oral cavity, requiring dental impressions to be taken in segments and the use of modified orthodontic appliances.

Recent evidence attributes some of the risk for orthodontic root resorption to genetic causes. In human patients, linkage of a chromosome 18 marker has been demonstrated.[3] Variability of root resorption between eight different inbred mouse strains also shows that genotype is a factor in the amount of root resorption occurring in response to orthodontic forces.[4] Some mouse strains are relatively resistant to root resorption and others are relatively susceptible. Likewise, idiopathic short roots are found in some Hispanics native to Mexico (unpublished data).

As medical treatment for systemic diseases improves, more patients seek quality of life improvements of the sort available through orthodontic treatment.[5] Some general concepts and precautions apply when considering orthodontic treatment for medically compromised patients. Since many conditions and/or their medical therapy are accompanied by susceptibility to infection, xerostomia, and depressed immune status, the orthodontist should take care to monitor periodontal health (Fig 11-4) and avoid using appliances that irritate the gingival or oral mucosa. Oral diseases should be treated before initiating orthodontic treatment (Fig 11-5). If orthognathic surgery is considered, anesthetic risks should be managed carefully. With careful planning and execution, most patients with medical conditions can undergo orthodontic treatment. A basic understanding of disease processes,

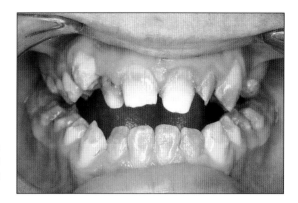

Fig 11-2 At best, brackets bond weakly to teeth in amelogenesis imperfecta. For tooth movement, teeth are banded; for surgical procedures, skeletal fixation is applied.

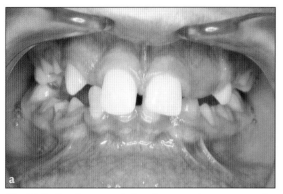

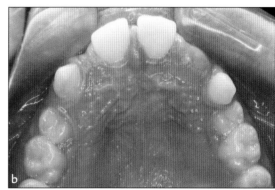

Fig 11-3 Tooth agenesis is a feature of many genetic syndromes.

access to a good library, and capable medical colleagues are basic requirements for providing orthodontic treatment to medically compromised patients. If the prognosis is uncertain, it is best to select a treatment plan that allows an early exit if needed. When patient responses to conventional treatment are unusual, the experienced practitioner will consider systemic disease as a possible cause.

Many conditions may already present in a patient seeking orthodontic treatment or may arise during orthodontic treatment, such as:

- Immunologic disorders
- Diseases of the blood and blood-forming organs
- Diseases of the respiratory system
- Nutritional and digestive disorders
- Disorders of the skin and subcutaneous tissues
- Disorders of the musculoskeletal system and connective tissues

- Endocrine and metabolic disorders
- Congenital anomalies, including genetic and acquired disorders

All of these categories may involve the craniofacial region. Some conditions or their treatment may increase patients' susceptibility to infection or carry degenerative and inflammatory risks. Generally, patients having medical conditions should not be denied orthodontic treatment, which can improve their lives greatly. A few conditions will be discussed in this chapter to illustrate management principles.

Mentally retarded children have a higher prevalence of severe malocclusion than physically handicapped or healthy control groups.[6–8] Down syndrome, trisomy 21, occurs in approximately 0.1% of births.[9] Most people with Down syndrome have a malocclusion, and many seek orthodontic treatment to help them integrate better into their school and work envi-

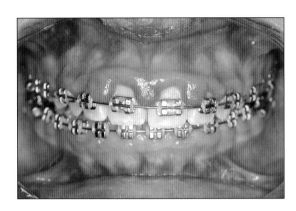

Fig 11-4 Even if patients are compulsive about oral hygiene, medications may cause gingival enlargement and may complicate orthodontic treatment.

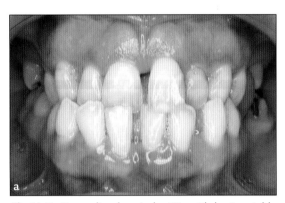
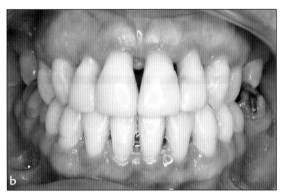

Fig 11-5 Generalized periodontitis with horizontal bone loss was treated before orthodontic treatment began.

ronments. For example, those who develop mitral valve prolapse require antibiotic prophylaxis for dental treatment. Immune characteristics include a reduced number of T cells, susceptibility to infection, and a high rate of periodontal disease. Mouth breathing also affects gingivitis, periodontal disease, fissured tongue, and halitosis. Muscle tone causes chewing problems, and abnormal tongue posture contributes to anterior open bite, Class III malocclusion, and sleep apnea. The eruption of teeth may be delayed by 2 or 3 years, and the teeth may have small conical roots. Oral hygiene must be strongly enforced.

Among the neurologic disorders influencing orthodontic therapy are epilepsy, Parkinson disease, and spinal cord injury. The diagnosis of epilepsy is of concern in orthodontic treatment. First, dilantin hyperplasia causes gingival overgrowth.[10,11] Also, seizures may lead to damage to protruding teeth[12] or aspiration of retainers.[13] Motor disorders such as Parkinson disease

and spinal cord injury must be considered in determining the level of compliance that can be expected of patients.

The neurofibromatoses are genetic disorders causing tumors of neural cells and leading to skin changes and bone abnormalities.[14] Craniofacial tumors may cause headaches, facial pain, facial numbness, loss of vision, and tinnitus, and may be disfiguring. Treatment is oriented toward controlling symptoms and may include surgical interventions. Sometimes, orthodontic consultations are sought regarding disturbances of the dental occlusion.

Diseases of bone are not common in orthodontic patients but are important to consider when planning orthodontic treatment. Conditions such as fibrous dysplasia,[15,16] osteogenesis imperfecta,[17] sclerosis, bone metabolism–altering thyroid diseases, and osteoporosis in postmenopausal women can complicate orthodontic treatment and affect prognosis. Fibrous dyspla-

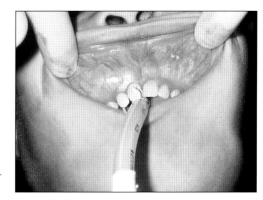

Fig 11-6 A patient with Paget disease undergoing surgical reduction of the enlarged maxilla.

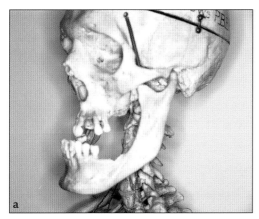

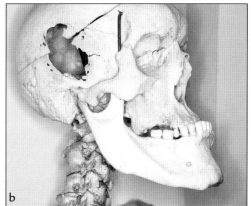

Fig 11-7 Two acromegalic skulls. (Courtesy of the Warren Museum, Harvard University.)

sia[15] and cherubism[16] lead to abnormal development of fibrous tissue, expansion deformities of bone, and sometimes pain, usually in children and young adults. McCune-Albright syndrome, a form of fibrous dysplasia, causes early onset of puberty and the formation of café-au-lait spots. A genetic basis for cherubism has been reported.[16]

A particularly poor prognosis accompanies Paget disease (osteitis deformans), which affects bone metabolism in adults and features abnormal osteoclasts (Fig 11-6).[18,19] Following osteoporosis, it is the most common bone disorder in individuals 50 years and older. When it occurs in the skull and jaws, characteristics of Paget disease include stages of excessive bone resorption followed by excessive formation of structurally disorganized bone, bone enlargement, deep severe bone pain, loosening of the teeth, nerve compression, and altered sensation, as well as headaches and loss of hearing.

Changes in jaw position may result from typical forms of unfavorable growth patterns in normal children as well as certain systemic and local diseases. Mandibular overgrowth is a feature found in acromegaly[20-23] (Fig 11-7) and condylar hyperplasia.[24] For both conditions, medical treatment of the disorder should be instituted as quickly as possible. Treatment of acromegaly involves halting the overproduction of growth hormone, either by radiation or through surgical approaches to the pituitary gland. That some acromegalics have sleep apnea is important to consider when planning treatment for their jaw disharmonies. Condylar hyperplasia is treated by removing the hyperplastic condylar cartilage. If the asymmetry accompanying condylar hyperplasia involves canting of the occlusal plane and compensation of the teeth, a surgical orthodontic plan involving both jaws is warranted. Juvenile rheumatoid arthritis (JRA)[25] and other degenerative conditions such as condylysis[26]

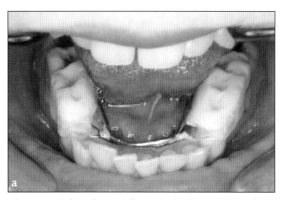
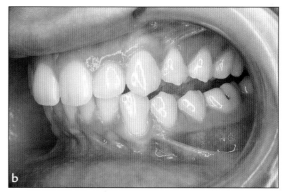

Fig 11-8 Splint therapy for TMJ dysfunction resulted in unwanted tooth movement.

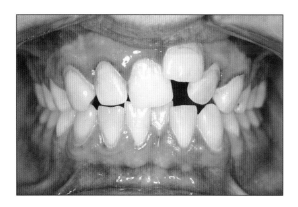

Fig 11-9 Trauma to the maxillary left central incisor at age 7 caused ankylosis; the tooth was left behind as the other teeth erupted to maintain occlusion as the face grew in height.

may be associated with progressive retrusion and open rotation of the mandible with the development of anterior open bite. Since effective treatment is not available, reconstruction of juvenile rheumatoid arthritis or condylysis is usually delayed until the degenerative condition stabilizes. Malocclusion in genetic syndromes such as achondroplasia[27,28] has been treated successfully.

There are more than 200 disorders of connective tissues linked to genetic mutations, including Ehler-Danlos syndrome, Marfan syndrome, epidermolysis bullosa, and various types of osteogenesis imperfecta. Some Marfan syndrome patients have transverse maxillary deficiency, anterior open bite, crowding, positive overjet, and early maturation.[29,30] Adolescent growth velocity was shown to peak more than 2 years prematurely in male and female Marfan patients com-

pared to a gender-matched general population. The genetic mutation involves fibrillin-1 and affects microfibrils, resulting in overgrowth of long bones and aortic dilatation. Orthodontic and orthognathic treatment are possible with medical management of vascular abnormalities and attention to gingival hyperplasia.

Chronic pain problems, such as fibromyalgia[31] and reflex sympathetic dystrophy/complex pain syndrome,[32] can interfere with orthodontic treatment. In reflex sympathetic dystrophy, for example, the constant, severe, burning pain can be disabling. Therapy may consist of physiotherapy, drugs, nerve blocks, hydrotherapy, acupuncture, transcutaneous electrical nerve stimulation (TENS), and machine application, and should be directed by a team of specialists, including neurologists, rheumatologists, physiotherapists, and psychologists. At all times, the orthodontist should be alert to complaints of pain that are beyond the usual level, work with a pain team when needed, and provide understanding to affected patients.

Patients may seek orthodontic correction of malocclusion after splint therapy for TMJ dysfunction or other pain complaints. For example, posterior bite blocks produce a posterior open bite (Fig 11-8). Patients are then advised to seek orthodontic or prosthetic treatment to regain occlusal function. Selective grinding to reduce the thickness of the splint and allow targeted eruption of teeth usually resolves the open bite satisfactorily.

Many patients who have had previous trauma will seek orthodontic treatment. The consequences include potential nonvitality and root resorption of teeth. Orthodontists may find that traumatized teeth are ankylosed (Fig 11-9) and not amenable to orthodontic tooth movement.

Orthodontic treatment and orthognathic surgery are possible in patients who have bleeding disorders if they are controlled by replacement of missing clotting factors. Patients with sickle cell anemia may have anesthetic risks, however, because of poor blood oxygen saturation.[5]

Acute lymphoblastic leukemia, the most common form of childhood cancer, now has a survival rate of 80%.[33–37] The preponderance of lymphoblasts with this condition results in red blood cell anemia, bleeding problems, and infections. Spontaneous bleeding in the mouth also occurs. The disease is treated by chemotherapy, although radiation or bone marrow transplantation may be used in some instances. The oral complications of chemotherapy are very painful. Oral mucositis occurs because the usual rapid regeneration of oral mucosa does not occur. Also, decreased saliva and salivary antibodies permit microorganisms to proliferate, producing periodontal disease. In young children, the cytostatic drugs affect skull, jaw, and dental development. Dental infections and caries must be eliminated before chemotherapy, and orthodontic appliances and intraoral devices must be removed. Surviving children may subsequently undergo orthodontic treatment; however, if chemotherapy is given during development of teeth, malformed teeth with short roots can complicate orthodontic treatment due to microdontia and enamel hypoplasia. Similar effects on dental development and caries occur when bone marrow transplantation is the treatment for aplastic anemia or other disorders, or when radiation treatment is delivered for treatment of retinoblastoma.

As drug therapy improves, the number of HIV-positive patients seeking orthodontic treatment is increasing rapidly. Orthodontic treatment can be successful in these patients under the supervision of the patient's physician but requires alertness to the susceptibility to infection.

Autoimmune and degenerative diseases are particularly difficult to manage because they are so poorly understood. Multiple sclerosis,[38–40] a neurologic condition of unknown origin, affects motor and sensory nerve transmission and vision; causes facial pain or trigeminal neuralgia, facial palsy, and paresthesia of the feet, legs, and hands; and leads to progressive disability and fatigue. The medications cause dry mouth, and the disability may affect the patient's ability to maintain adequate oral hygiene and health. Systemic lupus erythematosis[41–44] is a chronic autoimmune disease associated with joint and muscle pain, weakness, skin rashes, and in more severe cases, heart, lung, kidney, and nervous system problems. Treatment for lupus is symptom-dependent and may include aspirin, rest, steroids, and anti-inflammatory and other drugs, as well as dialysis and high blood pressure medication. Polymyositis is an inflammation of muscles treated with corticosteroids and immunosuppressants; symptoms include weakness, pain, and sometimes difficulty breathing and swallowing.[45]

Destruction of the TMJ in juvenile rheumatoid arthritis leads to mandibular retrusion, Class II malocclusion, anterior open bite, and a steep mandibular plane.[46,47] These changes may occur unexpectedly during routine orthodontic treatment if the condition flares up. Orthodontists should be alert to occurrences of abnormal growth. If it occurs, they should notify the patient and family and revise the course of treatment. Methotrexate has been suggested to minimize the potential for facial deformity in juvenile rheumatoid arthritis.

In Romberg syndrome,[48–50] patients experience progressive hemifacial atrophy with slow loss of subcutaneous fat and atrophy of skin, cartilage, connective tissue, muscle, and bone within the first decade. Both onset and cessation are spontaneous, and the condition eventually stabilizes. Dental effects include a decrease in mandibular ramus size, delayed eruption of teeth on the affected side, atrophic dental roots, canting of the occlusal plane, and malocclusion. After the condition stabilizes, orthodontic treatment may be involved in the reconstruction along with orthognathic surgery and surgical procedures for facial augmentation. The etiology of Romberg syndrome is unknown. Many different opinions have been expressed about a possible link to linear scleroderma localized to the face, although elastic tissue is preserved in Romberg syndrome. Other differential diagnoses of facial asymmetry include the effects of radiotherapy and fibrous dysplasia. It is distinguished from hemifacial microsomia by its acquired origin.

Lack of saliva and increased risk of oral infections, including caries, is characteristic of Sjögren syndrome, a common inflammatory disorder that affects mucous membranes throughout the body.[51] The cause is unknown, but it is most common in women over 50 years of age. Treatment with lubricants and saliva stimulants addresses the symptoms of dry eyes and dry mouth, respectively.

Pemphigus vulgaris, an autoimmune condition affecting the skin, begins as blisters in the mouth and is treated with immunosuppressive drugs.[52] It occurs in approximately 1 in 100,000 people usually between the ages of 40 and 60 years. The oral lesions can lead to dehydration and weight loss. When treating these patients, it is important to avoid using any sharp-ended orthodontic appliances.

Successful treatment of malocclusion has been documented for many syndromes and medical conditions, including Turner,[53] Aarskog,[54] and Apert[55] syndromes, as well as epidemolysis bullosa,[56] amelogenesis imperfecta,[57] and cystic fibrosis.[58,59] The consistent themes in these reports are thoroughness and caution. Particularly for those with chronic conditions, treatment may be timed for a period of remission. If a serious disease begins during orthodontic treatment, the appliances may be inactivated or removed as necessary.

In complex patients, efforts should be made to avoid lengthy continuous treatment and minimize the length of each phase of treatment. For example, orthognathic surgery procedures such as alveolar segmental osteotomies may be introduced to expedite movements of blocks of teeth. Surgical risks such as gingival defects (Fig 11-10), transsected roots (Fig 11-11), and fixation problems (Fig 11-12) can be minimized by working out the details of the intervention far in advance, maintaining open lines of communication with the other clinicians involved, and aligning the teeth properly during the orthodontic phase. Also, treatment alternatives such as prosthetics should be considered. The retention phase should address the potential for post-treatment relapse and adaptations, particularly when the initial etiology, eg, a large tongue, has not been eliminated. Likewise, orthodontic and orthognathic surgical procedures are possible in patients with vascular malformations,[60] but retention is difficult (Fig 11-13). Fixed and permanent retainers should be considered.

Sometimes, orthodontic appliances are involved in the treatment of systemic disorders. For example, orthodontic preparation for distraction osteogenesis of the maxilla and mandible may be sought for the treatment of sleep apnea.[61,62] Moving the jaws forward may be effective for increasing the volume of the nasopharynx and oropharynx as an alternative to tracheostomy in severe cases.

Oral appliances are also being advocated for improving general motor coordination in cerebral palsy.[63–65] Drooling and poor feeding skills are major problems. Drooling is caused not by the production of too much saliva, but rather because the patient does not swallow properly. Although short-term improvement has been noted with the Innsbruck Sensorimotor Activator and Regulator, 1-year follow-up reports show the same degree of improvement in children wearing the activator as in those who are allowed to mature without intervention.

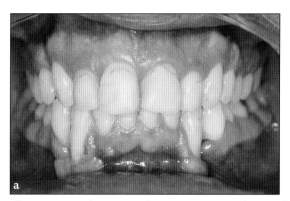
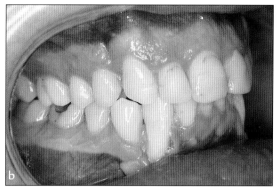

Fig 11-10 Less-than-optimal tissue contours and gingival defects after a mandibular anterior segmental osteotomy.

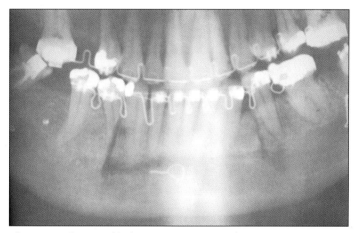

Fig 11-11 The mandibular anterior segmental osteotomy transsected a premolar root. The tooth remained vital.

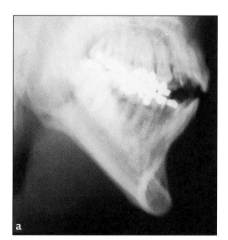
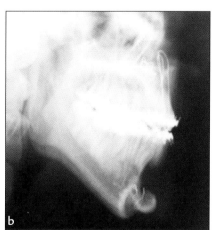
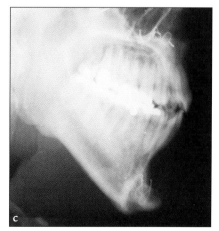

Fig 11-12 Iatrogenic displacement of mandibular incisor roots during intermaxillary fixation. (a) Before treatment, mandibular incisor roots were positioned within the alveolar process. (b) During intermaxillary fixation, heavy elastic force caused marked labial movement of the mandibular incisor roots outside the bone. (c) When the vertical elastics were removed from the anterior teeth, the roots recovered and the teeth remained vital.

Fig 11-13 Orthodontic treatment in the presence of a vascular malformation of the left face.

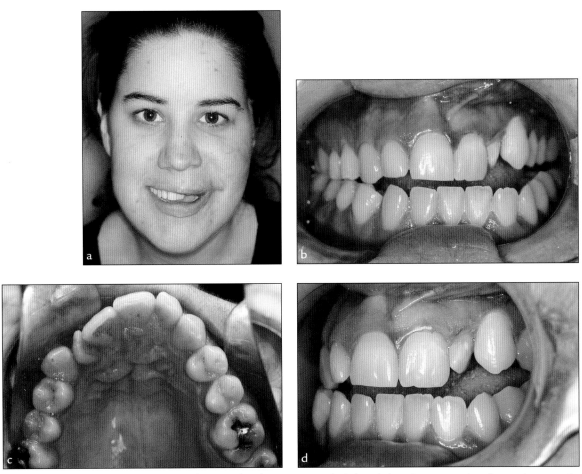

Figs 11-13a to 11-13d Pretreatment photographs demonstrating facial and dental asymmetries due to the mass in the left face.

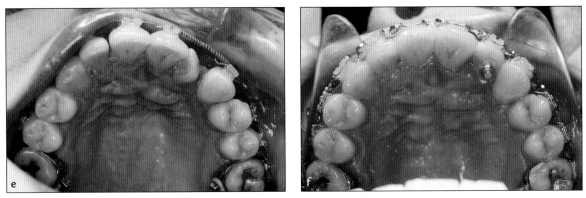

Figs 11-13e and 11-13f Alignment of the maxillary teeth after surgically assisted expansion following osteotomies to facilitate more expansion on the left than on the right.

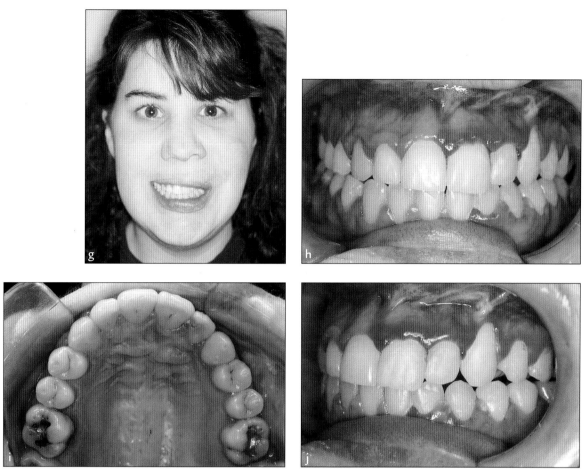

Figs 11-13g to 11-13j Localized gingival recession was present after completion of treatment and removal of the appliances. Permanent long-term retention was required.

Compliance

Compliance begins with patient education. Successful orthodontic treatment requires that patients and their families participate in the treatment; they must understand the procedures and what is expected of them. Today, families are stressed by day-to-day problems associated with jobs, school, and social predicaments. Family stability should be assessed; if it is found to be inconsistent, orthodontic treatment may have a low priority. Orthodontists can help their patients adopt healthy lifestyles by emphasizing excellent oral health care and educating them about healthy diets along with the dangers of tobacco, alcohol, and drug abuse.

Such an educational program should be sufficiently thorough that patients have realistic expectations about the treatment process and outcome. Prospective patients who maintain unrealistic expectations even after a discussion of treatment limitations and risks should not start treatment because they are likely to be disappointed. The orthodontist should use carefully chosen language in presenting treatment options.

Rather than saying that the treatment will "correct" a problem, one should use the word "improve." Rather than "eliminate" lip incompetence, use the word "reduce." Although most clinicians make it clear that revisions may be needed in the future, it is not commonly discussed during orthodontic consultations.

Alternative treatments should be considered when optimal compliance cannot be expected. Mental retardation and physical limitations that are found in conditions such as Down syndrome or cerebral palsy should not eliminate orthodontics as a treatment option for those patients, but the treatment must be designed around the limitations of the patient. For example, the spasticity of cerebral palsy does not infer low learning potential, but rather lack of motor control. It may be possible to place molar bands and bond brackets in the operating room at the same time that some other procedure is being performed. Also, family members may become actively involved in maintaining oral hygiene, or appliances may be chosen for their ease of insertion or attachment.

The uncooperative patient's orthodontic care should be terminated as quickly as possible. Every practice should have a structured dismissal program to deal with such patients. In addition, compliance in seeking adjunctive consultations or treatments should also be enforced. Requests for additional treatments or consultations should be written, documented in the patient record, and followed up. Many problems can be avoided by having written treatment requests and documented follow-up notes.

Sometimes, planning treatment in phases or stages will optimize compliance. For example, in the treatment of cleft lip/palate, care is provided in discrete steps with treatment-free periods between interventions. Even so, the treatment is lengthy, in terms of both number of appointments and duration of individual appointments. Providing treatment in steps also helps match fees with the overall degree of difficulty. When treatment is planned in stages, parents will realize that it is not appropriate to charge only the typical adolescent fee for multiphase complex treatments. When the prognosis of a stage is not clear, it is important to emphasize the likely need for re-evaluations and/or revisions when obtaining the informed consent.

Strategies for the Orthodontist

The standard of care in orthodontics for patients with medical issues is similar to that for the typical orthodontic patient. The practitioner must employ the same reasonable amount of skill and sound judgment as would other careful orthodontic specialists. Even so, some orthodontists refer patients with complex conditions to another practice because their management style makes it difficult to develop the necessary level of interaction with other professionals or to spend adequate time directly with the patient. Orthodontists who accept complex patients, however, should establish team-style working relationships with other clinicians before accepting very complex patients. Orthodontists should help patients understand that the choice of provider should not be made on the basis of location or cost alone. Patients should be aware of differences between providers in terms of their abilities and interest in managing complex problems.

Diagnosis and record keeping make a difference. Documentation consists not only of reports and notes, but also of the office operating procedures. A quality-assurance program is essential to make sure that careful and detailed records are routinely taken whenever appropriate. The orthodontist should not delegate responsibility for any portion of the clinical exam or diagnosis because a missed diagnosis could have adverse consequences on treatment outcome. Failure to detect an anomaly on a radiograph, or the misinterpretation of symptoms reported by the patient can lead to inappropriate treatment.

While the overall goal of orthodontic treatment is to provide high-quality, comprehensive treatment, the clinician may need to modify the treatment plan depending on the patient's condition. The orthodontist should be flexible and practical with the intent of minimizing iatrogenic sequelae. High-risk or high-relapse treatment plans should be presented as having a poor prognosis, and alternative treatments with better prognoses should be suggested.

The effective specialist detects adverse outcomes early. When treatment is not going as expected, the orthodontist must take time to reassess the problem.

Progress, whether good or poor, is reported to the patient without delay. Ongoing communication is important and includes listening to the patient's responses and concerns.

Research, education, and health legislation can improve the treatment available to patients. Orthodontists should promote well-designed research about treatment outcomes as well as publish their own experiences so others can improve their clinical skills. Education about medical conditions that may complicate orthodontic treatment should be included in orthodontic specialty training programs and also offered to practicing clinicians because all clinicians should be continual learners. Orthodontists should work with lawmakers to legislate funds for comprehensive health care because, at present, resources available to patients from third-party sources—namely government, insurance, and charities—are inadequate.

In summary, the orthodontist is obliged to:

1. Document that patients and families have been educated about the benefits of treatment, the associated risks, and treatment alternatives by having signed informed consents in the patient records
2. Implement behavioral strategies for both patients and parents so that treatment will progress as smoothly as possible
3. Recognize that failure to refer or to order necessary tests may have adverse consequences for the patient and the practitioner
4. Take time to re-evaluate the progress of treatment
5. Check that recommendations made by other clinicians have been followed
6. Document conversations and other communications with third parties in the treatment record
7. Explain disappointing outcomes and mistakes to the patient as soon as possible
8. Encourage second opinions
9. Recognize that therapy for patients with medical conditions is team treatment.

References

1. Vastardis H, Evans CA. Evaluation of cervical spine abnormalities on cephalometric radiographs. Am J Orthod Dentofacial Orthop 1996;109:581–588.
2. Arpino V, Giddon DB, BeGole EA, Evans CA. Presurgical profile preferences of patients and clinicians. Am J Orthod Dentofacial Orthop 1998;114:631–637.
3. Al-Qawasmi RA, Hartsfield JK Jr, Everett ET, Flury L, Liu L, Foroud TM, et al. Genetic predisposition to external apical root resorption in orthodontic patients: Linkage of chromosome-18 marker. J Dent Res 2003;82:356–360.
4. Al-Qawasmi RA, Hartsfield JK Jr, Everett ET, Flury LL, Liu L, Foroud TM, Roberts WE. Variable root resorption associated with orthodontic force among inbred mouse strains. J Dent Res 2003;82A:1189.
5. van Venrooy JR, Proffit WR. Orthodontic care for medically compromised patients: Possibilities and limitations. J Am Dent Assoc 1979;99:181–184.
6. Oreland A, Heijbel J, Jagell S. Malocclusions in physically and/or mentally handicapped children. Swed Dent J 1987;11:103–119.
7. Vittek J, Winik S, Winik A, Sioris C, Tarangelo AM, Chou M. Analysis of orthodontic anomalies in mentally retarded developmentally disabled (MRDD) persons. Spec Care Dentist 1994;14:198–202.
8. Taner T, Uzamis M. Orthodontic treatment of a patient with multiple supernumerary teeth and mental retardation. J Clin Pediatr Dent 1999;23:195–200.
9. Pilcher ES. Dental care for the patient with Down Syndrome. Down Syndrome Res Pract 1998;5:111–116.
10. Vandersall DC, Slade D. Periodontic/orthodontic management of diphenylhydantoin gingival hyperplasia: Case report. J Periodontol 1976;47:656–660.
11. Cunat JJ, Ciancio SG. Diphenylhydantoin sodium: Gingival hyperplasia and orthodontic treatment. Angle Orthod 1969;39:182–185.
12. Tsai TP. Extraction as a treatment alternative follows repeated trauma in a severely handicapped patient. Dent Traumatol 2001;17:139–142.
13. Klein AM, Schoem SR. Unrecognized aspiration of a dental retainer: A case report. Otolaryngol Head Neck Surg 2002;126:438–439.
14. Reynolds RM, Browning GG, Nawroz I, Campbell IW. Von Recklinghausen's neurofibromatosis: Neurofibromatosis type 1. Lancet 2003;361:1552–1554.
15. MacDonald-Jankowski D. Fibrous dysplasia in the jaws of a Hong Kong population: Radiographic presentation and systematic review. Dentomaxillofac Radiol 1999;28:195–202.
16. Lo B, Faiyaz-Ul-Haque M, Kennedy S, Aviv R, Tsui LC, Teebi AS. Novel mutation in the gene encoding c-Abl-binding protein SH3BP2 causes cherubism. Am J Med Genet 2003;15;121A:37–40.

17. Prince SE, Simpson MT. Osteogenesis imperfecta. Br J Oral Maxillofac Surg 2000;38:399–400. Comment in: Br J Oral Maxillofac Surg 2001;39:407.

18. Keen RW. The current status of Paget's disease. Hosp Med 2003;64:230–232.

19. Krane SM. Genetic control of bone remodeling—insights from a rare disease. N Engl J Med 2002;347:210–212.

20. Dostalova S, Sonka K, Smahel Z, Weiss V, Marek J. Cephalometric assessment of cranial abnormalities in patients with acromegaly. J Craniomaxillofac Surg 2003; 31:80–87.

21. Hochban W, Ehlenz K, Conradt R, Brandenburg U. Obstructive sleep apnoea in acromegaly: The role of craniofacial changes. Eur Respir J 1999;14:196–202.

22. Takakura M, Kuroda T. Morphologic analysis of dentofacial structure in patients with acromegaly. Int J Adult Orthodont Orthognath Surg 1998;13:277–288.

23. Chung KC, Buchman SR, Aly HM, Trotman CA. Use of modern craniofacial techniques for comprehensive reconstruction of the acromegalic face. Ann Plast Surg 1996; 36:403–408; discussion 408–409.

24. Bertolini F, Bianchi B, De Riu G, Di Blasio A, Sesenna E. Hemimandibular hyperplasia treated by early high condylectomy: A case report. Int J Adult Orthodont Orthognath Surg 2001;16:227–234.

25. Kjellberg H. Craniofacial growth in juvenile chronic arthritis. Acta Odontol Scand 1998;56:360–365.

26. Haers PE, Sailer HF. Mandibular resorption due to systemic sclerosis. Case report of surgical correction of a secondary open bite deformity. Int J Oral Maxillofac Surg 1995;24:261–267.

27. Dunbar JP, Goldin B, Subtelny JD. An American Board of Orthodontics case report. Correction of Class I crowding in an achondroplastic patient. Am J Orthod Dentofacial Orthop 1989;96:255–263.

28. Ohba T, Ohba Y, Tenshin S, Takano-Yamamoto T. Orthodontic treatment of Class II division 1 malocclusion in a patient with achondroplasia. Angle Orthod 1998;68: 377–382.

29. Erkula G, Jones KB, Sponseller PD, Dietz HC, Pyeritz RE. Growth and maturation in Marfan Syndrome. Am J Med Gen 2002;109:100–115.

30. Westling L, Mohlin B, Bresin A. Craniofacial manifestations in the Marfan syndrome: Palatal dimensions and a comparative cephalometric analysis. J Craniofacial Genet Dev Biol 1998;18:211–218.

31. Rhodos NL, Fricton J, Carlson P, Messner R. Oral symptoms associated with fibromyalgia syndrome. J Rheumatol 2003;30:1841–1845.

32. Wasner G, Schattschneider J, Binder A, Baron R. Complex regional pain syndrome—Diagnostic, mechanisms, CNS involvement and therapy. Spinal Cord 2003;41:61–75.

33. Oeffinger KC, Eshelman DA, Tomlinson GE, Tolle M, Schneider GW. Providing primary care for long-term survivors of childhood acute lymphoblastic leukemia. J Fam Pract 2000;49:1133–1146.

34. Massler CF. Preventing and treating the oral complications of cancer therapy. Gen Dent 2000;48:652–655.

35. Näsman M, Björk O, Söderhäll S, Ringdén O, Dahllöf G. Disturbances in the oral cavity in pediatric long-term survivors after different forms of antineoplastic therapy. Pediatr Dent 1994;16:217–223.

36. Näsman M, Forsberg CM, Dahllöf G. Long-term dental development in children after treatment for malignant disease. Eur J Orthod 1997;19:151–159.

37. Runge ME, Edwards DL. Orthodontic treatment for an adolescent with a history of acute lymphoblastic leukemia. Pediatr Dent 2000;22:494–498.

38. Fiske J, Griffiths J, Thompson S. Multiple sclerosis and oral care. Dent Update 2002;29:273–283.

39. Chemaly D, Lefrancois A, Perusse R. Oral and maxillofacial manifestations of multiple sclerosis. J Can Dent Assoc 2000;66:600–605.

40. Symons AL, Bortolanza M, Godden S, Seymour G. A preliminary study into the dental health status of multiple sclerosis patients. Spec Care Dentist 1993;13:96–101.

41. De Rossi SS, Glick M. Lupus erythematosus: Considerations for dentistry. J Am Dent Assoc 1998;129:330–339.

42. Romanides N, Marulli RD. Lupus erythematosus in an orthodontic patient. J Clin Orthod 1999;33:451–452.

43. Carrel R, Anderson R, Jackson T, Slawek S. Systemic lupus erythematosus: A teenage patient. J Clin Pediatr Dent 1990;15:55–59.

44. Hughes CT, Downey MC, Winkley GP. Systemic lupus erythematosus: A review for dental professionals. J Dent Hyg 1998;72:35–40.

45. Van Der Meulen MF, Bronner IM, Hoogendijk JE, et al. Polymyositis: An overdiagnosed entity. Neurology 2003; 61:316–321.

46. Kjellberg H, Kiliaridis S, Thilander B. Dentofacial growth in orthodontically treated and untreated children with juvenile chronic arthritis (JCA). A comparison with Angle Class II division 1 subjects. Eur J Orthod 1995;17: 357–373.

47. Ince DO, Ince A, Moore TL. Effect of methotrexate on the temporomandibular joint and facial morphology in juvenile rheumatoid arthritis patients. Am J Orthod Dentofacial Orthop 2000;118:75–83.

48. Pensler JM, Murphy GF, Mulliken JB. Clinical and ultrastructural studies of Romberg's hemifacial atrophy. Plast Reconstr Surg 1990;85:669–674.

49. Foster TD. The effect of hemifacial atrophy on dental growth. Br Dent J 1979;146:148–150.

50. Lehman TJ. The Parry Romberg syndrome of progressive facial atrophy and linear scleroderma en coup de saber. Mistaken diagnosis or overlapping condition? J Rheum 1992;19:844–845.

51. Steinfeld S, Simonart T. New approaches to the treatment of Sjögren's syndrome: Soon beyond symptomatic relief? Dermatology 2003;207:6–9.

52. Chan LS, Ahmed AR, Anhalt GJ, et al. The First International Consensus on Mucous Membrane Pemphigoid: Definition, diagnostic criteria, pathogenic factors, medical treatment, and prognostic indicators. Arch Dermatol 2002;138:370–379.

53. Vandewalle KS, Castro GW, Camm JH. Dental management of a patient with Turner syndrome. J Clin Pediatr Dent 1993;18:26–30.

54. Batra P, Kharbanda OP, Duggal R, Reddy P, Parkash H. Orthodontic treatment of a case of Aarskog syndrome J Clin Pediatr Dent 2003;27:229–233.

55. Rynearson RD. Case report: Orthodontic and dentofacial orthopedic considerations in Apert's syndrome. Angle Orthod 2000;70:247–252.

56. Goldschmied F. Orthodontic management of a patient with epidermolysis bullosa. Aust Orthod J 1999;15:302–307.

57. Rosenblum SH. Restorative and orthodontic treatment of an adolescent patient with amelogenesis imperfecta. Pediatr Dent 1999;21:289–292.

58. Kneezel RC, Tilghman DM. Orthognathic surgical correction of a dentofacial deformity in a patient with cystic fibrosis. J Oral Maxillofac Surg 1990;48:499–502.

59. Patel L, Dixon M, David TJ. Growth and growth charts in cystic fibrosis. J R Soc Med 2003;96 (Suppl43):35–41.

60. Mulliken JB, Young AE. Vascular Birthmarks, Hemangiomas, and Malformations. Philadelphia: WB Saunders, 1988.

61. Cohen SR, Holmes RE, Machado L, Magit A. Surgical strategies in the treatment of complex obstructive sleep apnoea in children. Paediatr Respir Rev 2002;3:25–35.

62. Cohen SR, Ross DA, Burstein FD, Lefaivre JF, Riski JE, Simms C. Skeletal expansion combined with soft-tissue reduction in the treatment of obstructive sleep apnea in children: Physiologic results. Otolaryngol Head Neck Surg 1998;119:476–485

63. Tahmassebi JF, Curzon ME. The cause of drooling in children with cerebral palsy—Hypersalivation or swallowing defect? Int J Pediatr Dent 2003;13:106–111.

64. Gisel EG, Haberfellner H, Schwartz S. Impact of oral appliance therapy: Are oral skills and growth maintained one year after termination of therapy? Dysphagia 2001; 16:296–307.

65. Gisel EG, Schwartz S, Haberfellner H. The Innsbruck Sensorimotor Activator and Regulator (ISMAR): Construction of an intraoral appliance to facilitate ingestive functions. J Dent Child 1999;66:180–187.

SECTION 2

Malpractice and Risk Management

Risk Management

Thomas M. Graber

The purpose of this section is to provide important information not only on patient protection, but also on malpractice litigation protection.

When I finished orthodontic specialty training a while back, the word "malpractice" was not even in our vocabulary. Today it is a different story. It has been a hobby of mine to testify in some of these cases; I find it exciting and challenging because the playing field is not level. The United States is fertile for litigation. However, other countries are not necessarily immune. In the lead article of the March 2001 issue of the *World Journal of Orthodontics*, Donald Woodside, eminent American Association of Orthodontics (AAO) leader from Toronto, reports on a local $4.4 million case award in litigation involving an orthodontist and an oral surgeon.[1] Malpractice litigation has become a worldwide phenomenon and continues to grow.

Recently, a *Chicago Dental Review* article entitled "Doctor, You Are Being Sued!" reported that the typical malpractice suit in Chicago lasts 2 or more years and is usually settled after significant trial prepara-

tion.[2] Since this article appeared, the risk management quicksand has become more treacherous. Elizabeth Franklin, claims manager for the AAO Insurance Company (AAOIC), says that about half of the cases filed are settled, and the other half go to court. You have about a 50% chance of defending yourself in such a suit because the jury is sympathetic to the poor patient, not the wealthy doctor and the successful insurance company. Because of potential jury bias, attorney David Thomas tells us elsewhere in this section, the job of defending someone is more difficult because the jury panel knows that the insurance company is going to take care of the cost. Mr Thomas has been highly successful in defending his clients, but nothing can repay you for the psychologic trauma that you suffer before, during, and after such an experience.

Rule number 1 about choosing your malpractice insurance company: These companies have become more cost conscious as a result of some astronomical awards, so make sure you have the ultimate decision to defend or settle your case. It is often much cheaper for the insurance company to settle the suit than to fight it, but your name then appears on the National Practitioner Data Bank, which should be avoided if at all possible.

Until 30 years ago, lawsuits were a last resort, but not anymore. We've seen one damage ceiling after another shattered. A recent *New York Times* editorial on silicone breast implants ("Trial by Science") and the class-action lawsuit by Marsha Angell, former editor of the venerable *New England Journal of Medicine*, provided a wake-up call.[3] The editorial states, "There is no scientific evidence that silicone implants cause any diseases at all in women." Nonetheless, the manufacturer paid out $2.5 billion dollars despite the fact that there was no evidence! The spurious claim of causing cancer could not be validated, but the jury still awarded $2.5 billion! The *New York Times* commented that this decision was a combination of greed, media sensationalism, judicial gullibility, and the cleverness of lawyers. The fact that the contingency-fee lawyers won is a kind of legal confiscation and obfuscation of several billion dollars, engineered by a gullible media, and a rejection of science.

For those of us in orthodontics, what we do may not be malpractice, but that does not mean a suit brought against us is going to come out in our favor. This section was written to let you know that there are ways to defend yourself. By the time you reach this part of the book, you should have a good idea of the potential iatrogenic sequelae in orthodontics. If you keep good records, follow the laws, and uphold the standard of care, your chances of being sued are infinitely reduced. As the Boy Scout motto says, "Be prepared!"

If, after serving as a defense expert in some 150 cases, I seem a bit biased, it's because I've seen so many things happen in which the dominant factor is a 5-letter word: *money*. (Others would substitute the word *greed*.) An extreme example is a recent tobacco case in Wisconsin. The plaintiff lawyers billed for 24,733 hours, most of it done by paralegals, at a rate of $3,782 per hour plus expenses![4] The irony is that even the defense attorneys who lost the case were amply paid, adding to the financial burden on the insurance companies.

In some of the cases in which I have been involved, the massive files, records, and depositions are a foot and a half thick. Too often, the records from many

orthodontists are not even half an inch thick, are incomplete, and/or are hard to decipher. Such problems are a magnet for contingency-fee lawyers. No doubt you've heard or seen their ads: "Sign right here. It won't cost you a penny. But if you win, you get two-thirds." Of course, by the time you pay the legal costs, it is far less. But it is still a lottery award for some patients.

There are many examples of this legal cancer, but I will cite only a couple. A Long Island hospital in New York was ordered to pay $40 million to a 39-year-old woman who lost a hand because of an IV needle that was improperly inserted during lung surgery. Sad for all concerned, except the lawyers. In Highland Park, Illinois, $21 million was awarded to a family because the doctor was late getting to the hospital when the child was being born and the child was later judged mentally retarded. The attorneys for the plaintiff blamed the late birth as the cause. Was it the cause? Inflation for a similar problem resulted in a payout of $35 million by Northwestern Memorial Hospital in early 2004.[4] The poor patient, the rich doctor, the rich hospital! Tragically, the public ultimately pays the doctor, who passes on the huge malpractice insurance premium.[5]

Like doctors, orthodontists have an affluent image, one that is likely to invite litigation. The public psychology is against us,[6] so you must protect yourself. The popular press has exposed this legal obfuscation with frequent articles, such as one that appeared in a recent issue of the *U.S. News and World Report*. The front cover showed the Statue of Liberty, the torch held high, with rats nibbling away at the statue base. As the legend below the figure stated, "The rats are no longer nibbling. They are devouring our very foundations!"[7] I have quite a collection of cartoons saying much the same thing.

As a result, malpractice premiums have skyrocketed, and insurance companies are suffering huge losses. In 2002, nine major companies stopped writing malpractice insurance because of their prodigious costs. St Paul Federal alone lost $1 billion, and some suits are still pending.[5] Ask any obstetrics/gynecology specialist how many medics have quit the specialty, not only because of the incredibly high insurance premiums but because of the psychologic trauma they suffer from frequent suits. There was a bill before

Congress, supported by President Bush, to put a $250,000 cap on awards for pain and suffering, but it was opposed by the trial lawyers lobby, the most powerful and well healed of all lobbies, and blocked in the Senate after passing in the House. The bill was defeated in late 2003. It will be re-introduced in 2004, but don't hold your breath. Ask your orthognathic surgery colleagues what their annual malpractice premiums are—at least $125,000 and climbing. No wonder so many are no longer doing orthognathic surgery. When I started in orthodontics, our malpractice fees were $72 annually. Now that is multiplied many times.

We must all take a proactive position to ward off the increasing financial burden that is being placed on our shoulders. It is no mere coincidence that the US has 5% of the world's population but 70% of the world's lawyers. The problem, as I see it, is that the lawyers make the laws, enforce the laws, and adjudicate the laws in all three branches of government. Among our representatives in Washington, how many are not lawyers? Your chances of being sued are much better if you live in a big city than if you are in a small town, since the greatest concentration of lawyers is in the big cities.

The risk-management section of this book provides some of the basic ways to defend yourself in the face of the exponential increase in the number of suits and the amounts paid out. In 1980, in Illinois, the total medical indemnity was $11 million; by 1995, it was $349 million; in 2000, it was $485 million! The number of annual claims has risen from 620 to 14,826! Dentistry has seen similar increases. The insurance companies are all very busy, though they are usually making less, not more, profit. Many have either gone out of business or stopped writing malpractice insurance altogether.

Another problem is that when one health service gets sued, it can have a machine-gun effect on all providers: Everyone is sued even if they have no direct involvement in the case. For example, it is highly likely for you to get sued in an orthognathic surgery case even if the problem is surgery-related. The only way to protect yourself is to keep complete, comprehensive written records of exactly what you have told all parties and to get records from other providers. Communication is the name of the game, as you'll read in this section again and again.

Contingency-fee lawyers have no monopoly on unethical behavior, so we have to keep our own house in order. Too many of our colleagues are ready to serve the ego-inflating role of "expert" in these cases. Some of them will take either side. Justice may not be the determining factor; the pecuniary reward is what is important to the self-styled expert, sometimes critically referred to in the press as "hacks for hire." These so-called experts are listed in a book organized by specialization. The advertising for one of these books trumpets, "This is the one book that defense lawyers do not want you to have!" I have faced one such "orthodontist" testifying on both sides of a question many times. We must protect our own ethics, our integrity, and our public image.

A recent Gallup poll surveyed the public on the relative honesty and integrity of various professions and trades.[6] Druggists were ranked highest at 64%, clergy at 56%, and college teachers and physicians both at 55%. Dentists were rated at 53%. Further down the list was lawyers at 17%, not far above used-car salesmen, at 8%. The public has an image of ethical behavior, and orthodontists do relatively well. But on a scale of 1 to 100, shouldn't our reputation be rated higher than 53%?

I'm not trying to argue that there is no malpractice; of course there is malpractice. But sometimes we think we see it much easier in a competing orthodontist's patient who comes to us, though it is not malpractice. We tend to be judgmental when we do not know all the facts. It is vitally important to know what has transpired. Why is it that dentistry is the most critical profession? I think maybe we sometimes have an inferiority complex, because we use the term *doctor* all the time, like podiatrists and chiropractors, in contrast to the medical profession, which instead uses the MD degree. Regardless of the cause, we tend to be too critical of our colleagues. Before delivering an opinion, the very first rule is to look at the patient, look at all the facts, know what has happened, determine the patient's level of cooperation. *Review the records.* It is amazing how few orthodontists ask for the records from the prior treating orthodontist.

In any event, "Do unto others as you would have them do unto you." If you have a patient who is unhappy for one reason or another, you should try to make sure that patient is taken care of by taking the time to consult with a colleague. Try to see that all the records go with the patient. The AAO can provide you with transfer or consultation forms. Call the subsequent orthodontist and do all you can to expedite the consultation and possible treatment. You and the patient will benefit from those actions. This is standard practice in medicine.

Make sure you do a comprehensive medical and dental history and functional and TMJ examination on every patient, preferably using one of the many excellent questionnaire sheets available. The AAO provides case history forms for patients under 18 and for adults (see Appendix). I have been involved in at least 24 TMD cases, and yet we don't even have any proof that TMD is a factor in orthodontics.[8] The 1996 National Institute of Health conference stated this categorically.[9,10] Nevertheless, the million-dollar Brimm case decision galvanized hundreds of copycat suits. The record shows that Ms Brimm had two third molars removed by the oral surgeon after orthodontics. It seems that her acute TMD symptoms developed afterwards. The surgeon who removed the third molars settled for $2,500, and the orthodontist got clobbered for $1 million. The orthodontist was a member of a university faculty and did the right thing. The so-called expert for the plaintiff was a general practitioner as well as a non-boarded specialist who I have faced a number of times in court. The expert supporting the orthodontist was a professor in a great university and a world-class orthodontist. None of us is immune. Moreover, the AAO appealed and lost on the appeal. Who says all decisions are fair?[11] Your records should reflect a functional exam, particularly of the TMJ and neuromusculature, before, during, and after treatment. Record nocturnal parafunctional activity, which is a leading cause of TMJ problems. If present, consider incorporating an anti-bruxism, anti-clenching modification in the patient's maxillary retainer, and instruct the patient about the probable need for indefinite wear at night.

If we get good records, it is harder for the plaintiff attorney and easier for your defense attorney. The AAOIC and other insurance companies work very hard to make sure you get the very best legal attention. In the past, malpractice cases were assigned to the junior members or partners of the firm, but this has changed. Now that more money is involved, the top people in the firm are handling malpractice cases. Retain the right to make a decision on court action in your insurance policy.

If you are a male dentist, you have a 2.8% chance of being sued; female dentists get sued only 0.7% of the time. Oral surgeons are sued much more often,[11] so you increase your chances of being sued if you are the orthodontist working on the case with the surgeon.

Communication is the name of the game. You must have informed consent forms signed by the patient or parent of a minor. Although the professional standard of care is the basis for judgment in many jurisdictions, there is a trend in this country to use what is known as the material-risk standard or the reasonable patient standard. Courts are more and more protective of the patient's rights and more hesitant about formulating a comprehensive standard. The feeling is that the dental and medical professions should not be allowed to dictate the standard for informed consent. The patient ultimately owns the right to determine what is to be done with his or her own body. This doctrine prevailed in Canterbury vs Spence.[12] We need to make sure consent forms are read by the patient (or parent of a minor), discussed personally with the doctor, and signed and even witnessed. After the patient (or parent) has read the informed consent document, ask him or her personally, "Have you any questions?" Then, have them sign and date the signature at the bottom of the document.[13] The AAO informed consent form (see Appendix) is available upon request.

You need a proactive staff as well as a patient ombudsman. The warmth of one staff person can be critical. A friendly patient is less likely to sue you if something goes awry. Of course, if you're going to be seeing 80 patients a day, it's more difficult to establish an optimal office rapport. You need somebody to represent you and represent the patient. You need to correspond with a referral source. Again and again, I have seen cases in which there is no correspondence with the referring dentist. There is no report letter to the general dentist, sometimes no diagnosis or summary of the patient's problems. I have seen malpractice cases with no models, no radiographs, no panoramic radiographs, no progress records, and no diagnostic summary or treatment plan—often not even a report letter to the patient. It's surprising how many clinicians don't do what they should do. This makes it hard for all members of our specialty.

In this era of malpractice mania, even the good samaritan sometimes suffers. If an orthodontist does a partial correction for an assistant, colleague, or relative of a referring dentist, it is often gratis or for a nominal fee as an expression of appreciation. If the treatment result doesn't meet the expectations of the patient, there is a distinct possibility that the orthodontist will face a malpractice suit. So often in such cases, full records are not taken, consent forms are missing, treatment notes are cryptic. This makes perfect litigious fodder to present to a jury. The experience is traumatic to the orthodontist even if the case is ultimately won and takes much time and money for the defense. Very simply, treat all cases with the same practice management details and goals, with no compromises at any level. Special "favors" can come back to haunt you.[14]

We need to follow these rules. In professional communication, use written records rather than the telephone, and always keep copies. Maintain continuous written communication with the orthognathic surgeon and with the general practitioner, not just with the referring dentist. You are not an island unto yourself. If you send something to an orthognathic surgeon or the pediatric dentist, stamp it on the records. It's better to send copies rather than originals. When you send a bill to the patient, put "Please see your dentist" at whatever interval you want—3 months, 6 months, whatever you prefer. Then, have your staff check that the patient followed through.

Use your trained auxiliary staff, but make sure they are qualified to perform the services you ask of them. Sometimes we have staff do things that are not legal. Ms Franklin refers to such a case, and the insurance company had to settle even though no damage was done. You do not face a friendly environment in court. I have been involved in a case where the auxiliary personnel took off the bonded brackets, polished the teeth, and took the impressions for final study casts. Is this legal in your state? In how many states is this legal? If it is not, try to change the law. This was done recently in Illinois, for example. Defensive practice is the name of the game for all health professions and surely applies to orthodontics.

Consider referring. Referral is necessary when a patient's treatment needs are beyond the ability of the treating dentist's skill, knowledge, and experience. Dr Vanarsdall stresses this again and again in his chapter on periodontal ramifications. We know that there's nothing wrong with referring. Have the patient get second opinions before or during treatment. Why are we so worried about referring to another orthodontist, particularly when patients or parents question one-phase versus two-phase treatment, extraction versus nonextraction therapy, expansion versus nonexpansion? Always say, "If this was my child, this is what I would do, but I want you to be sure." Get a second opinion if there is ever any question. Failure to refer is a legal goldmine now. In medicine, if a patient has a cardiac problem and you're treating the liver or some other area, then you're in trouble.

One of the most onerous problems is the cryptic, short-handed, inadequate, illegible written records that we keep to support each visit. I've gone over these records, and they look like hieroglyphics. Get yourself a little recorder or something that fits in your jacket breast pocket. When you've seen the patient, take the recorder out of your pocket and record some basic treatment notes: "Mary Jo Smith, 9-15-2003, retie archwire, torque incisors," etc. "Next time check mobility of incisors," etc. Have it typed into the record. Look at some medical records and then look at dental records. Ours are mediocre at best.

In 1996, the AAO councils developed an excellent statement of clinical practice standards of care. Request a copy of this document.[13] As orthodontists, our goal is well-aligned teeth, but that does not mean typodont perfection. Normal is not an ideal, it is a range based on morphogenetic skeletal pattern, muscle pattern, age, etc. Be sure to say, "Does this look good to you?" Have patients initial their reply. Few lawyers are going to accept a case with such evidence against a likely success. Remember, the lawyer gets nothing unless he or she wins.

There are controversial treatment objectives, such as canine-protected occlusion, that some clinicians try to attain. As the Greek aphorism says, "Everything in moderation." Lysle Johnston comments appropriately, "Gnathology is the science of how articulators chew!"[15] The jury is still out on this goal from a legal standpoint. Recording parafunctional habits is more important and a proven cause of some TMJ complaints.

Much has been written by eminent authorities in the first part of this book to emphasize what our biologic limitations are in spite of amazingly efficient orthodontic appliances. The informed consent must cover all potential iatrogenic sequelae as well as changes that may occur post-treatment. Do we cause damage? Is there something we can do? What price orthodontics? Missteps are potholes along the orthodontic highway. Ninety-nine percent of the cases that we treat have at least some minuscule degree of root resorption, according to a study from Ohio State University, although you may not see it on the periapical films or the panoramic radiograph.[7] Moreover, we lose some crestal bone with every extraction. We also must monitor the patient's periodontal response.

References

1. Woodside DG. The $4.4 million case. World J Orthod 2001;2:10–20.
2. Doctor, You Are Being Sued! [editorial]. Chic Dent Soc Bull May-June 2002.
3. Angell M. Trial by Science [editorial]. NY Times, December 9, 1998, p 29.
4. Chicago Tribune, February 15, 2004.
5. ADA News, February 12, 2004.
6. Honesty and ethics poll. Available at http://www.gallup.com. Accessed 14 January 2004.
7. Practice Management Forms. Updated 2003. American Association of Orthodontists, St Louis, Missouri.
8. National Institute of Health. Technology Assessment Conference: Management of Temporomandibular Disorders. NIH, Bethesda, April 29–May 1, 1996.
9. Kim MR, Graber TM, Viana MA. Orthodontics and temporomandibular disorders. Am J Orthod Dentofacial Orthop 2002;121:438–446.
10. Egermark I, Magnusson T, Carlsson GE. A 20-year follow-up of signs and symptoms of temporomandibular disorders and malocclusions in subjects with and without orthodontic treatment in childhood. Angle Orthod 2003;73:109–115.
11. Graber TM. Doctor, You Too Can Be Sued! American Association of Orthodontics, Orlando, May 4, 2004.
12. Canterbury v Spence, 464 F. 2d 772 D.C. Cir, 1972.
13. American Association of Orthodontists, 401 N Lindbergh Blvd, St Louis, Missouri 63141. Http://www.aaomembers.org.
14. Risk management review: Orthodontic "favors" can result in malpractice claims. AAO Bulletin January/February 2004; 22:10–11.
15. Johnston L. Seminar. Department of Orthodontics, University of Illinois, April 5, 2003.

13 Malpractice Aspects of Orthodontic Treatment in Patients with Periodontal Disease

Robert L. Vanarsdall

"Risk comes from not knowing what you're doing."
—Warren Buffet

Given the large number of claims related to periodontal treatment, orthodontists should be knowledgeable about the periodontal implications of orthodontic treatment. Knowledge and documentation are a clinician's best forms of protection. The greatest challenge for orthodontists as far as periodontology is concerned is in making the correct periodontal diagnosis *prior to initiating* orthodontic treatment.

The Role of Plaque and Bacteria in Periodontal Disease

The first step in diagnosis is understanding the parameters of plaque. There are many different types of supragingival and subgingival plaque. The types of pathogens that cause loss of attachment are well known and exist subgingivally, but it is the supragingival dental plaque that creates an environment for subgingival plaque to form. Some destructive subgingival plaque varieties are *Porphyromonos gingivalis*, *Bacteroides forsythus*, and *Prevotella intermedia*. Gingivitis produces reversible lesions: Individuals who have gingivitis can clean their teeth, have scaling performed, and reverse the gingival lesion. But adult periodontitis is an irreversible lesion. It causes loss of attachment and is the destructive process that clinicians often deal with. Periodontitis affects both adults and adolescents, and periodontal treatment response must be monitored to identify who the susceptible patients are *before* the destructive process can begin. For example, a 13-year-old boy who presented for orthodontic treatment (Figs 13-1a to 13-1d) had his teeth orthodontically aligned, whereas his older brother had been treated surgically because of his high susceptibility to periodontal disease. The 13-year-old was treated without the need for extraction, with some leveling and alignment. Note the gingival tissue and anatomic crowns following orthodontic

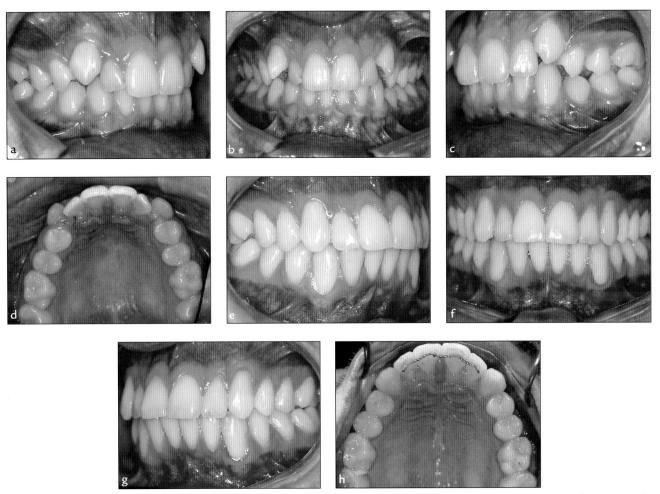

Fig 13-1 *(a–d)* Pretreatment photographs of a 13-year-old male patient. The tissue levels on the exposed anatomical crowns indicate increased periodontal susceptibility. *(e–h)* Post-orthodontic treatment photographs. Note the gingival recession and alveolar bone dehiscences throughout both arches. Facial movement resulted in reduced facial gingival dimensions.

treatment (Figs 13-1e to 13-1g). A significant price was paid to have his teeth aligned; he exhibited gingival recession on most of his teeth. He lost a significant amount of attachment at an early age during alignment and was treated to an unstable relationship. The teeth required bonding on the lingual of the maxillary incisors for permanent stabilization (Fig 13-1h). The maxillary anterior teeth were splinted in trauma, placing him in jeopardy of losing additional bone. It should have been obvious from the initial visit that this young child, exhibiting large clinical crowns and inflammation, was very susceptible to periodontal disease. This is an assessment that every clinician should make for all patients, both adolescent and adult: to identify the periodontally susceptible individuals *before* beginning orthodontic treatment. The ortho-

dontist must also be aware of any adverse change (increase in the size of the clinical crowns or gingival recession) while the teeth are being repositioned.

Paradoxically, the most challenging patient to treat is often the one who has the cleanest mouth (ie, no calculus or evidence of plaque and minimal local factors). Patients who show no treatment calculus on the roots and who clean their mouth meticulously require as much vigilance for adverse response as less cooperative patients. Figure 13-2 shows a model patient who took excellent care of her mouth and yet lost crestal bone during treatment. This patient had four premolars removed and the remaining teeth aligned. Note the spacing under the contacts in this photo taken several years later. The loss of attachment in the maxillary and mandibular anterior areas indicates

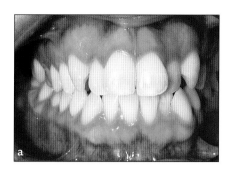
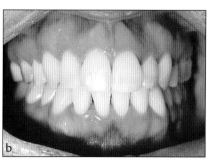
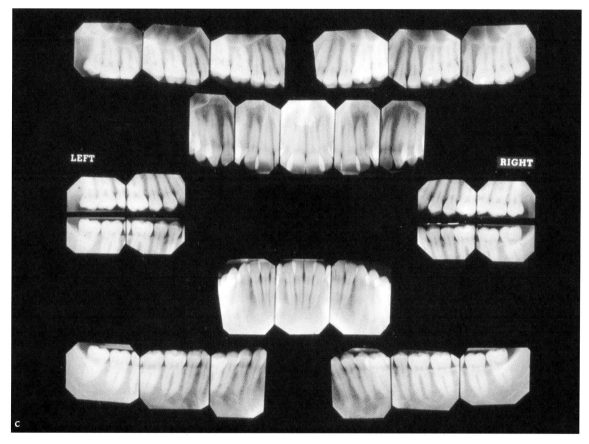
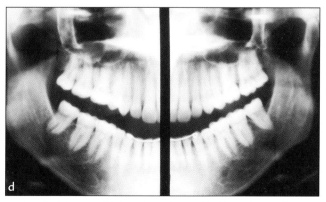

Fig 13-2 *(a)* Pretreatment photographs of a 28-year-old female patient with Class I bimaxillary protrusion. This patient had meticulous oral hygiene and received frequent professional cleanings. *(b)* Despite routine periodontal maintenance, this 2-year post-orthodontic treatment photograph reveals spaces below contacts, indicating bone loss during tooth movement. *(c)* Pretreatment periapical radiographs show no calculus present. *(d)* Post-treatment panoramic radiograph shows loss of bone on the anterior segments.

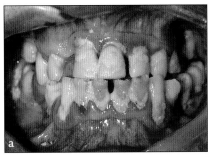 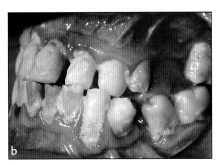 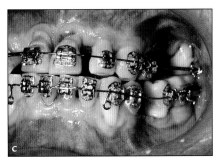

Fig 13-3 *(a,b)* Pretreatment anterior and left lateral views in an adult male patient, exhibiting poor oral hygiene prior to periodontal preparation for orthodontics. Dental records showed that the patient suffered no loss of attachment for more than 27 years despite the loss of teeth and evidence of gingival inflammation. *(c)* After scaling and root planing. No further attachment loss occurred during orthodontic treatment.

adverse change. Though her teeth were successfully aligned, a close comparison of the original radiographs and the post-treatment panoramic film reveals the loss of several millimeters of bone in the anterior segments.

The National Institute for Dental Research (NIDR) reported that about 80 to 90% of all adult patients presenting for treatment have the type of bacteria that can cause loss of attachment and lead to adult periodontitis.[1] Every patient who walks into the office has the potential to lose attachment because of the destructive power of periodontopathic bacteria, and it is essential for the orthodontist to evaluate every one of them for susceptibility. The periodontal status at initial inspection can be misleading; therefore, taking a history of prior orthodontic treatment as well as obtaining pretreatment intraoral radiographs, casts, and other records from the attending dentist are critical steps in determining if and when a patient has lost attachment. Such records also help determine whether the problem is stabilized or continues to be active. The records of the patient shown in Figs 13-3a and 13-3b indicated that he had not lost any attachment over a period of 27 years even though his oral hygiene was poor. After some scaling and soft tissue healing, fixed brackets were placed, and the teeth were moved without disarticulation (Fig 13-3c). Tooth replacement was successful, and the patient experienced no further loss of attachment.

It is important to recognize that there are different types of periodontitis.[2] Prepubertal *juvenile periodontitis* is rapidly progressive, whereas *adult periodontitis*

is the most common type. The type most frequently leading to litigation is *refractory periodontitis*, in which sites of active inflammation continue to be infected despite aggressive periodontal therapy, continuous root planing, curettage, and other forms of periodontal treatment. Other factors that can affect the periodontium include medication taken to control a systemic disease such as diabetes, cyclic neutropenia, etc; syndromes such as Down syndrome, Papillon-Lefèvre syndrome, Addison disease; and steroids taken for immunodeficiency diseases, which mask the patient's oral response to inflammatory elements in the periodontium. These factors should be recorded in the patient's record for the practitioner's protection.

Controlling Periodontal Disease Throughout Orthodontic Therapy

Greenwell et al[3] evaluated the best periodontal practices in the country. Patients were studied who came in for periodontal maintenance and to get their teeth professionally cleaned on a 3-month basis but still exhibited loss of attachment. About 30% of the patients who undergo regular scaling nonetheless continue to show evidence of progressive periodontal disease. This disease process must be controlled by more frequent maintenance visits, especially during orthodontic treatment. In adult periodontitis, 2 mm of

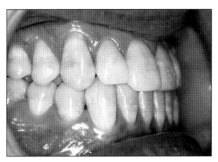

Fig 13-4a Post-orthodontic photograph of an 18-year-old female. Note the space under the first premolar–canine contact.

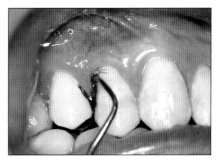

Fig 13-4b Gentle probing (just apical to the gingival margin) elicits significant bleeding, a risk predictor for bone loss in an orthodontic patient.

loss has been described as "mild," 50% bone loss is considered "moderate," and greater than 50% is "severe." These general classifications should be used to establish the severity of the disease at the initial presentation. Periodic periodontal assessments should be performed and recorded in the patient record throughout the course of orthodontic treatment.

A progress diagnosis must be made every time an orthodontic patient comes into the office. The diagnosis may be made by the orthodontist, the hygienist, or another staff member who has been appropriately trained to do so. Is the periodontal disease active or inactive? Is it stable, controlled, or advancing (resulting in bone loss)? If the patient is losing bone (nonresolution of recurrent disease) or teeth, he or she must be informed. Patient responsibility and compliance with prescribed care should be encouraged. For example, a recommendation to get scaling must be documented in the patient's record.

Bleeding indicates infiltration and inflammation of the tissue. A healthy gingiva is referred to as a *junctional* epithelium; when it becomes inflamed, it is called a *pocket* epithelium, and it is caused by an apical down-growth and infiltration of plaque and inflammatory cells into the connective tissue, resulting in bone loss. Figure 13-4a shows an 18-year-old female who had space under a contact upon the completion of orthodontic treatment. If the orthodontist were to gently probe this area, it would probably bleed. This is likely to become a periodontal problem if left uncorrected. If a hygienist, assistant, or clinician obtains bleeding upon probing in an orthodontic

patient (Fig 13-4b), the patient should be sent back to the referring dentist, since it is unlikely that orthodontic treatment can be completed without some loss of attachment. The condition and recommendations should be recorded in the chart, and the patient should be informed.

No studies have been reported to date on repopulation of subgingival bacteria in orthodontic patients. A study at the University of Pennsylvania in the early 1980s reported that bacteria will repopulate in 6 to 8 weeks after all subgingival bacteria have been removed.[4] Patients in the study were on periodontal maintenance and had regular recall visits. For active orthodontic patients, however, the bacteria may repopulate more rapidly; therefore, the standard 3-month recall may not be adequate for these patients. The radiographs in Figs 13-5a and 13-5b show no evidence of calculus on the teeth and apparently healthy roots, but no crestal dura is visible. Crestal dura is a sign that tissue is healthy; its absence usually indicates that the tissue is inflamed. Moving teeth in the presence of inflammation leads to bone loss. In this patient, there was a loss of 2 to 4 mm of bone after appliances were placed. Moreover, tooth mobility was exacerbated by a very heavy musculature.

Figure 13-6a shows a patient in the finishing stages of orthodontic treatment. More torque is still needed on the maxillary anterior teeth. The patient is experiencing the stress of both a divorce and trying to finish a postgraduate program and has begun to develop periodontal abscesses (Fig 13-6b). When this happens, a practitioner should immediately send the patient

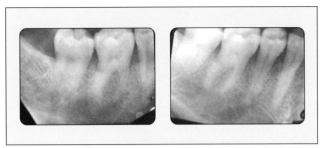

Fig 13-5a Pretreatment periapical radiographs of a female patient prior to placement of orthodontic appliances.

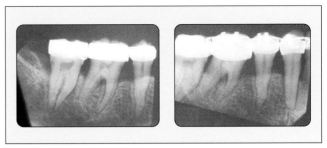

Fig 13-5b Progress films taken because of excessive tooth mobility several months later. Note the radiographic evidence of accelerated bone loss.

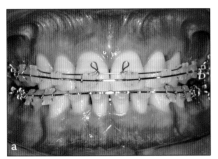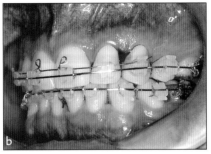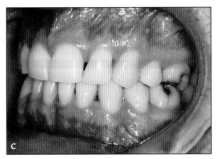

Fig 13-6 *(a)* Male patient in the final stages of treatment. Under stress of a divorce and a rigorous postdoctoral program, he experiences frequent periodontal abscesses. *(b,c)* Bleeding from the abscess between the left lateral incisor and canine, requiring the removal of appliances.

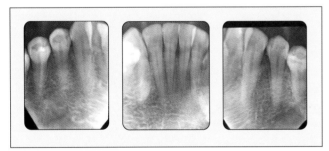

Fig 13-7a Pretreatment periapical radiograph of anterior mandibular area.

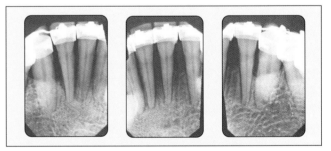

Fig 13-7b Progress radiographs reveal significant (3 to 6 mm) bone loss.

to a periodontist. Today, PerioChip (DexcelPharma, Edison, NJ), Atridox (CollaGenex, Newtown, PA), or another anti-inflammatory drug may be placed subgingivally. If the patient is irreversibly losing attachment, treatment must be terminated and all appliances removed. In this patient, it became impossible to control the inflammation in the left lateral incisor, and orthodontic therapy had to be discontinued (Fig 13-6c).

Figures 13-7a and 13-7b show the pretreatment and post-treatment radiographs of a patient who has undergone orthodontic therapy to align the teeth. The progress radiograph reveals the loss of 3 to 6 mm of bone. This adverse response does not occur slowly over a long period of time; it happens rapidly and therefore must be recognized as soon as it begins. When interdental contact points start moving away from the

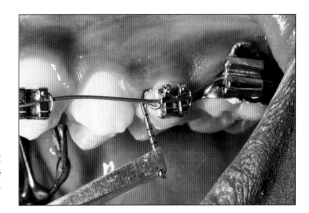

Fig 13-8 Probing of the maxillary left quadrant of a young patient with a pressure-sensitive probe to evaluate the effect of mobility on probing depths.

Table 13-1 Mean probing depth among bonded (test) and unbonded control teeth					
	Number of patients	Number of teeth	Mean PD at T1 (mm)	Mean PD at T-max (mm)	Mean PD DIF (mm)
Test	11	32	2.13 ± 0.54	3.20 ± 0.62	1.09 ± 0.53
Control	11	32	2.42 ± 0.42	2.34 ± 0.41	−0.08 ± 0.26

interdental papilla (commonly referred to as *black spaces*), photographs and radiographs should be taken and referred to a periodontist for evaluation. For this purpose, a growing number of orthodontic practices have invested in periapical radiography equipment. This is an efficient practice approach, and patients appreciate the convenience of not having to make another appointment elsewhere, spend more time, etc. Many orthodontists do not realize how often they would make use of such equipment until they have it.

Other Iatrogenic Factors

A study performed at the University of Pennsylvania provided documentation that when a tooth becomes mobile, the probing depths can deepen.[5] One control tooth in each quadrant was left unbonded (Fig 13-8) and demonstrated that the patient's periodontal health was maintained as the teeth were moved (Table 13-1). Test (mobile) teeth showed increased probing depths,

signifying a modification in response to periodontal susceptibility. Other studies have shown that changes in the environment can adversely affect an orthodontic patient.[6] In 1995, Grant et al[7] reported that tooth mobility may constitute a risk factor in periodontal breakdown because when a tooth becomes mobile, it causes the bacteria to shift. Mouthwashes designed to control plaque (such as Colgate Plax) or chlorhexidine gluconate are not adequate to destroy subgingival plaque. Plaque must be removed locally and subgingivally with a curette, and the subgingival bacteria must be controlled. During periods of increased tooth mobility, such as when leveling, aligning, or rotating a tooth, occlusal interferences can lead to increased probing depths. A patient often starts to brux once a tooth becomes mobilized; therefore, bruxing and other parafunctional activity become a major etiologic factor in tooth mobility. This only increases the possibility of loss of attachment. It is critically important to monitor severely rotated, malaligned teeth during the early stages of treatment. During pregnancy, a change in bacteria population within the second trimester requires these patients to undergo scaling more often during orthodontic therapy. This does not mean they cannot be treated, but merely that a few extra scalings are indicated in the second and third trimesters.

Recognizing Warning Signs

Problems must be detected during clinical visits, and a trained hygienist can be an invaluable member of the orthodontic team. Both gingival bleeding and excessive mobility in an orthodontic patient are warning signs that should be monitored throughout treatment. When a maxillary molar becomes so mobile that it can be pushed up and down (depressible mobility), adjusting the wire will not solve the problem because the bone will be lost from trauma in the furcation area. Occlusal grinding of the tooth can remove the trauma and allow it to restabilize; this can help prevent attachment loss.

When soft tissue becomes inflamed, it is slowly dissolved. As the gingival tissue thins, the root becomes exposed. Inflammation can be resolved before the tissue is dissolved. When bleeding is observed, inflammation can be controlled and loss of attachment avoided. For patients who have strong masseter and temporalis muscles and have a bruxing or other parafunctional habit, orthodontic treatment objectives must be modified. Strategies must be developed to prevent bone loss and gingival recession. Obviously, these patients are candidates for scaling and root planing, and orthodontic treatment should be delayed until inflammation can be controlled. It is not enough to accept the patient's intention to get the recommended pre-orthodontic periodontal treatment or scaling from their general dentist; if they fail to follow through and their appliances are placed, they may lose several millimeters of attachment within 8 to 10 weeks. The staff must make sure the patient received the needed care and note this in the patient's record.

Plaque control has only minimal effect on clinical indicators of periodontal disease.[8] The single most important element in controlling periodontal disease is scaling and root planing, and this is particularly true for the orthodontic patient. Patients are often given chlorhexidine gluconate 0.12% (Peridex, Proctor and Gamble, Cincinnati, OH) after scaling to control the supragingival plaque during the interval between scalings. However, because Peridex allows the bacteria that stain to discolor the teeth, it can be used for only 5 to 6 days. Sometimes it also helps patients to put Listerine (Pfizer, Morris Plains, NJ) on the toothbrush to help control the inflammation.

Patients with advanced periodontal disease accompanied by significant loss of attachment must be under occlusal and inflammation control when treatment with brackets and archwires is initiated. Posterior segment control is essential because the clinician minimizes tooth mobility during orthodontic leveling procedures. It is a good policy to insist that the patient be periodontally stable and prepared before orthodontic appliances are placed. Reluctance or refusal to have periodontal visits in referring offices or through the interdisciplinary care of a general dentist to ensure proper inflammatory control over the course of orthodontic treatment contraindicates orthodontic therapy. A defined protocol must be established among the referring general dentist, the periodontist, and the orthodontist.

Taking Preventive Measures Before Initiating Treatment

Some optional procedures should be considered before beginning the orthodontic phase of treatment. For example, gingival grafting may be indicated in a patient who has thin tissue. Figures 13-9a to 13-9c show a young female who needed her mandibular teeth aligned but did not want orthodontic appliances to be visible. Lingual appliances were placed on the anterior teeth (Fig 13-9d), and they were aligned in 3 weeks (Fig 13-9e). In the process, they were proclined 8 to 10 degrees. The right lateral incisor had pre-orthodontic recession on the labial aspect. To correct this, a graft was placed in that area and then overextended to the left lateral incisor (Fig 13-9f). When these teeth were aligned and proclined (Fig 13-9g), the patient had 4 to 5 mm of recession in the area of the left lateral incisor that had not been grafted. However, the gingiva that was placed actually crept over this tooth as it was being proclined (Fig 13-9h).

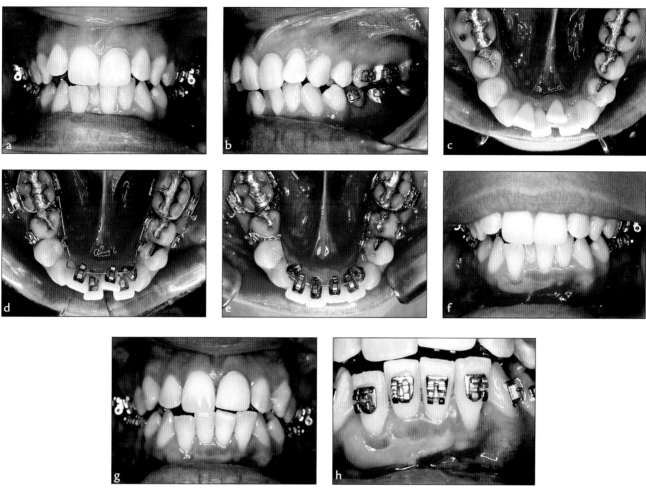

Fig 13-9 *(a–c)* Crowded anterior mandibular teeth in a 30-year-old female patient. *(d)* Occlusal view of lingual appliances placed to align mandibular incisors. *(e)* Occlusal view several weeks after proclination and alignment. *(f)* Pre-orthodontic labial view of teeth shows graft had been placed over the right lateral incisor due to recession before treatment. *(g)* As the incisors were proclined and aligned, the patient exhibited 4 to 5 mm of apical recession on the left lateral incisor, which had not been grafted. *(h)* The grafted tissue over the right lateral incisor actually crept incisally as the tooth was being moved labially. Labial appliances were then placed.

Therefore, the thickness of the gingival graft was increased and recession was prevented. Labial grafts have been proven to prevent recession in orthodontic cases.

Primate experiments performed in the early 1980s established that "a thin gingiva may serve as a *locus minoris resistentia* to soft tissue defects," especially in the presence of plaque.[9] Figure 13-10 shows a patient with thin gingiva in the mandibular anterior area. All patients have some bacterial plaque. As Maynard[10] once said, "After 20 years, I have never done a graft on a tooth for a pediatric patient (and most of them were orthodontically treated patients) and seen recession occur on the tooth." Figure 13-11 shows a 12-year-old boy who received a graft on the two mandib-

ular incisors prior to orthodontic treatment. Twenty-six years later (Fig 13-11b), these two teeth are the only ones that do not show gingival recession. Therefore, changes in the soft tissue can help to prevent the loss of attachment and gingival recession.

In some areas requiring gingival repair, the soft tissue can be thickened with a minimally invasive procedure that makes the patient more resistant to the loss of attachment and recession. Figure 13-12a shows the mother of a 9-year-old who presented for orthodontic treatment. During earlier orthodontic treatment, the mother had had a mandibular incisor removed because of severe labial recession; she exhibited recession on the other incisor years later.

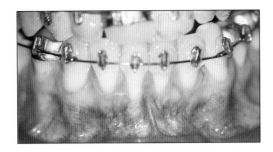

Fig 13-10 Very thin tissue in the labiolingual plane in an adult patient.

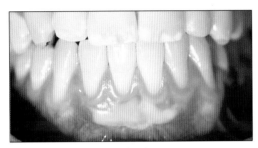

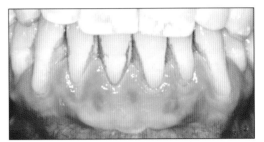

Fig 13-11a Before orthodontic treatment was initiated, this 12-year-old male patient received a graft on the two central incisors because of minimal keratinized tissue.

Fig 13-11b Twenty-six years after placement of the graft, it shows no evidence of recession, and the marginal tissue on the two central incisors appears to be stable, but recession has occurred around the lateral incisors, which were not grafted.

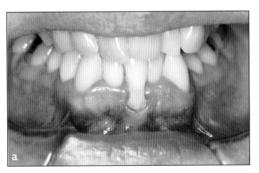

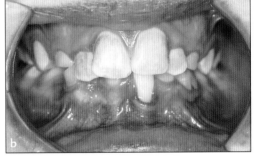

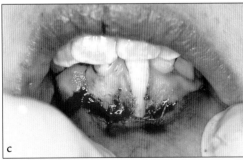

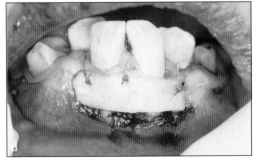

Fig 13-12 *(a)* This 28-year-old mother had her left central incisor removed because of recession during her orthodontic treatment. Recession on the right central incisor was present 20 years later. *(b)* Her 9-year-old daughter presented for orthodontic treatment exhibiting recession on her left central incisor. *(c)* The decision was made to graft the central incisor. Note the soft tissue bed preparation for an autogenous gingival graft. *(d)* A free donor tissue graft was placed on the prepared bed, and the tooth was maintained throughout orthodontic treatment.

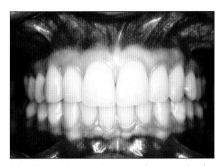

Fig 13-13 Normal gingival tissue thickness in an adult.

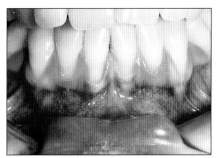

Fig 13-14 Thin keratinized tissue, which allows for gingival recession, and inflammation in an adolescent patient posttreatment. Thin tissue is a predisposing factor to recession.

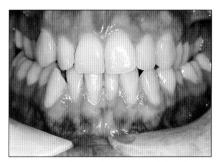

Fig 13-15 Thin soft tissue and thin bone predisposed this adult patient to recession. She is now undergoing retreatment.

Because of this, the mother asked if her daughter's incisor (Fig 13-12b), which showed recession also, should be removed. A decision was made to graft it instead (Figs 13-12c and 13-12d). The daughter went through treatment, and all incisors were maintained. It behooves the orthodontist to become more "soft tissue conscious" in the diagnostic assessment.

Generally speaking, children collect more plaque at 11 years of age than at any other time in their lives, a fact that has been substantiated by many studies.[11] Figure 13-13 shows an example of gingiva of normal thickness, the so-called Philadelphia norm. Figure 13-14 shows an example of thin gingival tissues. This patient had four premolars removed and the teeth retracted. Despite the retraction, there is significant recession throughout the mouth. Because the thickness of the tissues is a predisposing factor for recession, orthodontists must recognize the tissue type in the patients they treat. Some patients have thin soft tissue and thick bone, while others have thick soft tissue and thin bone. With a taurus, for example, there is very thin tissue over thick bone. With a cleft, there is thick soft tissue without bone. (With no bone, you get gingival recession.) The most challenging patient, however, is the one with thin soft tissue and thin bone. These patients are at risk regardless of the dental care being rendered and are good candidates for tissue- and bone-grafting procedures prior to beginning orthodontic therapy.[12] Teeth should not be moved into bony defects. The only way to change an infrabony defect predictably is with guided tissue regeneration, not by moving a tooth in different directions.

Identify susceptible patients and then adjust treatment as necessary to avoid adverse responses. Because of her thin tissue type, the patient shown in Fig 13-15 was advised to have a graft done on her two mandibular central incisors before treatment. She declined the graft and proceeded through treatment. Years later, she had an ulcer that caused the gingival tissue to strip off all the way to the apex of the two incisors. The following factors should be considered prior to initiating orthodontic therapy:

1. Growth and development
2. Tooth position
3. Oral physiotherapy
4. Type of hard and soft tissues
5. Inflammation
6. Integrity of the mucogingival junction
7. Mucogingival and osseous defects
8. Type and direction of anticipated tooth movement
9. Tissue changes associated with tooth movement
10. Profile considerations
11. Mechanotherapy to be used
12. Patient cooperation

Orthodontists should refer patients for prescription surgery or, at a minimum, for consultation with a periodontist. A wait-and-see approach could result in adverse effects for which the orthodontist may be held liable. As noted in chapters 14 and 15, we must learn to emulate our medical counterparts as far as referral is concerned for any periodontal, surgical, or restorative problem that arises.

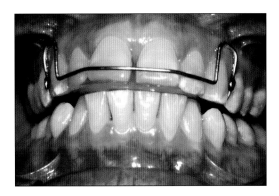

Fig 13-16 Periodontally susceptible adult with anterior Hawley bite plate that disarticulates the posterior teeth.

Identifying At-Risk Patients

In adult patients with susceptibility to periodontal disease, it is recommended that the teeth be disarticulated during posterior tooth movement. At the initial visit, full maxillary and mandibular appliances should not be placed in these patients. Figure 13-16 shows a patient under good periodontal supervision by a periodontist. A bite plate is being used to disarticulate the posterior teeth, and mechanotherapy was modified by delaying appliance placement on the anterior teeth. Bite plate therapy was also used successfully in the 30-year-old patient shown in Figs 13-17b and 13-17c. This patient had previously undergone orthodontic treatment, during which her teeth became mobile (Fig 13-17a) and she lost attachment. She had a 10-degree Frankfort–mandibular plane angle (FMA) and a strong musculature (Fig 13-17d). For these reasons, moving teeth in this patient is challenging. Moreover, the patient was traumatizing her teeth, making her very susceptible periodontally. In re-treatment, a bite plate was inserted for a period of time to allow the teeth to stabilize. Then sectional wires were placed in the posterior quadrants on the maxillary and mandibular teeth, with a bite plate to be worn 23 hours a day (the exception being during eating) (Figs 13-17e and 13-17f). The posterior teeth were aligned and leveled (Figs 13-17g and 13-17h), and only then were appliances placed on the anterior teeth (Figs 13-17i and 13-17j). The patient had some inflammation, but selective grinding allowed her to be treated without losing attachment. The restorations had been placed

to fit the malocclusion of her previous bite; therefore, when the teeth were aligned, the old restorations had to be recontoured (Figs 13-17k and 13-17l). She was re-treated orthodontically and has done well over the past 15 years.

In the patient shown in Figs 13-18a and 13-18b, a bite plate was used to separate the posterior teeth. This patient had some bite collapse, as indicated by the wear on the anterior segment (Fig 13-18c). Using the bite plate (Fig 13-18d), the posterior teeth were uprighted, after which appliances were placed on the anterior teeth and the maxillary incisors were bonded (Figs 13-18e and 13-18f). The posterior replacement was complete and the occlusion corrected without the loss of any attachment. As emphasized above, both the practitioner and the other staff must remain constantly vigilant regarding inflammation in the tissues and mobility of the teeth. The original radiographs show about 20% bone loss in the posterior segments (Fig 13-18g) after alignment and replacement of the mandibular teeth (Figs 13-18h to 13-18j).

Patients should be continually assessed for periodontal factors that place them at greater risk of developing disease during orthodontic treatment. A *risk marker* is a local predictive factor that identifies a patient who is likely to have periodontal disease. A *risk factor* is a characteristic behavioral aspect or environmental exposure that has been shown to be associated with periodontitis. Potential risk factors must be recorded in the patient's record as early as possible and the information communicated to the patient. This is the practitioner's best protection against litigation. Smoking, stress, diabetes and other medical conditions,

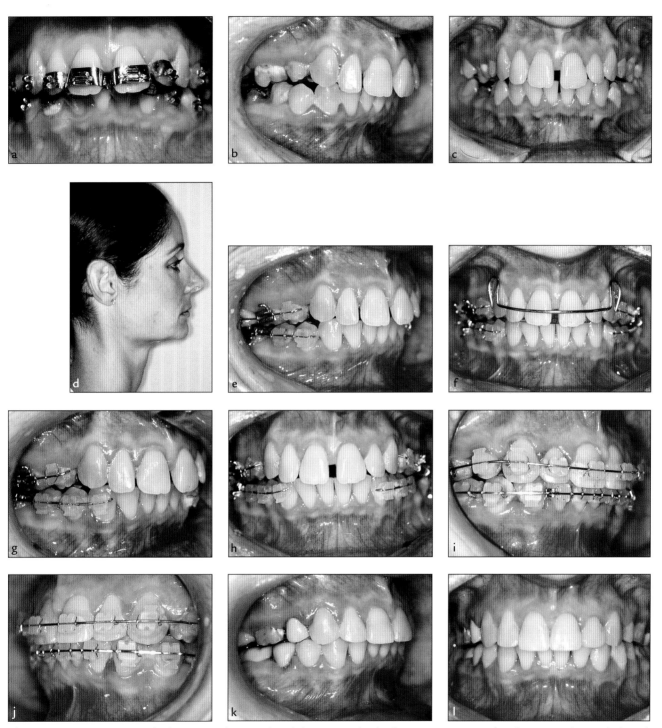

Fig 13-17 *(a)* Anterior view of edgewise appliances placed during initial orthodontic treatment in a female patient. *(b,c)* Right lateral and anterior views of the patient before retreatment at the age of 30 years. *(d)* Right facial view exhibiting heavy musculature and a 10-degree FMA angle. *(e)* Posterior sectional wires with the bite plate removed. *(f)* Anterior view with the bite plate. *(g,h)* Lateral and anterior views with bite plate removed prior to placement of anterior brackets. *(i,j)* Lateral views with full appliances and bite plate removed. *(k,l)* Lateral and anterior views of final result.

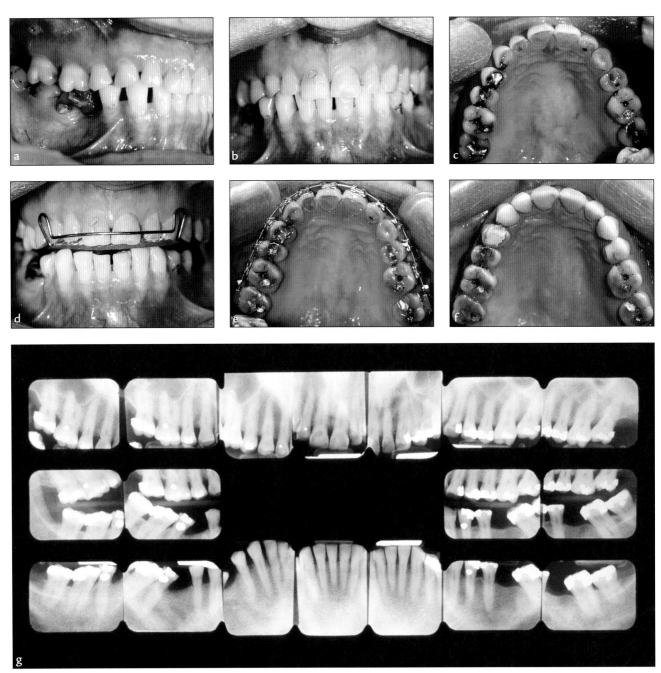

Figs 13-18a to 13-18g *(a,b)* Lateral and anterior pretreatment views of a 57-year-old female. *(c)* Pretreatment occlusal view. *(d)* Anterior view of bite plate used for disarticulation during posterior leveling and alignment. *(e)* Maxillary occlusal view with appliances. *(f)* Maxillary occlusal view, post-treatment. *(g)* Pretreatment periapical radiographs.

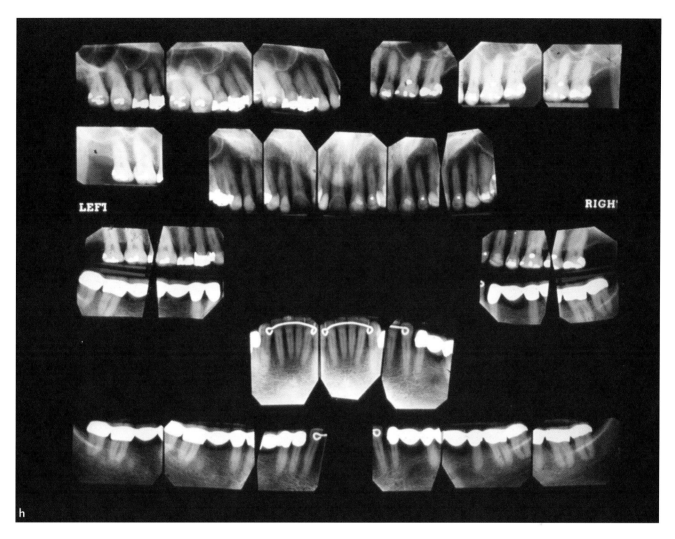

LEFT RIGHT

h

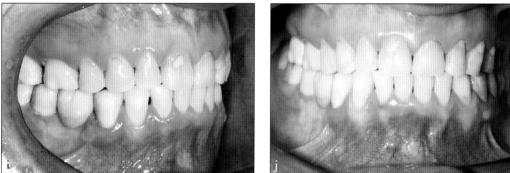

i j

Figs 13-18h to 13-18j *(h)* Post-treatment periapical radiographs. *(i, j)* Lateral and anterior post-treatment views.

and particularly a history of periodontal problems are all known risk factors. A patient with a loss of attachment will usually show advanced breakdown later.

Caution must be used when moving the teeth labially. Teeth moved beyond the envelope of the alveolar process may be predisposed to gingival recession. This applies to both anterior and posterior teeth. When considering expansion, it is important to remember that the bone on the facial surfaces is only 0.3 mm thick in the maxilla. In the mandible, the teeth are dentally compensated (leaning lingually to compensate the maxillary arch). In skull specimens where the mandibular teeth are dentally compensated, the facial surfaces of the teeth exhibit 50 to 60% loss of attachment.

Periodontal problems can develop around unerupted teeth as they are orthodontically positioned, particularly with the maxillary canines. Patients who consistently miss routine appointments are more likely to have periodontal problems. A young girl was noncompliant for about 1 year. When she finally came in, the roots were exposed on the labial aspect, and when the canine tooth was brought down into position, she bit on it every time she closed her mouth. With this type of trauma, teeth can come out of the palatal tissue, and significant attachment was lost.

Conclusion

As has been shown, periodontal problems often occur in routine orthodontic patients. Recognizing these problems and mastering the techniques to control them will improve the orthodontic prognosis and allow practitioners to provide better-quality care for their patients. Understanding the plaque and periodontal susceptibility of the individual patient, along with local factors of tooth mobility, heavy musculature, and inflammatory episodes (abscesses) are all critical to delivering optimal treatment. Risk markers must be recognized and recorded. Many techniques are available to cope with risk factors, such as scaling and root planing to eliminate inflamed areas, gingival grafting to change critically thin tissue, using a bite plate to control mobility, and selective grinding to remove

occlusal trauma and prevent problems with unerupted teeth. An initial periodontal diagnosis should be made at the initial visit and then followed by progress/response diagnoses throughout treatment. Such efforts must be clearly recorded on the patient's record. It is also a good idea to establish a hot line with the attending general dentist. In this litigious area, knowledge, documentation, and interceptive action are necessary to protect both the patient from adverse results and the orthodontist from liability.

References

1. Miller AJ, Brunell JA, et al. Oral Health of U.S. Adults. National Institutes of Health Pub. No. 97-1868, Bethesda, Maryland, 1987, National Institute of Dental Research.
2. Socransky SS, Haffajee AD, Goodson JM, Lindhe J. New concepts of destructive periodontal disease. J Clin Periodontol 1984;11:21–32.
3. Greenwell H, Bissada N, Whittwer J. Periodontics in general practice: Perspectives on periodontal diagnosis. J Am Dent Assoc 1989;119:537.
4. Mousques T, Listgarten M, Phillips R. Effect of sealing and root planing on the composition of the human subgingival microbial flora. J Periodontal Res 1980;15:144–151.
5. Vanarsdall R, Lemay J, Lindhe J. The effect of tooth mobility on probing depths. Compend Suppl 1988;12:S433–S437.
6. Vanarsdall R. Adult orthodontics: Diagnosis and treatment. In: Graber TM, Vanarsdall R (eds). Current Orthodontic Concepts and Techniques, ed 3. St Louis: Mosby, 2000.
7. Grant D, Flynn M, Slots J. Periodontal microbiota of mobile and nonmobile teeth. J Periodontol 1995;66:386–390.
8. Cercek J, Kiger RD, Garrett S, Egelberg J. Relative effects of plaque control and instrumentation on the clinical parameters of human periodontal disease. J Clin Periodontol 1983;10:46–56.
9. Lindhe J. Textbook of Clinical Periodontology. Copenhagen: Munksgaard, 1989.
10. Maynard JG. Mucogingival Considerations for the Adolescent Patient. Annual Meeting of the American Academy of Periodontology, New York, 1995.
11. Vanarsdall R. Management of the child and adolescent periodontium before and during orthodontic treatment. In: Richardson ER (ed). Periodontal Disease in Children and Adolescents: State of the Art. Nashville: Meharry Medical College, 1971:131.
12. Vanarsdall R. Periodontal/orthodontic interrelationships. In: Graber TM, Vanarsdall R (eds). Orthodontics: Current Principles and Techniques, 3rd ed. St Louis: Mosby, 2000:817.

Avoiding Malpractice Lawsuits:
Lessons Learned from Actual Malpractice Case Histories

Elizabeth Franklin

Malpractice claims are an unfortunate part of any professional practice. They take precious time to handle, and they often injure the doctor's self esteem by challenging the work product. The goal of any risk-management discussion is to share with others information that may minimize or avoid the initiation of new claims.

Drawing on actual case histories, this chapter provides information about the patient, the original diagnosis, the treatment plan, the problems that develop during treatment, and the final outcome, as well as some of the reasons malpractice claims are filed. To protect the privacy of those involved, no identifying information is disclosed for any case.

Early Termination of Treatment

The early termination of treatment is an important claim-prevention concept, as demonstrated by the fol-
lowing claim summary. It involves a 15-year-old male patient who began treatment with a Class II malocclusion, a posterior open bite, and crowding of the maxillary incisors. The orthodontist extracted the maxillary and mandibular first premolars and third molars, and appliances were placed in mid-1993. The treatment lasted 4.5 years. A significant reason for the protracted length of treatment was patient noncompliance; in 1995 and 1996, he changed appointments 11 times and missed appointments 15 times. He also had poor oral hygiene. The orthodontist advised him of the negative effect of his poor attendance and poor oral hygiene on the outcome of orthodontic treatment and documented the discussions in the records. In 1998, a general dentist examined the patient and found severe root resorption in the maxillary right central incisor. The appliances were immediately removed and the patient left the practice. At that point, the anterior teeth had been aligned, but the posterior open bite remained.

The patient filed a lawsuit against the orthodontist and three general dentists. He alleged that the root resorption on the maxillary right central incisor would result in its loss. He also had root resorption on the maxillary canines, the mandibular left premolar and first molar, and the mandibular right canine. He had root canal treatment on three of these teeth and was waiting to have root canal therapy on the other two. He also anticipated the eventual loss of the second premolar. In addition, he needed onlays to correct the posterior open bite.

The patient presented damages of more than $50,000 for past and future dental care and demanded $150,000 in his lawsuit. His allegation against the orthodontist was failure to monitor for root resorption during a protracted treatment period. Radiographs had been taken by general dentists in 1992 and 1994, and in 1997 the orthodontist had taken a panoramic radiograph. The plaintiff also alleged that the orthodontist was responsible for his posterior open bite. The doctor who provided subsequent treatment said ankylosis was the reason the open bite would not move and prescribed onlays to correct the problem.

The orthodontic expert witness for the defendant testified that no treatment was below the standard of care. He believed the root resorption was not caused by orthodontic treatment but that traumatic and idiopathic factors were the most likely cause. He concurred that there was some ankylosis in the posterior teeth.

Prior to trial, a maximum settlement offer of $25,000 was made on behalf of the orthodontist, and the codefendant general dentist offered $10,000. The plaintiff wanted to net $55,000 because he owed his attorney $22,000, and settlement was therefore not possible. The trial began in January 2001 and lasted 16 days; the orthodontist was present the entire time. Among the large number of witnesses were two endodontists and two orthodontists, who were retained as expert witnesses, an endodontist and orthodontist who provided subsequent treatment, several general dentists, and many others. After all the evidence was presented, the jury deliberated 1 hour and returned a verdict in favor of the dentists. For the defendant orthodontist, this was obviously a good outcome; however, his legal costs to achieve that outcome exceeded $100,000, not including his lost income for the 16 days of trial or for depositions and other time spent. Nor does this take into account the stress he suffered throughout the event.

When polled, the jurors indicated that they were not satisfied with the quality of the orthodontic treatment but did not believe it was the cause of the plaintiff's injuries. They felt the evidence indicated that science had not established a cause-and-effect relationship between the orthodontic movement and the external root resorption.

Would early termination of treatment have been appropriate in this case? Possibly so. Lack of compliance was compromising the treatment, and poor oral hygiene was jeopardizing the teeth. Early termination is appropriate when the result, for whatever reason, may be worse if treatment continues. Some patients are noncompliant. Some patients have poor oral hygiene. Some eat inappropriate foods that damage their appliances and cause caries and decalcification. In some rare cases, the patient's own physiology will undermine the treatment plan. If continuing the treatment will cause harm to the patient, then terminating treatment prematurely may be the best action to take.

The question of terminating treatment early in a patient who has failed to pay fees is more challenging because there can be no appearance of sacrificing the care of the patient for personal economic gain. Personality conflicts are another possible reason to end treatment early. The troublesome behavior of patients or parents can cause chaos in the office and disrupt the staff and/or other patients. In certain situations, the best solution to a difficult patient might be to terminate treatment rather than to allow the problem to develop to the point that the patient is so disgruntled he or she files a claim or lawsuit that will require significant time and energy to defend.

What are the risks of terminating treatment early? The primary risk is that the patient will feel abandoned and file either a dental board complaint or a professional negligence claim in retaliation. Each case must be considered on its own merits. What are the legal rights of the doctor? Provided that the contract does not prohibit it, early termination of treatment may be an option in some cases. A critical element to consider is the patient's condition. Previous litigation experience suggests that if the dentist has created an unnatural condition (eg, extraction spaces), juries and the law are less tolerant of early termination. On the other hand, if nature created the condition (eg, crowding), then the law will generally support early termination. The correct procedure would be to place retainers to preserve the progress to date and then proceed through the early-termination process.

It is important that the early-termination procedure be handled appropriately. The patient must be informed of the action, and treatment in another office may be recommended. There are patients for whom continued orthodontic treatment may be contraindicated. The presence of significant root resorption, for example, may preclude the viability of continued treatment. A particularly rebellious and noncooperative teenager may not benefit from continued care, even with another practitioner. Consider each situation on its own merits and advise the patient accordingly.

Even before the decision-making stage, it is important to make the patient and/or the parents aware of the problems that are developing and give them adequate time to correct them, if possible. Documentation of the relevant problems and of all discussions is an absolute necessity in such a case. When that effort has failed, the patient must receive written notification of the termination date at least 30 days in advance and a statement assuring cooperation with the other clinician in the transfer of records. Treatment of the patient on an emergency basis should be provided during that 30-day period. A summary of the treatment, emphasizing how far the patient has progressed, what additional treatment is required, and, if possible, an estimate of the additional time needed for treatment, must be placed in the record. Some lawyers refer to this letter as a "non-abandonment letter" because it clarifies for the patient all pertinent information and serves as evidence should the case later become a claim.

If the patient is a child, the orthodontist must contact the parents personally: Providing information to a teenager does not necessarily mean the information will reach the parents or be acted upon. In many claims, parents have denied any knowledge that their child has been noncompliant. When litigation is involved, memories can be selective; therefore, the orthodontist should not only convey the information regarding noncompliance to the patient and the parents, but document it as well.

Forgiving or Refunding Fees

Another important claim-minimizing step concerns the refunding of fees. Our claim department receives an average of a call per day from doctors asking about the merits of refunding fees. What are the advantages? If a fee refund is all the patient wants, it is quick and easy to do. A patient must sign a release that promises to absolve the doctor of liability for any claims arising from the treatment. The obvious disadvantage is the lack of payment for a therapy already provided. One could argue that it is not the amount of money but the principle of working without reward that is objectionable. However, dealing with a dental board complaint or a malpractice lawsuit may not be worth declining a small fee return. Once again, each situation must be considered on its own merits, taking into account the patient and/or parents involved, the treatment issues, the problems alleged, and the amount of money in question.

Another common concern doctors have regarding fee refunds is that the action will set a precedent, that the patient will tell his or her neighbor whose children are also in treatment, and they too will request a fee refund. To avoid this problem, the release should contain a confidentiality agreement that prohibits the patient from discussing the matter.

The following case demonstrates some of the unexpected problems involved in collecting for nonpayment of fees. A young patient had a rapid palatal expander appliance in her mouth for 1 year. The fees incurred, approximately $1,000, remained unpaid at the end of the treatment. Before he would remove the expander, the doctor demanded that the fee be paid. The mother took the child to another dentist, who removed the appliance. The doctor then filed an action in a small claims court for the payment of the fees; he received an award in his favor. The mother retaliated by filing a malpractice claim alleging practice below the standard of care. A claim was filed with the insurance company, and defense counsel was retained. Some legal discovery was completed. The doctor took time to answer interrogatories, complied with requests for production, and submitted his records to the plaintiff for review. A year later, mediation was arranged. After 7 hours of negotiations, the doctor forgave the fees and the mother agreed to dismiss her malpractice claim. The costs associated with this fee-related issue included $15,000 in legal expenses and several days of lost orthodontic practice time. When the issue presents itself, the practitioner must consider not only the fees, but also the time and aggravation involved.

Reputation in the community is another concern related to nonpayment and/or reimbursement of fees. Some doctors believe that reputation is important in their practice and usually try to reimburse fees if possible. This decision often depends on the practice location. Is it in a small town or a large city? What are the potential consequences in the community if fees are refunded? Doctors in smaller population areas often feel they need recommendations and good community support to operate a successful practice. They may be more motivated to offer a refund. In a large city, where population is plentiful, practitioners may be less inclined to do so.

Since it takes a great deal of time to attend legal proceedings and even dental board hearings, it would be simpler to refund some or all of the fees if the situation so merits. However, a release must be signed to clarify that the refund is not an admission of liability. It also must state that the refund is confidential and thus may not be discussed with others.

Another factor to consider regarding the refunding of fees is that it will not be reported in the National Practitioner Data Bank. The NPDB is a repository of information about medical and dental malpractice payments and adverse actions taken against a practitioner's license and clinical privileges. It can be accessed by state licensing boards, hospitals and other healthcare entities, professional societies, and federal agencies. Fee returns are not reported to this data bank, whereas a malpractice settlement or judgment is.

Patient Records

An orthodontist's patient records are very important. The primary function of patient records is of course to document treatment plans and patient care, not only for those working within the orthodontic office but for other orthodontists who may provide treatment should

that be necessary. They are used not only to facilitate the patient's care, but they also protect one against dental board complaints, malpractice claims, and lawsuits. Good records contain all information critical to patient care, including some or all of the following: chart notes, radiographs, casts, any information from the appointment books regarding the patient, correspondence to and from the patient or the patient's parents, phone records, medical history forms, the contract, the signed informed consent, interoffice memos related to the patient, and anything else that might be pertinent. All of this information must be legible.

How long should records be retained? This must be determined according to state dental board or society regulations. The statute of limitations for minors usually extends for a period beyond the age of majority, and records should be retained at least that long. Many defense attorneys recommend keeping records indefinitely if possible, since occasionally there have been claims on treatment rendered 20 years earlier.

Any requests for records should be made in writing, and permission to release them must be signed by the patient or parents. It is important that the procedure for obtaining records is understood by every member of the staff. One doctor related an interesting record-related incident. While he was away from the office the father of one of his patients, a very aggressive attorney, appeared in person and badgered the office manager into giving him several original radiographs. This man eventually filed a lawsuit, and the original radiographs had to be retrieved through the litigation process. The fact that the original radiographs were missing was a disadvantage to the doctor's defense during the early evaluation stage of the case.

If the patient requires the records, the doctor is entitled to charge for the duplication process. Usually that charge is a few cents per page for photocopying, reasonable costs for reproducing radiographs and casts, and a nominal administration fee. Overcharging for the records may create ill will.

Informed Consent

Like the written records, the informed consent document is a critical tool for discouraging the filing of malpractice claims and for defense in the event a claim is made. It is, simply stated, the process by which the patient is provided with enough information to make a reasonably informed decision regarding the proposed treatment. It is primarily necessary because it provides with the patient important information on which to base the decision to have treatment. Secondarily, it will serve as proof that you provided this information to the patient. Despite having signed an informed consent document, plaintiffs often allege lack of informed consent: They take the position that the issues described in the document were not adequately explained. Having the signed informed consent document will substantiate the doctor's claims. Thus, in a case involving the temporomandibular joint (TMJ) in an adult female, the insured doctors prevailed because she clearly had signed an informed consent that specifically addressed the TMJ issue.

The contents of an effective informed consent include a description of the nature of the action, the necessity for the treatment, its benefits, projected length, and cost (see Appendix). It should discuss alternatives, specialty referrals, the ramifications of not having treatment, and the possible consequences of the treatment.

There are various methods for conveying informed consent. The most common is a written format, which can be found in several books. Some doctors prefer to use a videotape accompanied by a form that is signed and placed in the records verifying that the tape was viewed and understood. There are also CDs available for practices that are highly computerized.

If the treatment changes, the original informed consent document must be amended. For example, if root resorption or periodontal disease that was not present at the beginning is discovered during the course of treatment, this issue and any others should be addressed in the consent form. Likewise, if the treatment is extended significantly beyond the originally projected time, the patient must sign an updated document.

Office-Related Issues

Claims often can and do develop from activities of the staff. One such claim was filed against a registered dental assistant, who allegedly used a high-speed drill to remove excessive bonding agents from several anterior teeth. The lawsuit was settled prior to trial. In that particular state, a registered dental assistant is not permitted to perform such an activity. Depending on the contractual language, malpractice coverage may be jeopardized if staff members are allowed to perform activities beyond the scope of the Dental Practices Act. In addition, the doctor could be subject to sanctions from the state dental board. All processes performed by your employees must be approved, and the staff performing the tasks must be adequately trained.

Practice size and the number of patients per day can influence not only the filing of a claim but its outcome as well. Often the plaintiff's lawyer will allege that the dentist is seeing too many patients per day and could not possibly have enough time to give adequate attention to each one.

Practice organization is another important factor. Doctors often practice in the offices of general dentists in different towns, visiting offices on different days of the week. Thus, if the doctor was unable to work in a particular office, the patient was encouraged to travel to another office for the appointment. If that was not possible, the appointment was missed altogether. In the past there have been lawsuits filed against doctors who perform as above, and all three plaintiffs alleged inadequate attention to their needs. One young patient testified that he was seen at 6- to 8-week intervals. During the deposition, the doctor was asked about the adequacy of the visits and, of course, answered affirmatively. In fact, the treatment was protracted and ineffective, which may have been at least partially a result of the practice organization situation.

Orthodontic clinics also can be a significant source of claims. Some doctors join clinics when they are beginning practice and leave when they are ready to invest in their own practice. Another orthodontist is then hired to take over the doctor's cases, and this revolving-door process repeats itself. Often at such clinics, a large number of doctors will treat the same patient depending on the day the patient visits and the rotation schedule. Having multiple doctors involved with one treatment can lead to a "deep-pocket" theory of legal liability: if one doctor creates a problem or a perception of a problem, all doctors involved with the patient are likely to be named in any claim or lawsuit. Sometimes doctors receive claims involving patients for whom no treatment was rendered; they were employees or independent contractors in the facility during the patient's treatment. There have also been lawsuits against doctors who could not recall the patient because so much time had elapsed that the doctor had forgotten the case. Thus, exposure to other doctors or staff can lead to malpractice claims that are not based on the treatment but the result of association with others. Exposure to such lawsuits can be minimized by carefully reviewing all patient records and by taking new records to document the status of the treatment, both when a new doctor takes over treatment and when he or she leaves the facility.

Another disadvantage sometimes associated with clinic employment occurs when the director establishes office procedures and the orthodontist has little control over staff activities. One claim involved the adjustment of a child's wires by an assistant. She allowed the patient to leave the facility without first having the work checked by the doctor, as was the appropriate procedure. When the young patient returned for her next visit, her teeth were significantly flared and the parents were upset. The parents filed a lawsuit against the clinic and the orthodontist.

Accidental Injuries

Accidents in the office are a reality of any practice. The following cases illustrate some examples of common accidents that occur.

In the first case, a small amount of etchant was dripped on the side of the patient's mouth and she was burned slightly. Another very traumatic case involved the laceration of a child's cornea when the chairside assistant clipped a wire that flew under the child's glasses. In both of these cases, the orthodontist made certain the patient received immediate emergency medical care and agreed to pay all costs associated with that emergency care. They were concerned but did not smother the family during the crisis. Both cases later developed into claims, but the damages were contained because of the effective initial response by the doctors.

If an accident occurs in the office, the patient must receive whatever medical care is needed, whether in an emergency room or by the dentist or doctor who

practices across the hall. If the patient requires transportation, it should be arranged by the doctor. The family must be aware that the billing for the emergency treatment will be covered by the doctor. Financial concerns can create animosity that encourages claims and litigation.

Empathy is an important factor in these incidents. Several claimants have complained that the doctor never called to inquire about their well-being. The doctor must call and ask how they are and if he or she can be of assistance in any way. On the other hand, the doctor should not call so often that the patient is bothered during a difficult period. Not only is that disruptive to the patient's schedule, but it may also be interpreted as guilt and liability and thus encourage a malpractice action. Above all, when the incident occurs, remember that emotions are high, including the orthodontist's. At that stage, the orthodontist may not be clear about all the facts that precipitated the incident and should not admit liability under any circumstances. The insurer must investigate and determine liability once the claim is reported. Sometimes there are issues involved about which the clinician is unaware, and if the investigation indicates no liability, it is difficult later for the insurer to handle the claim if the doctor has earlier admitted liability.

Extraction Issues

Extracting the wrong tooth

Tooth extractions can become malpractice issues and are usually classified into three categories. The first is the extraction of the wrong tooth. One such case was caused when the doctor completed a prescription form improperly. In the far right corner at the top of the form were directives to the general dentist, and the doctor had checked the box labeled "restorations." He wanted the general dentist to restore tooth number 27, and so he circled number 27 in the box located in the middle of the page. However, printed immediately above the grid with the tooth numbers were the words "Please extract the following permanent teeth," and the general dentist did just that. This claim was settled for the price of an implant and some pain and inconvenience. The lesson is to exercise extreme caution and to be accurate.

Making an erroneous decision

A similar case involved the orthodontist misreading an initial radiograph and making an erroneous decision to extract a tooth. The patient was congenitally missing a maxillary right second premolar. The doctor prescribed the extraction of the maxillary right first premolar. After he discovered his mistake, the doctor failed to inform the family. For almost 10 months an attempt was made to fill the space. When that was unsuccessful, the parents were finally advised. They were understandably angry, filed a lawsuit, and eventually settled the matter for $40,000 at mediation.

To extract or not to extract?

The third type of extraction claim involves the treatment plan itself. Some doctors believe extraction is appropriate for orthodontic treatment and others do not, as illustrated in the following case. A young adult female patient with a Class II tendency, a slight maxillary retrusion, facial asymmetry, abnormally shaped teeth, midline deviation, and partially impacted third molars sought orthodontic treatment. The doctor was going to slenderize the abnormally shaped incisors to create space and, at the end of treatment, extract the third molars. After 3 years, when the braces were removed, the teeth were significantly flared; the patient was unable to close her lips. The new orthodontist proceeded to extract eight teeth. After another 2-year treatment period, the patient was very satisfied with her result. She filed suit against the first orthodontist, alleging improper treatment. The expert witness retained to review the defendant orthodontist's records agreed with the doctor's treatment plan. He believed that root resorption, crestal bone loss, and periodontal problems could have resulted from the extraction of the premolars. It appeared as though extraction also might result in a profile flattening. The fact is, however, that after the teeth were extracted, the patient was happy with her appearance. The appropriateness of the treatment plan was therefore

questionable. Communication difficulties between the original orthodontist and the patient may have contributed to the unsuccessful result; she was so upset, she left his practice before he could complete the case. The damages alleged included the cost of extractions and subsequent orthodontic treatment. The case was settled at mediation for $38,000.

Pre-existing and Developing Pathology

Periodontal disease

Pre-existing and other oral pathology are rapidly becoming costly claims in terms of settlement dollars. Periodontal disease leading to bone loss is one such problem. Adult patients generally have a higher incidence of this, although children are not immune. To protect themselves from claims arising out of this issue, doctors must perform a thorough initial examination. Orthodontists are trained first as general dentists and therefore are qualified to determine if a patient should be referred to a specialist or back to his or her general dentist for clearance to begin orthodontic treatment. Some orthodontists report that they have all adult patients examined by a general dentist for periodontal disease prior to initiating treatment. Responsibility for recognizing the problem cannot be abdicated.

If a doctor refers a patient to a specialist, he or she must verify compliance. Do not assume patients are following instructions and carry on your work. Juries are holding orthodontists accountable. In one case, the doctor had taken over the patient's care from another who had left the practice. He recognized periodontal disease and referred the patient to see a specialist. In the meantime, he continued orthodontic treatment. Several months later, the patient called with severe periodontal problems, including mobile teeth. She needed intensive periodontal treatment and expected to lose several teeth. The orthodontist had never determined that this patient actually saw a specialist, and in fact she did not. She was an attractive single mother in her 30s, had little money and less time, and was more interested in esthetics than pathology. After her problem developed, she filed a lawsuit against both orthodontists and the clinic. Taking into account her own comparative negligence, the settlement from all parties approached $100,000. The issue was not recognition, it was the failure to determine whether continuing treatment under certain dangerous conditions was appropriate.

Root resorption

Root resorption is another dental condition that frequently results in claims with serious damages. A 27-year-old female patient was diagnosed with a Class II, division II malocclusion with a deep overbite, maxillary protrusion, and mandibular overcrowding. The orthodontist planned to extract the maxillary first premolars and two mandibular second premolars. Brackets were placed in August 1996. In August 1997, the orthodontist suffered a series of strokes, and substitute doctors treated the patient until May 1998, when the practice was sold. In July 1998, the new orthodontist removed the braces, sent the patient for cleaning, and formulated a new treatment plan. He noted loose teeth and recommended a hold on all future orthodontic treatment. The patient saw the periodontist in October 1998 for root scaling. The maxillary central incisors showed severe root resorption. The overbite continued, and the patient expected to lose four anterior maxillary and four anterior mandibular teeth. She sued her general dentist and the orthodontist, who was by that time deceased. She alleged practice below the standard of care and lack of informed consent. (There is often more than one problem in a case.) The patient's expert witness was also her subsequent treating orthodontist. He criticized the insured orthodontist's record keeping as inadequate and unclear. He also criticized the treatment plan, the extraction of the premolars, the direction of the tooth movement, and the gauge of the wire used to move the teeth. He saw root resorption in the initial radiographs, which indicated a need for interim radiographs. His opinion was that orthognathic surgery had been required. The plaintiff alleged damages approximating $60,000, including the cost for implants, orthognathic surgery, continued orthodontic

care, and past dental bills of $5,000. The demand was $350,000. Pretrial settlement negotiations were unsuccessful, so the case proceeded to trial. The venue was conservative, not prone to awarding excessive verdicts against professionals. The codefendant general dentist was dismissed from the lawsuit on a technicality, which left the deceased orthodontist as the sole defendant. The jury returned a verdict of $300,000.

Caries and decalcification

Caries and decalcification are other forms of pathology that can create claims with substantial damages for orthodontists. Patients must be advised of their needs, doctors' expectations, and the consequences of noncompliance, as illustrated in the following case. The young male patient was 10 years old when treatment began. The treatment continued for 5 years. He needed correction of a severe overbite. He was noncompliant and, over the course of treatment, had 62 loose bands, many missed appointments, and poor oral hygiene, all documented in the records. He also had significant tooth decay. He alleged damages in excess of $20,000 for restorations. He also needed veneers for discoloration and possible root canals. An important element of this case was the patient's use of the drug Accutane for acne at age 15. This drug is known to cause xerostomia, a dry mouth condition that leads to infection and tooth decay in cases of poor oral hygiene. The doctor denied any knowledge of the patient's drug usage; the patient contested the denial. A factor that contributed to the defense difficulties in this case was the doctor's frequent absence from his practice for personal reasons over the years of the patient's treatment. The patient alleged improper use of dental assistants due to the extraordinary absence of the doctor. All of the patient's teeth had decay, much of it visible to the eye. The expert witness who reviewed the case for the orthodontist opined that the depth of the decay indicated it had been present for many years. The location was behind the bands, which he believed indicated failed cementing. There were 62 loose bands, which, in his opinion, also indicated failed cementing. The case notes were inadequate, and it appeared that the staff handled much of the treatment. The original demand in this case was $250,000. It was settled prior to trial for an amount in excess of $100,000.

Temporomandibular disorders

Temporomandibular disorders (TMD) seem to be resurging as an allegation against orthodontists at this time, despite the fact that evidence tying it to orthodontic treatment purportedly disappeared almost 10 years ago. Usually there are no substantial damages coming from TMD allegations, but defense costs are often necessary and significant. In one case, the patient was a 33-year-old female who was being treated for crowding and crooked teeth. She had pre-existing TMD problems, along with headaches and myriad other complaints. She continued to have pain issues, left the care of the insured orthodontist, and sued him, alleging his orthodontic treatment caused her TMJ pain. The case was tried and won by the doctor. The doctor had excellent records and had had the patient sign an informed consent which clearly listed TMD as a potential problem for adults, especially adult females.

Interim Radiographs

Radiographs are often significant elements of malpractice claims. Have a sufficient number been taken? Were they properly interpreted? In the root resorption case involving the 27-year-old woman who was losing her maxillary and mandibular anterior teeth, much of the trial evidence surrounded the question of adequate interpretation of the initial radiographs, which clearly indicated the presence of root resorption. In addition to problems developing from original radiographs, the failure to take interim radiographs seems to be a major factor if problems like root resorption or periodontal disease develop during treatment, especially if the treatment is protracted.

One such case involved a young male patient who began treatment at age 11. Treatment lasted 22 months. The diagnosis was a Class II malocclusion with a 20% overbite, 2-mm overjet, and maxillary crowding with a displaced canine. Projected treatment

time was 2 years. After the treatment ended, a general dentist discovered significant root resorption in eight anterior teeth as well as an open bite. The case was settled for $30,000, not because it appeared that the orthodontic treatment actually caused the root resorption or that the evidence indicated that the teeth would eventually be lost, but because, without radiographs to document what was happening to the roots, it was difficult to defend against those allegations.

Miscellaneous Treatment Issues

Surgery

Documentation of surgical recommendations and a patient's decision to decline that option is important. If surgery is the preferred treatment, the doctor must clearly record that fact in the records along with a copy of a letter clarifying the issue to the patient. Frequently, when a claim is made because results were not as expected, patients will deny that the doctor recommended surgery as the preferred option for treatment and make a claim for inappropriate diagnosis.

Jaw growth

Jaw growth after treatment can pose a problem, especially in males. This problem usually unfolds as follows. The child has orthodontic treatment, which may or may not be completed; he or she grows and renders the treatment ineffective or even counterproductive. The parents allege poor orthodontic diagnosis and treatment and sue the doctor for additional treatment, usually including the cost of surgery necessitated by the growth. It is good practice to take careful records at the conclusion of treatment so as to prove the treatment outcome before the growth took place. It is also important to notice any growth occurring during the course of treatment; claims develop when the parents are not adequately apprised of all aspects of their child's dental care, especially if it relates to the need for surgery.

Patient transfers

In situations involving patient transfers, good records must be transferred to the new doctor. The doctor can easily follow the existing treatment plan if it is clearly documented. Effective communication with the patient or parents and the new doctor serves to minimize problems. It is surprising how many malpractice claims develop from criticism of one orthodontist by another. No direct criticism of the previous treatment plan should ever be made.

Additional fees

Charging additional fees for a transfer case is another source of claims. One doctor had 13 claims, all based on the fact that the doctor who purchased his practice charged the transferring patients a new and full orthodontic fee.

Conclusion

Today, malpractice claims against professionals are common. It is difficult for any orthodontist to practice an entire career without having at least one claim made against him or her. Some of the claims are legitimate; not all orthodontists do good work all the time. Others are the result of poor communication between the patient and the doctor and probably would not have developed had there been better information, explanation, and rapport. Many of the claims are not deserved. When there is no evident practice below the standard of care, it appears the disgruntled patient is trying to "get something for nothing." No matter what the source of the claim, most orthodontists are unhappy at the prospect of being the recipient of malpractice allegations. Responding to a claim is unfamiliar territory and uncomfortable because it is a confrontational situation which criticizes the work product.

15 Practical Legal Advice for Avoiding Malpractice Lawsuits

CHAPTER

David Thomas

I have had the privilege, for the last 20 years, of limiting my practice of law to professional liability work, and I have yet to lose my first professional liability trial. Despite the doom and gloom associated with risk management, the fact that you get sued does not mean that you have done something wrong, or that you are going to lose, or that you need to reallocate your assets. What it does mean is that you need to be an active participant in your legal defense. Next week I will be taking my daughter to the orthodontist for the first time, and I don't know whether I'll be the best parent or the worst parent, but I'll certainly be an informed parent, and I'll try my best to help her health care provider. By the same token, when you are in my office, you need to be the best client you can be. The more information you give me about yourself and your problem, the better I will be able to defend you. Previously, health care providers could be comfortable knowing that even if there was a case of malpractice or malfeasance or simply a bad result, it could usually be resolved for a nominal sum, but not anymore. Today, you must participate in your own

defense. I will share with you practical information about steps you should be taking so that you will be successful in defending your practice.

The All-Important Patient Record

The first thing that I do when I get a lawsuit is to read the doctor's records. If they are illegible to me, if the shorthand or the hieroglyphics are so unique that I cannot understand them, it is more likely than not that a jury, which is composed of laypersons, unsophisticated more often than not, is also not going to have the benefit of understanding the record. In my experience, the clinician is usually a person who has practiced successfully and has a sterling reputation in the community. Often, the clinician's initial response is indignation at being sued by this particular patient of all patients, because he or she was noncompliant and that's why the treatment was not successful from a clinical perspective. The reality, however, is that the record does not demonstrate the patient's noncompliance. This places the lawyer in a position of wanting to blame the patient for the outcome, but the lawyer does not have adequate records upon which to lay that foundation to rescue the clinician from what is currently a bad result. It is absolutely imperative that you take pretreatment records and maintain them.

What records do you need? If you don't have any pretreatment radiographs, I can assure you no lawyer is going to be able to defend you successfully in a court of law. The same holds true if you do not have pretreatment casts or progress notes. Today I see the exact same mistakes being made by orthodontists and other health care professionals that I saw 20 years ago. But for these mistakes, I would be unemployed, so I'm a third-party beneficiary of those who choose not to follow my advice. How can you compare whether the patient's periodontal status has changed from 3-mm pockets to 8-mm pockets if you don't have any records of what they were at the commencement of treatment? Yet I see cases like this in my law practice with some degree of regularity.

The biggest sin I see is one of omission. That happens when the orthodontist does not consult with the referring general dentist and does not correspond with the referring general dentist and does not obtain the patient's chart from the referring general dentist. I think it is incumbent upon you to do that. I too am in private practice. I have my own overhead just like most practicing orthodontists, so I understand that the time I spend doing administrative tasks is nonprofessional, nonbillable time. However, there is a trade off in the minutes of time it takes in a day to do these things as opposed to the actual weeks you would spend with a lawyer dealing with a lawsuit, not to mention all the emotional and psychological trauma you would suffer. If you fail to document your treatment, you cannot blame your patient. I know full well that many patients are noncompliant; they act in contravention to your specific written and verbal instructions. However, juries are not sympathetic to us as professionals versus our clients, your patients. So you have to document what they are not doing. You have to document what your instructions were, particularly when you know that the patient is not compliant. If my daughter had missed the last three appointments

because I was too busy to get her there, that should be my problem, it should not be a problem of your practice. But if you don't document it and there is a bad result, I am certainly going to try to share that blame with you if you do not place that blame upon us. So protect yourself. Take a moment to write in the chart what it is that the patient is doing or not doing. Having a parent initial this comment in the record can't hurt.

Get Informed About Informed Consent

Every lawsuit I have defended during the past 20 years has had one common allegation: informed consent. Informed consent has nothing to do with clinical skills and everything to do with mental skills, that is, what steps were taken to prepare the patient for the course of treatment. Without informed consent, wrongful treatment is the easiest claim for a patient's lawyer to prove because it is the clinician's word against the patient's word. I can assure you that I will be able to recall the meeting I'm going to have at 1 o'clock with my daughter and her orthodontist 2 years from now a lot better than the orthodontist. Why? Because it is going to be the only orthodontist to whom I will have entrusted my daughter's care. The orthodontist, conversely, will have met a thousand parents and had a thousand conversations over that same 2-year period of time, so it is not even fair to expect him or her to recall the conversation to the extent that I will. And that is why records save you. The AAO informed consent form is an excellent form (see Appendix). For that matter, most forms that I have seen are excellent or at least sufficient for their purpose, but they are nonetheless inadequate to defend someone who is being sued.

Let us imagine that you, an orthodontist, receive a summons and complaint, and you send me the lawsuit along with a copy of the patient's signed informed consent form. This will not make the lawsuit disappear, and the reason is that the law requires that you, individually, obtain informed consent, not a form. Your average patient is not a trial attorney who specializes in professional liability work but a real person with a real job who does not understand most of the language in those forms. If you think they do, then have an honest conversation with a parent someday and ask them what they really understood about those informed consent forms. That is what happens inside the courtroom. I say to the patient, "You were given this form." The patient replies "yes." "Did you read it?" "Yes." "Did you sign it?" "Yes." "Did you understand it?" "Not a word." You see, the consent form is written *by* lawyers *for* lawyers. It is not written by orthodontists for patients because its purpose is to provide legal protection. But the ultimate protection is to obtain the patient's informed consent, and that is done simply by giving them a booklet, giving them the opportunity to read it and then asking the simple question "Do you have any questions?" and documenting their answer. Two years from now, when you are confronted with a summons and complaint, you will have a good record as to what did and did not occur: "Mr and Mrs Smith did not have any questions at that time." My job over the past 20 years would have been much easier had I had the benefit of that simple statement in all of my clients' records. You must obtain your patients' informed consent, and furthermore, *you must be there when they sign that document.* I see case after case where the document was provided to the parent by an administrative person within the practice who asked them to "take this home and read it." The parent brings it back and gives it to that same administrative person, who files it in the chart because now we are "protected." You are not protected at all because you, the doctor, the health care provider, did not obtain the patient's informed consent. It does not take long, but it will eliminate 50% of the potential areas of a malpractice claim if you simply take a few seconds and ask that question and then document that you have asked that question. Getting periodic initialed recognition of treatment progress is another act of informed consent that will protect you even more, and I strongly recommend it.

Don't Pay for Your Principles

Another area where lawsuits are generated and proliferated is when practitioners get into an economic battle with their patient over a fee for the record. At least 10% of all the lawsuits that I have defended were pre-cipitated by an action wherein the orthodontist requested a fee for duplication of the patient's records or instituted a collection action. One or the other of those prompted the patient to consult a lawyer, who then turned that built-in animosity between the two into a lawsuit. I am not telling you not to pursue collection of your claims. I do it myself against insurance companies. I work hard and I expect to get paid for the services I perform, but one must exercise judgment in following their principles. If it is a case that is a bad result and it is a nominal sum, ask yourself if the money is worth all the time and emotional expense associated with working with an attorney on a trial that may take up to 2 weeks of your professional time. The answer is clearly "no." When patients want records, the lawyers they consult are not unsophisticated. They get records from all of the client's health care providers, and if they think that one of them is engaging in some form of gouging, they are going to go after them. Trial lawyers are competitive people by definition, and if you are entering the legal turf, it can be a traumatic experience, especially when you realize that it is an arena in which the lawyer is more comfortable. If you get into a verbal volleyball match with a trial lawyer, you may end up on the losing side, so do not enter that arena if you can avoid it.

When in Doubt, Refer

In what areas are lawsuits filed? This should come as no surprise to you: failure to diagnose periodontal disease, failure to make referrals, and taking action outside the scope of your practice. As a trial lawyer, I cannot probate your estate because I do not have the skills to do that; I would refer you to a probate attorney. You need to do the same thing within your practice. The number one area where people get into trouble is the failure to refer. We are all successful at what we do and therefore our egos say, "I can do this. I can help this patient." The reality is that maybe we can't and maybe there's someone more qualified to undertake that task for that patient. The other area where orthodontists get into trouble is with temporomandibular disorders (TMDs), and again, that goes back to your initial records. If you do not at least make some notation—"TMJ is fine," for example—your case is flawed. If that patient develops a TMD problem, you are certainly going to be blamed as the etiology of that condition. If the patient didn't have TMD when starting treatment but has it at the end of treatment, you will be blamed for causing it. So if you don't have a record of the status of the temporomandibular joint, you aren't going to have a very good chance of defending yourself.

Be Careful What You Say . . .

What is it like to face a malpractice lawsuit? First of all, your assets will be in jeopardy. Your practice will be affected. Your spouse will not know you during the 2 or 3 weeks of the trial, and it will have a profound effect on you for a very significant period of time. It can also have a very rewarding effect when you are vindicated and you validate what you believed in and what you know to be the truth. I encourage everyone who faces the unpleasant circumstance of receiving a summons and complaint to critically analyze the situation and, if they did nothing wrong, if they adhered to the standard of care, to continue to believe in their care and treatment. However, if there *is* something wrong in your treatment of a patient, tell the risk manager that you think there is a problem and the reason why you think so. But do not tell your patient. I say this keeping in mind my conversation next week with my daughter's own orthodontist. There is a difference between telling the patient that you aren't achieving the results you want or that you're achieving a result that was unintended, and saying, "I committed malpractice." That statement is a knife through the heart, legally speaking, and I have a hard time extracting it without leaving some scar tissue. The classic case occurs when a second orthodontist says to a patient, "I would never have implemented that treatment plan." All the patient hears is, "The other doctor committed malpractice." If half the orthodontists would do treatment plan A and the other half would do treatment plan B, who is right? Who is wrong? The answer is, everyone is right as long as they are doing what is reasonable. But when you criticize your predecessor, in the patient's mind you are indicating that you think he or she committed malpractice, and more often than not they run off to the lawyer's office and tell the

contingency-fee lawyer the magic words he or she wants to hear, "My doctor told me the other doctor committed malpractice." That trial immediately gets moved to the top of their work pile. They do not have to hire an expert. They do not have to find someone who lacks credibility to testify against you. They have a ready-made expert witness. As a defense lawyer, I find it very difficult to find a secondary health care provider who lives within the same community and who is very critical of what you did or did not do. So when you're evaluating someone else's work, be careful how you express yourself to that patient because they absorb all the negatives and they throw out all the modifiers like, "I may have done things differently." All they heard was, "I would have done this differently," and that leads to lawsuits. Although we can successfully defend such suits, there is a lot of time and a lot of emotion and a lot of effort involved. Being judicious in how you select your words to express yourself on those critical issues will eliminate the lawsuit entirely.

Standard of Care: "Do What Is Right"

When it comes to questions about standards of care, my clients tell me, "I didn't do anything wrong." My response is always, "I'm sure you didn't." But I am an attorney, not an orthodontist, so I can't tell whether a client adhered to the standard of care or not. All I can tell them is what I think a jury is going to conclude based on the evidence. To do that, I consult two sources: expert witnesses and people within the local community. During the course of a trial, jurors are inundated with technical information. They have the records of the general dentist before them. They have the orthodontist's records before them. And they probably have some records of a medical health care provider as well. In the course of a week, we lawyers are trying to educate them in these various fields. This is an enormous task. Therefore, jurors do what they think is right. Time and time again, when you get the right jurors on a jury, they will tend to want to do what is right. In fact, in every closing argument I give to a jury, after explaining all the orthodontics involved in the case and after attempting to succinctly summarize the law that is applicable to that situation, I tell them that when they get back into that jury room and they are trying to remember all the instructions and law, simply do what is right. This is peer review. The same applies to you in your practice. When you're treating my daughter, all I ask is that you do what is right. It's a pretty easy standard if we apply it. How you go about doing that is the key.

One final word of advice: chairside manner dictates the number of lawsuits a health care provider receives. This is a maxim that I have learned over 20 years. If the patient thinks you're a reasonable orthodontist who cares about their time constraints, does not keep patients waiting in the reception room for an hour and a half or apologizes and explains why, the likelihood of creating risk-management problems is greatly reduced. No one has time to waste. This is true in your own life, and it is also true in your patients' lives. If I have to wait an hour and a half, I know I will not be pleased. The average layperson will not be pleased either. This has been brought out time and time again. Whether you are an attorney, an orthodontist, or another professional, we are all perceived as making far more money than we do, working far less than we do, and enjoying what we do. To the extent that you have a good chairside manner when there is an opportunity to bridge a problem, take 30 seconds to do so, because the patient will leave feeling good about you, and it is a fact that people do not sue people they like. I cannot stress enough how important that is, in addition to all the risk-management control factors covered elsewhere in this book. Be yourself, be warm and human, and treat patients as individuals, not as cogs in your practice.

Appendix: Patient Information Forms

Obtaining a comprehensive medical and dental history and providing the patient with enough information to make an informed decision regarding the proposed treatment are both critical steps that all orthodontists need to take to protect themselves against the threat of a malpractice lawsuit. The forms presented in this appendix were designed specifically for use by orthodontists and are available for purchase through the American Association of Orthodontists (www.aaomembers.org).

DRAFT

American Association of Orthodontists
MEDICAL DENTAL HISTORY FORM FOR
PATIENTS UNDER 18 YEARS OF AGE

American Association of
Orthodontists

CONFIDENTIAL

Date: _____

Patient's Last Name: _____ First Name: _____ Middle Name/Initial: _____

Birth Date: _____ Age: _____ Sex: Male ☐ Female ☐ I Prefer To Be Called: _____

S.S.N./S.I.N.: _____ Home Phone No.: _____

Patient's Address: _____

City: _____ State/Province: _____ Zip/Postal Code: _____

Attends School At: _____ Grade: _____

Musical Instruments Played: _____

Sports And/Or Hobbies: _____

No. of brothers and sisters: _____ Ages: _____

Other family members treated here: _____

Birth Father's Height _____ ft. _____ in.   Birth Mother's Height _____ ft.____ in.

Patient's Birth Weight _____ lbs.____ oz.   Patient's Present Weight _____ lbs.   Height _____ ft. _____ in.

Custodial Parent(s) or Guardian(s): _____

Phone No. (if different than patient's): _____

Address (if different than patient's): _____

City: _____ State/Province: _____ Zip/Postal Code: _____

E-mail address: _____ Cell phone/pager: _____

Name of Patient's Dentist: _____ Phone No.: _____

Dentist's Address: _____

City: _____ State/Province: _____ Zip/Postal Code: _____

Date Last Seen: _____ Reason: _____

Name of Patient's Physician(s): _____

Phone No(s): _____

Physician's Address: _____

City: _____ State/Province: _____ Zip/Postal Code: _____

Date Last Seen: _____ Reason: _____

Who Is Financially Responsible For This Account?

Last Name: _____ First Name: _____ Middle Name/Initial: _____

Address (if different from patient's): _____

City: _____ State: _____ Zip: _____ Years at this address: _____

If less than five years, previous address: _____

City: _____ State: _____ Zip: _____

1

History Form – Child 6/03

Fig 1a Medical Dental History Form for patients under 18 years of age. (Courtesy of the American Association of Orthodontists.)

Phone No. (if different than patient's): _____ S.S.N/S.I.N.: _____

Employer: _____ How many years? _____

Insurance Coverage for Dental Treatment? Yes ☐ No ☐   Insurance Coverage for Orthodontic Treatment? Yes ☐ No ☐

Primary Policy Holder's Name: _____ S.S.N./S.I.N.: _____

Birth Date: _____ Employed By: _____

Dental Insurance Company: _____ Group No.: _____

Secondary Policy Holder's Name: _____ S.S.N./S.I.N.: _____

Birth Date: _____ Employed By: _____

Dental Insurance Company: _____ Group No.: _____

Medical Insurance Company: _____ Group No.: _____

Who suggested that your child might need orthodontic treatment? _____

Why did you select our office? _____

For the following questions mark yes, no, or don't know/understand (dk/u). The answers are for office records only and will be considered confidential. A thorough and complete history is vital to a proper orthodontic evaluation.

PATIENT PROFILE

☐yes ☐no ☐dk/u   Does patient follow directions well?

☐yes ☐no ☐dk/u   Does patient brush his/her teeth conscientiously?

☐yes ☐no ☐dk/u   Does patient have learning disabilities or need extra help with instructions?

☐yes ☐no ☐dk/u   Is patient sensitive or self-conscious about teeth?

MEDICAL HISTORY

Now or in the past, have you had:

☐yes ☐no ☐dk/u   Birth defects or hereditary problems?

☐yes ☐no ☐dk/u   Bone fractures, any major accidents?

☐yes ☐no ☐dk/u   Rheumatoid or arthritic conditions?

☐yes ☐no ☐dk/u   Endocrine or thyroid problems?

☐yes ☐no ☐dk/u   Kidney problems?

☐yes ☐no ☐dk/u   Diabetes?

☐yes ☐no ☐dk/u   Cancer, tumor, radiation treatment or chemotherapy?

☐yes ☐no ☐dk/u   Stomach ulcer or hyperacidity?

☐yes ☐no ☐dk/u   Polio, mononucleosis, tuberculosis, pneumonia?

☐yes ☐no ☐dk/u   Problems of the immune system?

☐yes ☐no ☐dk/u   AIDS or HIV positive?

☐yes ☐no ☐dk/u   Hepatitis, jaundice or liver problem?

☐yes ☐no ☐dk/u   Fainting spells, seizures, epilepsy or neurological problem?

☐yes ☐no ☐dk/u   Mental health disturbance or depression?

☐yes ☐no ☐dk/u   Vision, hearing, tasting or speech difficulties?

☐yes ☐no ☐dk/u   Loss of weight recently, poor appetite?

☐yes ☐no ☐dk/u   History of eating disorder (anorexia, bulimia)?

☐yes ☐no ☐dk/u   Excessive bleeding or bruising tendency, anemia or bleeding disorder?

☐yes ☐no ☐dk/u   High or low blood pressure?

☐yes ☐no ☐dk/u   Tired easily?

☐yes ☐no ☐dk/u   Chest pain, shortness of breath or swelling ankles?

☐yes ☐no ☐dk/u   Cardiovascular problem (heart trouble, heart attack, angina, coronary insufficiency, arteriosclerosis, stroke, inborn heart defects, heart murmur or rheumatic heart disease)?

DRAFT

☐yes ☐no ☐dk/u   Skin disorder?

☐yes ☐no ☐dk/u   Does the patient eat a well-balanced diet?

☐yes ☐no ☐dk/u   Frequent headaches, colds or sore throats?

☐yes ☐no ☐dk/u   Eye, ear, nose or throat condition?

☐yes ☐no ☐dk/u   Hayfever, asthma, sinus trouble or hives?

☐yes ☐no ☐dk/u   Tonsil or adenoid conditions?

Allergies or reactions to any of the following:

☐yes ☐no ☐dk/u   Local anesthetics (Novocaine or Lidocaine)

☐yes ☐no ☐dk/u   Aspirin

☐yes ☐no ☐dk/u   Ibuprofen (Motrin, Advil)

☐yes ☐no ☐dk/u   Penicillin or other antibiotics

☐yes ☐no ☐dk/u   Sulfa drugs

☐yes ☐no ☐dk/u   Codeine or other narcotics

☐yes ☐no ☐dk/u   Metals (jewelry, clothing snaps)

☐yes ☐no ☐dk/u   Latex (gloves, balloons)

☐yes ☐no ☐dk/u   Vinyl

☐yes ☐no ☐dk/u   Acrylic

☐yes ☐no ☐dk/u   Animals

☐yes ☐no ☐dk/u   Foods (specify) _____

☐yes ☐no ☐dk/u   Other substances (specify) _____

☐yes ☐no ☐dk/u   Is the patient taking medication, nutrient supplements, herbal medications or non prescription medicine? Please name them.

Medication _____ Taken for _____

Medication _____ Taken for _____

Medication _____ Taken for _____

2

History Form – Child 6/03

Fig 1a (*cont*)

□yes □no □dk/u   Does the patient currently have or ever had a substance abuse problem?

□yes □no □dk/u   Does the patient chew or smoke tobacco?

□yes □no □dk/u   Operations? Describe: _____

_____

□yes □no □dk/u   Hospitalized? Describe:_____

_____

□yes □no □dk/u   Other physical problems or symptoms? Describe: _____

_____

_____

□yes □no □dk/u   Being treated by another health care professional?

For: _____

Date of most recent physical exam? _____

Are there any other medical conditions that we should be aware of?

_____

GIRLS ONLY

□yes □no □dk/u   Has the patient started her monthly periods?
If so, approximately when?_____

□yes □no □dk/u   Is the patient pregnant?

FAMILY MEDICAL HISTORY

Do the patient's parents or siblings have any of the following health problems? If so, please explain.

Bleeding disorders _____

Diabetes_____

Arthritis_____

Metabolic disturbances _____

Severe allergies _____

Unusual dental problems _____

Jaw size imbalance _____

Any other family medical conditions that we should know about?

_____

DRAFT

DENTAL HISTORY

Now or in the past, has the patient had:

□yes □no □dk/u   Started teething very early or late?

□yes □no □dk/u   Primary (baby) teeth removed that were not loose?

□yes □no □dk/u   Permanent or "extra" (supernumerary) teeth removed?

□yes □no □dk/u   Supernumerary (extra) or congenitally missing teeth?

□yes □no □dk/u   Chipped or otherwise injured primary (baby) or permanent teeth?

□yes □no □dk/u   Teeth sensitive to hot or cold; teeth throb or ache?

□yes □no □dk/u   Jaw fractures, cysts or mouth infections?

□yes □no □dk/u   "Dead teeth" or root canals treated?

□yes □no □dk/u   Bleeding gums, bad taste or mouth odor?

□yes □no □dk/u   Periodontal "gum problems"?

□yes □no □dk/u   Food impaction between teeth?

□yes □no □dk/u   Thumb, finger, or sucking habit? Until what age_____?

□yes □no □dk/u   Abnormal swallowing habit (tongue thrusting)?

□yes □no □dk/u   History of speech problems?

□yes □no □dk/u   Mouth breathing habit, snoring or difficulty in breathing?

□yes □no □dk/u   Tooth grinding or jaw clenching?

□yes □no □dk/u   Any pain in jaw or ringing in the ears?

□yes □no □dk/u   Any pain or soreness in the muscles of the face or around the ears?

□yes □no □dk/u   Difficulty encountered in chewing or jaw opening?

□yes □no □dk/u   Aware of loose, broken or missing restorations (fillings)?

□yes □no □dk/u   Any teeth irritating cheek, lip, tongue or palate?

□yes □no □dk/u   Concerned about spaced, crooked or protruding teeth?

□yes □no □dk/u   Aware or concerned about under or over developed jaw?

□yes □no □dk/u   "Gum boils", frequent canker sores or cold sores?

□yes □no □dk/u   Taking any forms of fluoride?

□yes □no □dk/u   Any relative with similar tooth or jaw relationships?

□yes □no □dk/u   Had periodontal (gum) treatment?

□yes □no □dk/u   Would you object to wearing orthodontic appliances (braces) should they be indicated?

□yes □no □dk/u   Any serious trouble associated with any previous dental treatment?

□yes □no □dk/u   Ever had a prior orthodontic examination or treatment?

□yes □no □dk/u   Been under another dentist's care?

Specialist _____

Other _____

How often does your child brush: _____ floss: _____

What is your primary concern? Why are you here? _____

I have read and understand the above questions. I will not hold my orthodontist or any member of his/her staff responsible for any errors or omissions that I have made in the completion of this form. If there are any changes later to this history record or medical/dental status, I will so inform this practice.

Signed: _____ Date Signed: _____
            (Parent or Guardian)

Signed: _____ Date Signed: _____
            (Dental staff member)

History Form – Child 6/03

Fig 1a (cont)

MEDICAL HISTORY UPDATE OR CHANGES

Comments: _____
_____
_____

Signed: _____ Date Signed: _____
     (Parent or Guardian)

Signed: _____ Date Signed: _____
     (Dental staff member)

MEDICAL HISTORY UPDATE OR CHANGES

Comments: _____
_____
_____

Signed: _____ Date Signed: _____
     (Parent or Guardian)

Signed: _____ Date Signed: _____
     (Dental staff member)

DRAFT

MEDICAL HISTORY UPDATE OR CHANGES

Comments: _____
_____
_____

Signed: _____ Date Signed: _____
     (Patient)

Signed: _____ Date Signed: _____
     (Dental staff member)

MEDICAL HISTORY UPDATE OR CHANGES

Comments: _____
_____
_____

Signed: _____ Date Signed: _____
     (Patient)

Signed: _____ Date Signed: _____
     (Dental staff member)

    4   History Form – Child 6/03

Fig 1a *(cont)*

American Association of
Orthodontists

DRAFT

Date: _____

CONFIDENTIAL

American Association of Orthodontists
MEDICAL DENTAL HISTORY FORM – ADULT

Patient's Last Name: _____ First Name: _____ Middle Name/Initial: _____

Birth Date: _____ Age: _____ Sex: Male ☐ Female ☐ I Prefer To Be Called: _____

S.S.N./S.I.N.: _____ Home Phone No.:_____ E-mail address: _____

Cell phone number: _____ Pager number:_____

Patient's Address: _____

City: _____ State/Province: _____ Zip/Postal Code:_____

Years at above address: _____

If less than 5 years at current address, previous address: _____

Years at previous address: _____ Patient is: Single ☐ Married ☐ Widowed ☐ Separated ☐ Divorced ☐

Occupation: _____ Employer: _____ Years with Employer: _____

Business Phone No.: _____

Name Of Spouse/Closest Relative: _____ Phone No.: (if different than yours) _____

Relationship To You: _____

Address (if different than yours): _____

City: _____ State/Province: _____ Zip/Postal Code:_____

Name Of Patient's Dentist: _____

Phone No.: _____

Dentist's Address: _____

City: _____ State/Province: _____ Zip/Postal Code: _____

Date Last Seen: _____ Reason: _____

Name Of Patient's Physician(s): _____

Phone No(s).:_____

Physician's Address: _____

City: _____ State/Province: _____ Zip/Postal Code:_____

Date Last Seen: _____ Reason: _____

Who suggested that you might need orthodontic treatment? _____

Why did you select our office? _____

Who Is Financially Responsible For This Account?

Last Name: _____ First Name: _____ Middle Name/Initial: _____

Address (if different than patient's)_____

Phone No.: _____

City: _____ State/Province: _____ Zip/Postal Code:_____

1   History Form – Adult 6/03

Fig 1b Medical Dental History Form for adult patients. (Courtesy of the American Association of Orthodontists.)

DRAFT

Insurance Coverage For Dental Treatment? Yes ☐ No ☐

Insurance Coverage For Orthodontic Treatment? Yes ☐ No ☐

Primary Policy Holder's Name: _____ S.S.N./S.I.N.: _____

Birth Date: _____ Employed By: _____

Dental Insurance Company: _____ Group No.: _____

Secondary Policy Holder's Name: _____ S.S.N./S.I.N.: _____

Birth Date: _____ Employed By: _____

Dental Insurance Company: _____ Group No.: _____

Medical Insurance Company: _____

For the following questions mark yes, no, or don't know/understand (dk/u). The answers are for office records only and will be considered confidential. A thorough and complete history is vital to a proper orthodontic evaluation.

MEDICAL HISTORY

Now or in the past, have you had:

☐yes ☐no ☐dk/u Birth defects or hereditary problems?

☐yes ☐no ☐dk/u Bone fractures, any major accidents?

☐yes ☐no ☐dk/u Rheumatoid or arthritic conditions?

☐yes ☐no ☐dk/u Endocrine or thyroid problems?

☐yes ☐no ☐dk/u Kidney problems?

☐yes ☐no ☐dk/u Diabetes?

☐yes ☐no ☐dk/u Cancer, tumor, radiation treatment or chemotherapy?

☐yes ☐no ☐dk/u Stomach ulcer or hyperacidity?

☐yes ☐no ☐dk/u Polio, mononucleosis, tuberculosis, pneumonia?

☐yes ☐no ☐dk/u Problems of the immune system?

☐yes ☐no ☐dk/u AIDS or HIV positive?

☐yes ☐no ☐dk/u Hepatitis, jaundice or liver problem?

☐yes ☐no ☐dk/u Fainting spells, seizures, epilepsy or neurological problem?

☐yes ☐no ☐dk/u Mental health disturbance or depression?

☐yes ☐no ☐dk/u Vision, hearing, tasting or speech difficulties?

☐yes ☐no ☐dk/u Loss of weight recently, poor appetite?

☐yes ☐no ☐dk/u History of eating disorder (anorexia, bulimia)?

☐yes ☐no ☐dk/u Excessive bleeding or bruising tendency, anemia or bleeding disorder?

☐yes ☐no ☐dk/u High or low blood pressure?

☐yes ☐no ☐dk/u Tired easily?

☐yes ☐no ☐dk/u Chest pain, shortness of breath or swelling ankles?

☐yes ☐no ☐dk/u Cardiovascular problem (heart trouble, heart attack, angina, coronary insufficiency, arteriosclerosis, stroke, inborn heart defects, heart murmur or rheumatic heart disease)?

☐yes ☐no ☐dk/u Skin disorder?

☐yes ☐no ☐dk/u Do you have a well-balanced diet?

☐yes ☐no ☐dk/u Frequent headaches, colds or sore throats?

☐yes ☐no ☐dk/u Eye, ear, nose or throat condition?

☐yes ☐no ☐dk/u Hayfever, asthma, sinus trouble or hives?

☐yes ☐no ☐dk/u Tonsil or adenoid conditions?

☐yes ☐no ☐dk/u Osteoporosis?

Allergies or reactions to any of the following:

☐yes ☐no ☐dk/u Local anesthetics (Novocaine or Lidocaine)

☐yes ☐no ☐dk/u Aspirin

☐yes ☐no ☐dk/u Ibuprofen (Motrin, Advil)

☐yes ☐no ☐dk/u Penicillin or other antibiotics

☐yes ☐no ☐dk/u Sulfa drugs

☐yes ☐no ☐dk/u Codeine or other narcotics

☐yes ☐no ☐dk/u Metals (jewelry, clothing snaps)

☐yes ☐no ☐dk/u Latex (gloves, balloons)

☐yes ☐no ☐dk/u Vinyl

☐yes ☐no ☐dk/u Acrylic

☐yes ☐no ☐dk/u Animals

☐yes ☐no ☐dk/u Foods (specify)_____

☐yes ☐no ☐dk/u Other substances (specify)_____

☐yes ☐no ☐dk/u Are you taking medication, nutrient supplements, herbal medications or non prescription medicine? Please name them.

Medication _____ Taken for _____

Medication _____ Taken for _____

Medication _____ Taken for _____

Medication _____ Taken for _____

Medication _____ Taken for _____

Medication _____ Taken for _____

Medication _____ Taken for _____

☐yes ☐no ☐dk/u Do you currently have or ever had a substance abuse problem?

☐yes ☐no ☐dk/u Do you chew or smoke tobacco?

☐yes ☐no ☐dk/u Operations? Describe:_____

☐yes ☐no ☐dk/u Hospitalized? Describe:_____

☐yes ☐no ☐dk/u Other physical problems or symptoms? Describe: _____

☐yes ☐no ☐dk/u Being treated by another health care professional?

For: _____

Date of most recent physical exam? _____

Do you have any other medical conditions that we should know about?

_____

2

Fig 1b (cont)

WOMEN ONLY

☐yes ☐no ☐dk/u   Are you pregnant?

☐yes ☐no ☐dk/u   Are you anticipating becoming pregnant?

FAMILY MEDICAL HISTORY

Do your parents or siblings have, or have ever had any of the following health problems? If so, please explain.

Bleeding disorders _____

Diabetes_____

Arthritis_____

Severe allergies _____

Unusual dental problems _____

Jaw size imbalance _____

Any other family medical conditions that we should know about?

_____

DENTAL HISTORY

Now or in the past, have you had:

☐yes ☐no ☐dk/u   Permanent or "extra" (supernumerary) teeth removed?

☐yes ☐no ☐dk/u   Supernumerary (extra) or congenitally missing teeth?

☐yes ☐no ☐dk/u   Chipped or otherwise injured primary (baby) or permanent teeth?

☐yes ☐no ☐dk/u   Teeth sensitive to hot or cold; teeth throb or ache?

☐yes ☐no ☐dk/u   Jaw fractures, cysts or mouth infections?

☐yes ☐no ☐dk/u   "Dead teeth" or root canals treated?

☐yes ☐no ☐dk/u   Bleeding gums, bad taste or mouth odor?

☐yes ☐no ☐dk/u   Periodontal "gum problems"?

☐yes ☐no ☐dk/u   Food impaction between teeth?

☐yes ☐no ☐dk/u   "Gum boils", frequent canker sores or cold sores?

☐yes ☐no ☐dk/u   Thumb, finger, or sucking habit? Until what age_____?

☐yes ☐no ☐dk/u   Abnormal swallowing habit (tongue thrusting)?

☐yes ☐no ☐dk/u   History of speech problems?

☐yes ☐no ☐dk/u   Mouth breathing habit, snoring or difficulty in breathing?

☐yes ☐no ☐dk/u   Tooth grinding or jaw clenching?

☐yes ☐no ☐dk/u   Any pain, clicking or locking in jaw or ringing in the ears?

☐yes ☐no ☐dk/u   Any pain or soreness in the muscles of the face or around the ears?

☐yes ☐no ☐dk/u   Difficulty in chewing or jaw opening?

☐yes ☐no ☐dk/u   Have you ever been treated for "TMD" or "TMJ" problems?

☐yes ☐no ☐dk/u   Aware of loose, broken or missing restorations (fillings)?

☐yes ☐no ☐dk/u   Any teeth irritating cheek, lip, tongue or palate?

☐yes ☐no ☐dk/u   Concerned about spaced, crooked or protruding teeth?

☐yes ☐no ☐dk/u   Aware or concerned about under or over developed jaw?

☐yes ☐no ☐dk/u   Any relative with similar tooth or jaw relationships?

☐yes ☐no ☐dk/u   Any wisdom tooth problems?

☐yes ☐no ☐dk/u   Had periodontal (gum) treatment?

☐yes ☐no ☐dk/u   Had any serious trouble associated with any previous dental treatment?

☐yes ☐no ☐dk/u   Been under another dentist's care?

Specialist _____

Other _____

☐yes ☐no ☐dk/u   Ever had a prior orthodontic examination or treatment?

☐yes ☐no ☐dk/u   Would you object to wearing orthodontic appliances (braces) should they be indicated?

DRAFT

How often do you brush: _____ Floss: _____

What is your primary concern? Why are you here? _____

I have read and understand the above questions. I will not hold my orthodontist or any member of his/her staff responsible for any errors or omissions that I have made in the completion of this form. If there are any changes later to this history record or medical/dental status, I will so inform this practice.

Signed: _____   Date Signed: _____
(Patient)

Signed: _____   Date Signed: _____
(Dental staff member)

MEDICAL HISTORY UPDATE OR CHANGES

Comments: _____

_____

_____

Signed: _____   Date Signed: _____
(Patient)

Signed: _____   Date Signed: _____
(Dental staff member)

History Form – Adult 6/03

Fig 1b (cont)

MEDICAL HISTORY UPDATE OR CHANGES

Comments: _____

_____

_____

Signed: _____ Date Signed: _____
    (Patient)

Signed: _____ Date Signed: _____
    (Dental staff member)

MEDICAL HISTORY UPDATE OR CHANGES

Comments: _____

_____

_____

Signed: _____ Date Signed: _____
    (Patient)

Signed: _____ Date Signed: _____
    (Dental staff member)

MEDICAL HISTORY UPDATE OR CHANGES

Comments: _____

_____

_____

Signed: _____ Date Signed: _____
    (Patient)

Signed: _____ Date Signed: _____
    (Dental staff member)

MEDICAL HISTORY UPDATE OR CHANGES

Comments: _____

_____

_____

Signed: _____ Date Signed: _____
    (Patient)

Signed: _____ Date Signed: _____
    (Dental staff member)

DRAFT

© American Association of Orthodontists 2003   4   History Form – Adult 6/03

Fig 1b *(cont)*

Notes

Record

DRAFT

ACKNOWLEDGEMENT OF INFORMED CONSENT

I hereby acknowledge that the major treatment considerations and potential risks of orthodontic treatment have been presented to me. I have read and understand this form and also understand that there may be other problems that occur less frequently or are less severe, and that the actual results may be different from the anticipated results.

Dr(s). _____

has(have) discussed the orthodontic treatment

for _____

with me. I have been asked to make a choice about that treatment. I have been presented information to aid in the decision-making process, and I have been given the opportunity to ask the above doctor(s) all questions I have about the proposed orthodontic treatment and information contained in this form.

CONSENT TO UNDERGO ORTHODONTIC TREATMENT

I hereby consent to the making of diagnostic records, including x-rays, before, during and following orthodontic treatment, and to the above doctor(s) and, where appropriate staff providing orthodontic treatment described by the above doctor(s) for the above individual. I fully understand all of the risks associated with the treatment.

AUTHORIZATION FOR RELEASE OF PATIENT INFORMATION

I hereby authorize the above doctor to provide other health care providers with information regarding the above individual's orthodontic care as deemed appropriate. I understand that once released, the above doctor(s) and staff has(have) no responsibility for any further release by the individual receiving this information.

SURGICAL SUPPLEMENT

If the orthodontic treatment plan includes correction of the malocclusion by orthodontic appliance (braces) therapy in conjunction with orthognathic (corrective jaw) surgery, I understand that oral surgery is necessary in conjunction with the above patient's orthodontic treatment. I authorize the office(s) of the above doctor(s) to communicate with the surgeon and release information from the above patient's treatment record to the designated surgeon. I acknowledge that expenses incurred from the surgery are separate from orthodontic treatment expenses, and I will be responsible to the surgeon and hospital for all such expenses.

I understand that if I do not complete the surgical component of the treatment plan that I may have a compromised treatment result and other complications. I hereby agree not to hold the above doctor(s) and staff liable for any compromised treatment resulting from my failure for any reason to follow the treatment plan.

OFFICE COPY

SIGNATURE

_____ _____
Signature/Patient, Parent or Guardian   Date

_____ _____
Signature (Orthodontist)   Date

_____ _____
Witness   Date

PATIENT'S AUTHORIZED REPRESENTATIVE

If you are consenting to the care of another: I have the legal authority to sign this on behalf of _____

_____
Relationship to Patient

_____ _____
Signature   Date

_____ _____
Witness   Date

OPTIONAL

CONSENT TO USE OF RECORDS

I hereby give my permission for the use of orthodontic records, including photographs, made in the process of examinations, treatment, and retention for purposes of professional consultations, research, education, or publication in professional journals.

I have the legal authority to sign this on behalf of

_____
Relationship to Patient

_____ _____
Signature   Date

_____ _____
Witness   Date

Fig 2 Acknowledgement of Informed Consent Form. (Courtesy of the American Association of Orthodontists.)

Index